# INTRODUCTION TO COMMUNITY-BASED NURSING

# INTRODUCTION TO COMMUNITY-BASED NURSING

## THIRD EDITION

Roberta Hunt, RN, MSPH, PhD

LIPPINCOTT WILLIAMS & WILKINS
A **Wolters Kluwer** Company
Philadelphia • Baltimore • New York • London
Buenos Aires • Hong Kong • Sydney • Tokyo

*Senior Acquisitions Editor:* Margaret Zuccarini
*Developmental Editor:* Deedie McMahon
*Managing Editor:* Amy Dinkel
*Editorial Assistant:* Carol DeVault
*Production Editor:* Diane Griffith
*Senior Production Manager:* Helen Ewan
*Manufacturing Manager:* William Alberti

*Senior Art Director:* Carolyn O'Brien
*Interior Design:* Holly Reid Mclaughlin
*Cover Design:* Christopher Shea
*Indexer:* Michael Ferreira
*Compositor:* Lippincott Williams & Wilkins
*Printer:* RR Donnelly–Crawfordsville

3rd Edition

Library of Congress Cataloging-in-Publication Data is available on request.
ISBN 0-7817-4505-5

Care has been taken to confirm the accuracy of the information presented and to describe generally accepted practices. However, the authors, editors, and publisher are not responsible for errors or omissions or for any consequences from application of the information in this book and make no warranty, express or implied, with respect to the content of the publication.

The authors, editors, and publisher have exerted every effort to ensure that drug selection and dosage set forth in this text are in accordance with the current recommendations and practice at the time of publication. However, in view of ongoing research, changes in government regulations, and the constant flow of information relating to drug therapy and drug reactions, the reader is urged to check the package insert for each drug for any change in indications and dosage and for added warnings and precautions. This is particularly important when the recommended agent is a new or infrequently employed drug.

Some drugs and medical devices presented in this publication have Food and Drug Administration (FDA) clearance for limited use in restricted research settings. It is the responsibility of the health care provider to ascertain the FDA status of each drug or device planned for use in his or her clinical practice.

## DEDICATION

*To my daughters, Megan Davis and Jackie Smith, with love.*
RJH

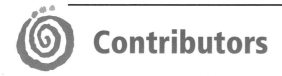

# Contributors

**Paula Swiggum, MS, RN**
Assistant Professor of Nursing
Gustavus Adolphus College
Saint Peter, Minnesota

**Marva Thurston, MS, RN**
Clinical Nurse Specialist
Hennepin County Mental Health Center
Minneapolis, Minnesota

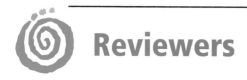

# Reviewers

**Christine Brosnan, RNC, DrPH**
Assistant Professor and Lead Faculty for Community Health Nursing
University of Texas—Houston Health Science Center
Houston, Texas

**Mary Emily Cameron, RN, PhD**
Assistant Professor of Nursing
Rutgers, the State University of New Jersey
Camden, New Jersey

**Karen Cassidy, RN, EdD**
Associate Professor of Nursing
Bellarmine College
Louisville, Kentucky

**Katherine A. Conroy, RNC, MS**
Assistant Professor of Nursing
West Chester University
West Chester, Pennsylvania

**Grace P. Erickson, RNC, MPH, MSN, EdD**
Assistant Professor of Nursing
University of South Florida
Tampa, Florida

**Lucille C. Gambardella, RN, CS, APN, PhD**
Chair and Professor, Division of Nursing
Wesley College
Dover, Delaware

**Ruth N. Knollmueller, RN, PhD**
Clinical Associate, School of Nursing
University of Connecticut
Hamden, Connecticut

**Carol M. Patton, CRNP, DrPH**
Director, RN to BSN and Second Degree Programs
Director, Family Nurse Practitioner Program
Assistant Professor of Nursing
Duquesne University
Pittsburgh, Pennsylvania

# Preface

The changing health care delivery system presents new challenges for contemporary nurses. Schools of nursing are struggling with the best way to restructure curriculum to meet current needs and to give students experiences in a variety of clinical situations and settings that will prepare them for their careers in the increasingly diversified field of nursing. This textbook is designed to fill such a need. *Introduction to Community-Based Nursing*, third edition, is a textbook about community-based nursing. The foundational concepts in this text spring from my experience of more than 25 years of teaching community health nursing and working in community settings. These concepts are articulated with careful attention to the National League for Nursing competencies.

## Purpose of the Text

As *Introduction to Community-Based Nursing*, third edition, was developed, four major goals were considered:

1. *To give an informative and experiential introduction to nursing care in the community.*

   Before now, most schools of nursing have focused on preparing students to provide care in the hospital. Under the new health care delivery system, much of nursing care has moved out of these acute care settings into a variety of settings and specialties throughout the community. This book presents fundamental aspects of community-based care and builds a knowledge base that the nurse can use in any community setting.

2. *To illustrate the variety of settings and situations in which the community-based nurse gives care.*

   Because of the variety of settings in which a nurse may practice and the limitation of time in the curriculum of schools of nursing, it is often difficult to schedule sufficient diversified clinical experiences. One of the purposes of this text is to address this problem by using a variety of clinical applications. This is accomplished in several ways. First, representative examples of different settings and situations are scattered throughout the body of the text. Second, one of the features of the text, *Client Situations in Practice*, integrates and synthesizes chapter concepts, showing the student step-by-step how the theory in the chapter relates to the reality of clinical practice. Third, additional *Care Studies* appear in *Learning Activities* at the end of each chapter and in the Instructor's Manual. Such client care situations give the student an opportunity to practice skills while applying chapter concepts. Last, *questions for reflection* for use with a *clinical journal* or *individual assignments* are found in the *Learning Activities* at the end of each chapter.

3. *To clarify the cultural diversification of the community in which nurses provide quality care.*

   Another important emphasis of *Introduction to Community-Based Nursing,* third edition, is its cross-cultural approach. Our society is diversified with many racial, ethnic, and minority groups. The community-based nurse will care for clients from many diverse cultures and must be prepared to give quality and culturally competent care. Chapter 3, Cultural Care, is written by Paula Swiggum, who has extensive experience in cross-cultural nursing in both recruiting and providing academic support for students from diverse cultural backgrounds, as well as in curriculum development. She is a member of the Transcultural Nursing Society as well as a Certified Transcultural Nurse. Consideration of cross-cultural issues is woven throughout the text.

4. *To integrate the importance of the individual to the family and the family to the individual throughout the text.*

   Most clients will be part of a family. The client's health and the client's care during illness are influenced by the family. At the same time, the client's health status and outlook will influence the continuous growth and development of the family. This symbiotic relationship plays a prominent role in *Introduction to Community-Based Nursing.* Special attention is given to nursing support of the lay caregiver.

## Organization of the Text

*Introduction to Community-Based Nursing* is divided into five units: basic concepts, nursing skills, application, settings, and implications for future practice.

▸ *Unit I, Basic Concepts in Community-Based Nursing,* includes essential elements of community-based nursing. An introductory chapter discusses definitions of a community and a healthy community, components of community-based nursing, and nursing skills and competencies needed to give quality care in the community. The unit also includes information on health promotion and disease prevention, cultural considerations, and family implications.

▸ *Unit II, Skills for Community-Based Nursing Practice,* reviews basics of assessment, teaching, case management, and continuity of care, and addresses those skills specific to community-based settings.

▸ *Unit III, Community-Based Nursing Across the Life Span,* provides assessment guides, teaching materials, and strategies for addressing health promotion and disease prevention across the life span.

▸ *Unit IV, Settings for Practice,* discusses a wide sampling of practice settings and opportunities and practice specialties. One chapter discusses home health care in depth. Two new chapters have been added to this section in the third edition. Specific roles for home health care nurses are outlined in the chapter on specialized home care nursing. Mental health nursing in community-based settings is the topic of the second new chapter.

▸ *Unit V, Implications for Future Practice,* discusses trends in health care and implications on community-based nursing.

Consistency of approach was one of the goals in the development of the text. Many chapters include a short section giving a historical perspective on the chapter subject. Most chapters address nursing skills and competencies. These sections may include information on the nursing process or on such things as communication, teaching, and management. Seeming repetition of any information is for the purpose of reinforcing knowledge or skills in light of the chapter's subject. Documentation is covered in many chapters because of its importance to community-based nursing. All chapters end with *Learning Activities.*

## Key Features of the Text

The following features of the book were developed as pedagogical aids for the student. They help clarify text information, give the student guidelines for actions, or require the student to use critical thinking.

- ▶ Learning Activities: three to more than five activities at the end of every chapter form a compact study and application guide. These contain the following exercises:
  - ▶ Journaling: to be used for a clinical journal or as individual assignments to assist the student in applying theoretical content to clinical situations to become a reflective practitioner.
  - ▶ Client Care: at least one in most chapters. A client situation is described and followed by critical thinking exercises.
  - ▶ Practical Applications: appear in many chapters. Not related to a specific client, these include activities to prepare the student for clinical application.
  - ▶ Critical Thinking Exercises: at least one in every chapter. A problem is presented in a sentence or two with directions for critical thinking.
- ▶ Community-Based Nursing Care Guidelines: boxed information that includes specific interventions for the community-based nurse.
- ▶ Community-Based Teaching: boxed lists of information to give clients and their families.
- ▶ Research in Community-Based Nursing Care: boxed information that includes short paragraphs of descriptive research.
- ▶ Assessment Tools: many chapters provide sample assessment forms to be used in community-based nursing care.
- ▶ Healthy People 2010: Health promotion and disease prevention material: plentiful materials in Chapters 9, 10, and 11 for health teaching and addresses of Web sites from which numerous additional materials can be downloaded.
- ▶ Glossary: helps the student review terminology or understand new terminology used in the book.
- ▶ Other pedagogical aids: Objectives, Key Terms, Chapter Topics, References, and Bibliography.
- ▶ What's on the Web: Found in most chapters, these features contain addresses and descriptions of Web sites related to the chapter material and providing additional resources. Chapter 16 includes a list of general Web sites helpful in community-based nursing.

We have tried to avoid sexist terms for the nurse and clients. Throughout the text we have used the term "family" for consistency. However, the term refers to anyone who is concerned about and supportive of the client and can signify a relative or significant other.

## Instructor's Manual

The Instructor's Manual was prepared with an ongoing emphasis on practical application of the student's knowledge base. More than 50 assignments, test questions, and additional client care studies are designed to develop skills and knowledge essential for the unique role of the associate-degree nurse in community-based nursing. Suggestions of how to identify, develop, and structure community-based clinical experiences are also found in the manual. Many of the assignments have been used and improved over years of teaching community health nursing.

*Roberta Hunt, RN, MSPH, PhD*
*hunthean@comcast.net*

# Acknowledgments

I am grateful to many individuals, especially family, friends, and colleagues, for their encouragement and assistance in the development of this textbook. It is impossible to acknowledge everyone, given the limitations of memory and space.

To all my colleagues who have given encouragement and validation and who have made the teaching of nursing an exciting and stimulating profession—you have contributed to this project. The more than 2,000 students whom I have had the pleasure of working with in the classroom and in clinical settings in the community, who have provided feedback and suggestions about my teaching and assignments, you have each made an invaluable contribution to this book.

There are several people in the Nursing Education department of Lippincott Williams & Wilkins who have provided invaluable expertise and assistance. Margaret Zuccarini, Senior Acquisitions Editor, has given professional guidance to craft and redefine the focus of this text. Carol Devault has been terrific with her quick, competent assistance. Jackie Smith made important contributions with her valuable editorial assistance.Thanks to Deedie McMahon, whose congenial personality has made the last leg of this journey pleasant and painless. Thanks to Amy Dinkel, for her quick response time and her kind and sweet temperament. She made the last of the "dirty details" quick and easy.

To my dear friend of many years, Paula Swiggum, I owe an enormous thanks for writing Chapter 3, Culture Care. This expertly crafted and beautifully written chapter adds a great deal to the overall message of the importance of respectful care, which is the central premise of *Introduction to Community-Based Nursing*. To my former colleague and dear friend, Marva Thurston, an enormous thanks for writing Chapter 15 while starting a new job. In this chapter she shares her knowledge and sensitive approach to care that she has gained through over 20 years of working with individuals with mental health issues. This chapter makes an important contribution in highlighting that mental and physical health are both essential to comprehensive community-based care.

Finally, I am grateful to my family and friends who provide day-to-day support and encouragement. To all of my former colleagues at the College of St. Catherine—the most professional and supportive faculty group an educator could ever hope to work with—thanks for the opportunity to work with all of you. I especially want to thank Meg Carolan, Joann O'Leary, Sue Larson, and Susan O'Conner-Von for their ongoing friendships and listening ears. Thanks to my family, especially Becky Hunt Carmody, John Harris, and Steve Hunt, for your continuing encouragement. To Andrew and Mark, you guys are the most terrific young men, you make your Dad and me so proud of you. To my terrific son-in-law, David, and darling granddaughter, Josie, you both really brighten up my life. To my wonderful daughters—Jackie, for your cheerful attitude plus valuable editorial assistance prodding me forward, and Megan, for your thoughtful advice and balanced view of the world—a heartfelt thank-you. Most of all, I am grateful to my loving husband, Tim Heaney—your committed attitude towards me and all that I do has helped me become more than I ever imagined.

*Roberta Hunt*
School of Nursing
University of Minnesota

# Contents

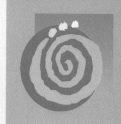

# BASIC CONCEPTS IN COMMUNITY-BASED NURSING

Before you practice nursing in a community-based setting, you must understand the basic concepts behind community-based health care. Unit I introduces these concepts as a knowledge base for further exploration as you begin to apply what you have learned.

Chapter 1 gives an overview of community-based nursing, beginning with a brief historical perspective. Health care reform and health care funding, which have taken health care out of the hospital and into the community, are discussed, along with the definition of a community, especially a healthy community. Components of community-based care and nursing skills and competencies round out the introductory chapter.

Health promotion and disease prevention, as outlined by the federal government's *Healthy People 2010* (U.S. Department of Health and Human Services, 2000), is the focus of Chapter 2.

Chapter 3 discusses the ever-changing makeup of our society and asks you to look at your own cultural background and attitudes about diversity. The chapter promotes culturally competent care.

Chapter 4 discusses family involvement, an important consideration in community-based care.

The remainder of the book will use these concepts to build your knowledge base and relate it to practical experiences.

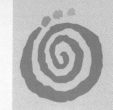

## CHAPTER 1

# Overview of Community-Based Nursing

Roberta Hunt

1. Identify major issues leading to the development of community-based nursing.
2. Discuss the current reimbursement system for health care services and its impact on nursing.
3. Describe the factors that define community.
4. Indicate the relationship between health and community.
5. Compare acute care nursing, community-based nursing, and community health nursing.
6. Discuss components of community-based care.
7. Examine the skills with which you perform necessary competencies.

## KEY TERMS

acute care
advance directives
community
community-based nursing
continuity of care
demographics
diagnosis-related groups (DRGs)
extended family

health maintenance organizations (HMOs)
living will
nuclear family
preferred provider organizations (PPOs)
prospective payment
self-care
vital statistics

## CHAPTER TOPICS

- **Historical Perspectives**
- **Health Care Reform**
- **Health Care Funding**
- **The Community**
- **Community Nursing Versus Community-Based Nursing**
- **Focus of Nursing**
- **Components of Community-Based Care**
- **Nursing Skills and Competencies**
- **Conclusions**

## THE NURSING STUDENT SPEAKS

In general, having clinical in the community has broadened my horizons of what I am able to do as a nurse. Before this community experience, my mind-set was that you had to work in a hospital or a nursing home when you graduated. Acute care was the only setting that I could think about working in, and now I realize that these people in the community need me too. Public health, I have noticed, is short staffed too, just like hospitals. They only have one nurse at the shelter to see all of the families. It seems to be overwhelming. This experience has broadened my horizons to see the different roles that I can play as a nurse, most of which I have never seen myself in.

Before this experience, I could not believe that we had to do a community rotation. Once I was out there, I was shocked at how my views of community health were distorted. After the rotation was over, I was glad that we were able to experience the community setting. Working in the homeless shelter helped me to look at people in a more holistic way, which I now believe is the only way to look at people. Before this experience, it [my focus] was always the physical aspects of a person, such as blood pressure and pain. Now I can see the whole person—the physical, the mental, and the spiritual aspects. These are all of the parts that need to be healed. I appreciate what I have learned from the community experience. It is all coming together.

— **Kristin Ocker, RN**
    Student completing a BSN
    College of St. Catherine

Changes in settings for nursing practice have occurred over the last 25 years as a result of public concern regarding our health care system. Concerns center on quality of, access to, and cost of health care, as well as fragmentation of health care. These concerns and the resultant changes give nurses an opportunity to help shape health care at the beginning of the 21st century. In 1999, the National League for Nursing (NLN) predicted 10 trends in health care that will affect nursing education and practice (Box 1–1).

These trends and the implications for nursing educational preparation and quality nursing practice are the focus of this book. This chapter provides an overview of nursing care and its historical background, introduces the reader to the community and community-based nursing, and describes components of community-based nursing practice, skills, and competencies.

 **HISTORICAL PERSPECTIVES**

During most of the 20th century, nursing care was associated primarily with hospital settings (Bellack & O'Neil, 2000). However, historically, the setting for nurs-

> ▶ **Box 1-1** The Future of Nursing Education: ◀
> Trends to Watch

1. Changing demographics and increasing diversity
2. The technology explosion
3. Globalization of the world's economy and society
4. Educated consumers, alternative therapies and genomics, and palliative care
5. Shift to population-based care and increasing complexity of client care
6. Higher costs of health care and challenges of managed care
7. Effects of health policy and regulation
8. The growing need for interdisciplinary education for collaborative practice
9. Nursing shortages, opportunities for lifelong learning, and workforce development
10. Significant advances in nursing science and research

Source: Heller, B., Oros, M., & Durney-Crowley, J. (1999). The future of nursing education: Ten trends to watch. New York: National League for Nursing. Retrieved on March 3, 2003, from http://www.lnl.org/infotrends.htm.

ing care was the home. The first written reference to care of the ill in the home is found in the New Testament, in which mention is made of visiting the sick at home to aid in their care.

Florence Nightingale, credited as the mother of modern nursing, developed a classic model for educating nurses in hospital-based programs. Nightingale's curriculum also included the first training programs to educate district nurses, with 1 year of training devoted to promoting self-care and the health of communities (Monteiro, 1991).

William Rathbone, a resident of Liverpool, England, in the 1850s, established the modern concept of the visiting nurse (Kalish & Kalish, 1995). Lillian Wald and Mary Brewster began a program for visiting nurses in the United States in the early 1900s (Frachel, 1988). Wald, the founder of public health nursing, drew on contemporary ideas that linked nursing, motherhood, social welfare, and the public. Her work was designed to respond to the needs of those populations at greatest risk by nursing the sick in their homes and providing preventive instructions to reduce illness. Wald argued that the nurse, through her "peculiar introduction to the patient and her organic relationship with the neighborhood," could be the "starting point" for wider service in the community. Wald believed that nurses could reach and educate their clients in the broadest sense, drawing on diversity of cultural beliefs and societal demands of the populace (Reverby, 1993).

## Shift From Community to Hospital

In 1910, approximately 90% of all nursing care was provided in the home. After World War I, care of the sick started to shift to the hospital. Early in the 1950s, the growing complexity in health care technology resulted in an increased need for hospital care. During the 1960s and 1970s, a person typically stayed in the hospital for 7 to 10 days for uncomplicated conditions or for surgery (Craven & Hirnle, 2000).

This trend continued until the early 1980s, when escalating health care costs prompted changes in the health care delivery system and its financing. In brief, nursing care provided in the home in the 1800s migrated to the acute care hospital in the middle of the 20th century and then back to the home in the 1980s. From 1980 to 2000, this trend intensified as the number of nurses working in public and community health, ambulatory care, and other institutional settings increased rapidly (Health Resources and Services Administration [HRSA], 2000).

## An Era of Cost Containment

President Reagan signed the Tax Equity and Fiscal Responsibility Act (TEFRA) in 1982 and the Social Security Amendments in 1983. This legislation changed the way Medicare and Medicaid services were reimbursed, initiating a service called the **prospective payment** system. The prospective payment system calculates reimbursement to hospitals based on the client's diagnosis according to federally mandated **diagnosis-related groups (DRGs)**. The client's diagnosis is categorized according to the federal DRG coding system, and payment is bundled into one fee, which is then paid to the hospital. Payment by client diagnosis, therefore, was an attempt to contain Medicare and Medicaid costs.

Gradually, many insurance companies, health maintenance organizations (HMOs), and other third-party payers adopted the DRG method of payment. As the reimbursement system for health care changed, the average length of stay for a hospitalized client decreased substantially. In fact, it became financially advantageous for the hospital if clients had shorter stays. As a result, a scenario was created in which clients were discharged "quicker and sicker." With this transition, it became evident that it was more cost-effective to provide services outside the hospital.

## Shift From Hospital to Community

### Acute Care Setting

Acute care became the term used for people who were receiving intensive hospital care. The term is used today for the setting in which this care is provided. An acute care setting contrasts with the hospital setting, which also can be used as an ambulatory clinic or day surgery unit. In general, individuals in acute care settings are very sick. Many are postsurgical clients or need highly technical care. Many of these clients have life-threatening conditions and require close monitoring and constant care. The care given these clients is specialized and requires considerable expertise in physical caregiving. Acute nursing care is very different from community-based nursing care, as evidenced by differences between hospital and home environments shown in Table 1–1.

### Community Setting

Clients affected by the transition into community-based health care were not in need of fewer services. Rather, the focus of services simply shifted from the hospital to the community. Care that once was considered safe only within the hospi-

**TABLE 1-1** • Differences Between Hospital and Home

| Factors | Hospital | Home |
|---|---|---|
| **Practice** | | |
| Resources | Predetermined | Variable |
| Environment | Predictable | Highly variable |
| Locating client | Simple | Requires planning |
| Access to client | Routine | Determined by client's family |
| Focus | Individual | Client in family system |
| Family support | Helpful | Critical |
| Client role | Relatively dependent | Highly autonomous |
| **Instruction** | | |
| Student safety | Awareness | Central concern |
| Supervision of practice | Mostly direct | Mostly indirect |
| Teaching style | Often teacher-directed | Collaborative problem-solving |

Source: Reed, F. C., & Wuyscik, M. A. (1998). Community health strategies: Teach what? Reflections on the transition from hospital teaching to teaching in the community. *Nurse Educator, 23*(3), 11–13.

tal became routine in outpatient settings, such as ambulatory care centers, surgical centers, dialysis centers, rehabilitation centers, walk-in clinics, physicians' offices, and the home.

The change in health care services resulted in changes in nursing care as well. Settings changed to the community, especially the home; services relied on more technically complicated and high-tech procedures. In the past decade, the number of nurses working in every employment setting has increased. However, the rate of increase in hospitals is less than in previous years. The greatest increase occurred in community-based settings (Fig. 1-1).

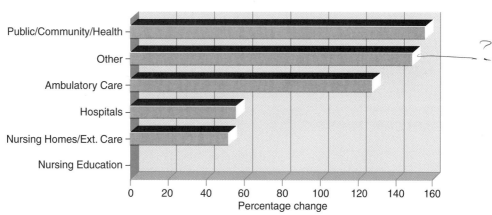

***Figure 1–1.*** ▶ Percent change between 1980 and 2000 in RNs employed in selected settings. Source: Health Resources and Services Admininstration. Bureau of Health Professions. (2000). The registered nurse population: Findings from the national sample survey of registered nurses.

The Bureau of Labor Statistics estimates that increases in health care services in the last decade account for 3.1 million jobs. Nursing is one of the five occupations with the greatest number of jobs in the next decade. In 2000, national supply of registered nurses was estimated at 1.89 million while the demand was estimated at 2 million. Based on what is known about trends in the supply of RNs and their anticipated demand, the shortage is expected to grow relatively slowly until 2010 when it is expected to reach 12%. Unlike nursing shortages in the past, this shortage will be driven by a permanent shift in the labor market that is unlikely to reverse in the next few years (Buerhaus, Staiger, & Auerbach, 2000). Demand will exceed supply at an accelerated rate, and by 2015 the shortage is anticipated to quadruple to 20% and grow to 29% by 2020 (HRSA, 2002).

These changes make it imperative for nursing educators to prepare graduates for positions outside the walls of the acute care setting and for roles in the community. The NLN (2000a) recommends that all nursing education undergo a shift in emphasis to continue to ensure that all nurses from all education levels are prepared to function in a community-based, community-focused health care system. This means that nurses must be competent to practice in varied settings across the continuum of care (American Organization of Nurse Executives [AONE], 2000).

 ## HEALTH CARE REFORM

Health care in general is in transition. The United States is in the midst of reviewing and revising its health care system, and few people deny that some changes must occur. Legislation on state and national levels may result in the most dramatic changes of all. *Healthy People 2010* (U.S. Department of Health and Human Services, 2000), which lists government goals (discussed further in Chapter 2), has stirred our imagination about meeting the needs of all Americans. Particular populations are targeted for care. The question has been raised: Is health care a right or a privilege? Who gets health care and who pays for this health care will be at the center of the debate for some time. These issues present challenges and opportunities for the nurse in the first decade of the new century.

Nurses fit into health care reform first by being prepared for practice in community settings. Further, nurses must understand the business aspects of health care. Last of all, nurses in community settings need highly developed skills in assessment, communication, interdisciplinary collaboration, and working with culturally diverse populations.

 ## HEALTH CARE FUNDING

Health care is extremely expensive, and costs continue to rise. Increasing health care costs have affected many health care agencies and organizations. They must now find funds, in addition to fee-for-service charges, in the form of voluntary donations and state and federal programs.

Few individuals can afford to pay their health care costs out of their own pockets. Many individuals belong to HMOs or rely on government-funded health care such as Medicare and Medicaid. Insurance plans, HMOs, and government programs provide a variety of coverage plans. Many, however, do not cover preventive care, psychiatric treatment, outpatient support services, and medications. Many limit the amount of service paid for a particular type of care, such as home health care visits.

## Federally Funded Health Care

Primary government funding comes through Medicare and Medicaid. Under Medicare, home health care is an important service for the elderly, and concern about it will continue to grow as the elderly population increases in the United States. Medicare covers nursing; physical, speech, and occupational therapies; home care aides; medical social services; and some medical supplies. With the Balanced Budget Act in 1997, changes were made to Medicare's payment system to contain cost. These changes have affected and will continue to affect the role of the nurse in the delivery of home care services (Jitramontree, 2000).

## Group Plans

Group plans include HMOs, preferred provider organizations (PPOs), and private insurance. **HMOs** are prepaid, structured, managed systems in which providers deliver a comprehensive range of health care services to enrollees. **PPOs** allow a network of providers to provide services at a lower fee in return for prompt payment at prenegotiated rates. Private insurance may be obtained through large, nonprofit, tax-exempt organizations or through small, private, for-profit insurance companies. This type of insurance is called third-party payment. Long-term care insurance may also be obtained through private insurance companies.

 **THE COMMUNITY**

Nurses who practice community-based nursing need to understand the community within which they practice. Knowledge of the community helps nurses maintain quality of care.

## Defining Community

**Community** can be defined in numerous ways, depending on the application. This text uses the definition of community as "a people, location, and social system" (Josten, 1989).

### People: Families, Culture, and Community
The variety of individuals, families, and cultural groups represented in a community contributes to the overall character of that community. The simplest way to understand a community is through **vital statistics** and **demographics.** These data may be thought of as the community's vital statistics, similar to an individual's vital signs. A community consisting primarily of senior citizens has a totally different personality from a community of young, unmarried adults.

The characteristics of the families living in a community contribute to the overall complexion of that community and, in turn, the community health care needs. In communities where families are strong and nurturing, there is an opportunity for a strong and caring community. In communities where families are nonexistent or fail to provide an adequate basis for individual growth, problems with physical abuse, neglect, substance abuse, and violence may arise. A strong family unit is the basic building block for strong communities.

Culture contributes to the overall character of a community and, in turn, its health needs. In most of the world, a scarcity of resources necessitates **extended family** residences. Included in the extended family are grandparents, aunts, uncles, and other relatives. When living together in one household, many members may be involved with child care and care of the sick or injured. In these communities, there are different needs related to child and health care than in communities such as those in the United States and Western Europe, where the **nuclear family** is the norm. In the 6% of the world where nuclear family structures prevail, isolation and self-reliance affect the design and delivery of services. A client, then, who has a nuclear family and no extended family often has different needs from the client with numerous extended family members living in the same household or close by it.

The role of individuals according to their ages is often dictated by culture. In some cultures, the older people are retired from leadership and governing responsibilities, whereas in other cultures, these members are considered essential to the governing structure of the community. In this situation, the more prestigious positions of authority and responsibility are assigned to the older members of the community.

Health is affected by culture. Madeleine Leininger (1970) observed that "health and illness states are strongly influenced and often primarily determined by the cultural background of an individual." The culture of the individual and his or her family has an impact on the community's definition of health and on the service needs of that community.

### Location: Community Boundaries

A community usually is defined by boundaries. Boundaries may be geographic, such as those defined as a city, county, state, or nation. Boundaries may be political; precincts and wards may determine them. Boundaries to a community may also emerge as the result of identifying or solving a problem. Consequently, a community may establish a boundary within which a problem can be defined and solved. Figure 1–2 depicts this variety of community boundaries.

Community boundaries are important because they often determine what services are available to individuals living within a particular geographic area. Eligibility for services may be limited, or denied, depending on whether one resides within a certain geographic area. It is important for the nurse to realize that community boundaries limit availability of, and eligibility for, services. For example, suppose you are a nurse working at Ramsey County Hospital. Your patient is from Hennepin County. You will refer the client to services in Hennepin County. The client, however, may also be eligible for services with a home health care agency that serves multiple counties but is not located in Hennepin County. It is helpful for you to be familiar with eligibility requirements of a variety of community organizations.

It is important to have a working knowledge of service restrictions for agencies in a geographic area. In some counties, the first assessment visit by the county nurse is free; in other areas this may not be the case. Not only should the nurse be familiar with boundaries and basic eligibility criteria and restrictions, the nurse also needs to know about the available resources within the area.

A community defined by its problems and solutions has a fluid boundary. The problems and those who are affected by those problems determine this boundary. This allows all those who may be affected by the problems to participate in the solutions and the resulting outcome. Thus, a more fluid boundary may allow for greater eligibility or opportunity for service.

The problem of air pollution in one community provides us with an example of a community solution where the boundary is fluid. In the suburbs of Rosie Mountain and Awful Valley (Fig. 1–2), two school nurses in different elementary schools notice that the percentage of children they are seeing with symptoms of asthma is increasing. The school nurses talk to each other and note that most of the children with asthma in both school districts live west of a large oil refinery. The school nurses contact the Department of Health. The parents of the children from both schools are invited to a public meeting to discuss the issue of air pollution and the incidence of asthma. After several meetings, a group of parents from both schools forms a constituency devoted to the identification of the problem and potential solutions. The theoretical boundaries of this community are shown in Figure 1–2. Established school boundaries become fluid in this scenario when a problem arises.

### Social Systems

Social systems have an impact on a community and, consequently, the health of that community. Social systems include a community's economy, education, reli-

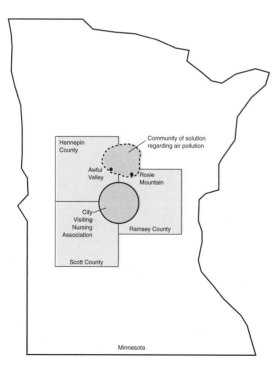

***Figure 1–2.*** ▶ A community's boundaries may be many things: geographic, political, problematic. These boundaries are used in the example in this chapter.

gion, welfare, politics, recreation, legal system, health care, safety and transportation, and communication systems. Depending on the infrastructure, these systems may have a beneficial or detrimental impact on the health of individuals living in a given community. Where recreational facilities provide opportunities for health promotion activities, for instance, the health of the citizens will be enhanced.

It is a documented fact that the infant mortality rate is lower in communities where prenatal care is available and readily accessible to all pregnant women. Here is a social system at work within a community; it has a profound impact on the quality of health of its individual members.

## A Healthy Community

Just as there are characteristics of healthy individuals, so are there characteristics of healthy communities. These include the following:

▶ Awareness that "we are community"
▶ Conservation of natural resources
▶ Recognition of and respect for the existence of subgroups
▶ Participation of subgroups in community affairs
▶ Preparation to meet crises
▶ Ability to solve problems
▶ Communication through open channels
▶ Resources available to all
▶ Settling of disputes through legitimate mechanisms
▶ Participation by citizens in decision making
▶ Wellness of a high degree among its members

A dynamic relationship exists between health and community. In this relationship, health is considered in the context of the community's people, its location, and its social system (Fig. 1–3). Healthy citizens can contribute to the overall health, vitality, and economy of the community. Similarly, if a large portion of individuals in a community is not healthy, not productive, or poorly nourished, the community can suffer from a lack of vitality and productivity (Fig. 1–4).

Location also influences the health of a community. If a toxic landfill or refinery contaminates the earth, water, or air, the health of the people in the area will obviously be detrimentally affected. Figure 1–5 illustrates the relationship between the location and the level of health in a given community.

Social systems and public policy also affect health. Figure 1–6 shows how a community's social systems affect its health. For example, there will be fewer smokers in communities where smoking is not allowed in public buildings or the sale of cigarettes to minors is restricted and strictly enforced. In a community where all pregnant women receive prenatal care, the infant mortality rate will be lower. In a community where immunizations are available and accessible to all children, the immunization rate will be higher and the communicable disease rates low. The array of social systems that affect health is shown in Figure 1–6.

The public sees lowering crime rates, strengthening families and their lifestyles, improving environmental quality, and providing behavioral or mental health care as critical elements to creating healthy communities. A Healthcare Forum survey in 1993 pointed out " . . . the emergence of public recognition that one's health is somehow related to the health of one's neighbors; suggesting that perhaps, the

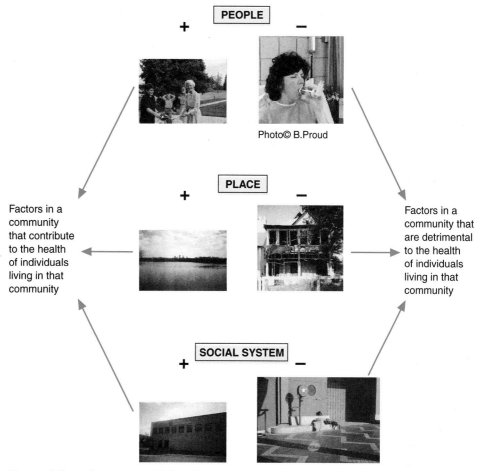

**Figure 1–3.** ▶ A community's health is considered in the context of its people, its location, and its social system.

most practical approach to pursuing a healthier life is the pursuit of a healthier community."

## COMMUNITY NURSING VERSUS COMMUNITY-BASED NURSING

More opportunities are created for nurses in the community as the setting for nursing care moves outside the acute care setting. Many of these settings, positions, and opportunities are discussed in Chapter 12. The prominent nursing role in the community in the past was that of public health or community health nurse, but this has changed with the current health care delivery system. Although a monumental need for provision of nursing care in the community has resulted

**PEOPLE**

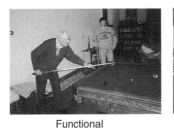

|                          | Functional               | Nonfunctional            |                          |
| ------------------------ | ------------------------ | ------------------------ | ------------------------ |

High level of
health in
a community

Productive

Able to:
• Work
• Care for self
  or others
• Volunteer
• Pay taxes

Nonproductive

Unable to:
• Work
• Care for self
  or others
• Volunteer
• Pay taxes

Low level of
health in
a community

***Figure 1–4.*** ▶ Functional and dysfunctional individuals affect the health of the community.

**PLACE**

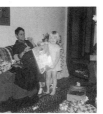

High level of
health in
a community

Enhancement
of health
――――――――
Clean air, water,
and land

Detrimental
to health
――――――――
Environmental
pollution

Low level of
health in
a community

Lower incidence
and prevalence of
• URI
• Asthma
• COPD
• Lung cancer
• Infertility
• Congenital anomalies

Higher incidence
and prevalence of
• URI
• Asthma
• COPD
• Lung cancer
• Congenital anomalies

***Figure 1–5.*** ▶ Location affects the health of the community.

from the changes in the health care delivery system, this increase for nurses has been not for community health nurses but for community-based nurses.

While community health nursing practice includes nursing directed to individuals, families, and groups, the predominant responsibility is to the population as a whole (American Nurses Association [ANA], 1999). Thus, community, or public, health nursing is defined by its role in promoting the public's health. Community health nursing is a subset of community-based nursing. Community health nursing has a definitive philosophy of practice and requires specific knowledge and skill.

Community-based nursing is not defined by the setting or by the level of academic preparation but by a philosophy of practice (Hunt, 1998). It is about *how* the nurse practices, *not where* the nurse practices. Community-based nursing is based on the following concepts (NLN, 2000a):

► The individual and the family have primary responsibility for health care decisions.
► Health and social issues are acknowledged as interactive.
► Treatment effectiveness, rather than the technologic imperative, drives decisions.

**Community-based nursing** care can be defined as nursing care directed toward specific individuals and families within a community. It is designed to meet needs of people as they move between and among health care settings. The emphasis is on a "flowing" kind of care that does not necessarily occur in one setting.

High-technology care that previously was available only in acute care settings is now provided in the home. The community-based nurse must teach clients and families how to manage highly technical equipment and to be responsible for complex self-care.

##  FOCUS OF NURSING

Nursing, in any setting and with any nursing theory, involves a focus of four components: the client, the environment, health, and nursing (Fawcett, 1984). Each area is approached differently depending on whether the care is provided in the acute care setting or in the community-based setting (Table 1–1).

In the acute care setting, the client is typically identified by the medical diagnosis and is separated from the family. The environment is controlled by the facility with restriction of the family's access to the client and a limitation on the client's freedom. Health and illness are seen as separate and apart from one another. If the client is discharged, the goals of acute care are met. Nursing functions are largely delegated medical functions that center on treatment of illness.

In community-based nursing, the client is in his or her natural environment, in the context of the family and community. Illness is seen as merely an aspect of life, and the goals of care are focused around maximizing the client's quality of life. Nursing in the community is an autonomous practice, for the most part, with nursing interventions decided on by the client, family, and health care team and based on the values of the client or family and the community. The community model of care reflects the principles of community-based nursing where the goal of care is to encourage self-care in the context of the family and community with a focus on illness prevention and continuity of care.

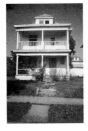
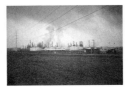
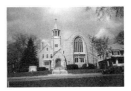
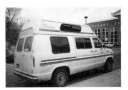

High level of health     **Systems**     Low level of health

Stable economy, ◄— Economic —► Unstable economy, lack —► No insurance
sufficient well-paying     of jobs     No preventive
employment     care

Quality public ◄— Education —► Low quality public —► Difficulty getting
schools, affordable     education, non-     well-paying jobs
post-secondary     affordable post-
education     secondary education

Services that assist ◄— Welfare —► Lack of assistance for
with job training     job training

Programs that ◄— Recreation —► Lack of programs and —► Higher incidence
provide health     facilities     of obesity, high
promotion     blood presure,
opportunities     heart disease

Information ◄— Communication —► Lack of assimilation of —► Services not
available regarding     information on health     utilized
health care services     programs

Support for ◄— Religious —► Religious community not
community needs     involved in health issues

Public policy ◄— Political —► Lack of public policy
supporting community     supporting community
health issues     health issues

Available ◄— Transportation —► Inaccessible health care, —► Noncompliance,
transportation to     and     unsafe streets     higher crime:
health care facilities,     available safe     homicide, rape
safe neighborhoods ◄— housing —►

Adequate legal ◄— Legal —► Lack of adequate legal
assistance for all     assistance for all
members of the     members of the
community     community

Available, ◄— Health care —► Lack of accessible and
accessible, and     quality primary,
quality primary,     secondary, and tertiary
secondary, and     health care
tertiary health care

**Figure 1–6.** ► Social system and public policy affect the health of the community.

**COMPONENTS OF COMMUNITY-BASED CARE**

Transitions in health care settings and consumer participation have brought about some changes in the directions of health care. Several components make up community-based care: self-care, preventive health care, care within the context of the community, continuity of care, and collaborative care. These are described here and expanded on throughout the text.

## Self-Care: Client and Family Responsibility

The consumer movement within the past several decades has led to self-care awareness. Consumers are becoming aware that it is better to take care of themselves and remain healthy than to neglect their health and have to treat an illness or injury. Programs on stress management, nutrition, exercise and fitness, and smoking cessation and substance abuse prevention are examples of this health-seeking behavior on the part of consumers. As a further result, political and government factions have promoted such things as seatbelt use, motorcycle and bicycle safety, pollution control, and handgun control.

The first component of community-based nursing is self-care. **Self-care** charges the individual client and the family with primary responsibility for health care decisions and actions. Because more and more health care is provided outside the acute care setting, by design this care must be provided by the client, family, or other caregiver, such as a friend or neighbor, rather than a health care professional. It has become too expensive to do otherwise.

Empowering individuals to make informed health care decisions is an essential component of self-care. One example is the recently introduced federal mandate for advance directives. **Advance directives** allow clients to participate in decisions about their care, including the right to refuse treatment. One type of advance directive is the **living will,** which is the client's statement regarding the medical treatment he or she chooses to omit or refuses in the event the client is unable to make those decisions for himself or herself.

Although community-based nursing affords the opportunity for direct intervention, it also requires self-care teaching for the client and caregiver. The nurse's participation in self-care requires use of the nursing process. In other words, assessment, planning, implementation, and evaluation revolve around this question: How much care can the client and other caregivers *safely* provide themselves?

## Preventive Health Care

Treatment efficacy rather than technologic imperative promotes nursing care that emphasizes prevention. Community-based nursing considers all three levels of prevention (discussed in Chapter 2). Unlike community health nursing, community-based nursing focuses primarily on tertiary prevention. This emphasis is evident in all settings of community-based nursing.

For example, a nurse in the emergency room considers not only the impact of the child's poisoning, but also what preventive nursing interventions will maximize recovery and prevent a repeat of the incident. Careful teaching about wound care to avoid infection is an important preventive intervention for the client who is having a laceration sutured. Likewise, referral of a client for substance abuse assessment is an appropriate preventive nursing intervention for an intoxicated person who presents at the urgent care center after a fall.

## Care Within the Context of the Community

Another component of community-based nursing recognizes that health and social issues are interactive. Nursing care is provided while considering the culture, values, and resources of the client, the family, and the community. If the client requests a particular religious or social ceremony before tube feeding, then the nurse attempts, within the constraints of safety, to comply with the client's request. In situations where family members want to participate in the client's care but their psychomotor skills restrict their ability to do so, the nurse will accommodate the desire within the constraints of time and safe care. If the client lives in a community where older individuals enjoy the social functions of religious services every week, the visiting nurse honors that community value by careful scheduling of visits.

Care in the context of the client, family, and community is affected by the location and social systems of each community. Location often defines eligibility for health care services. Consequently, access and availability of services affect the health of the community. For instance, access to care is impeded by location when an adolescent who does not drive lives in the suburbs where there is no public transportation and seeks information about family planning services offered only in the nearby metropolitan area. In such a case, the social systems of the community affect access to care.

## Continuity of Care

Fragmentation of care has long been a concern of health care professionals. For instance, a client with a variety of problems may be seen by several physicians: the family physician, cardiologist, endocrinologist, consultants, and surgeon. A variety of other health care providers may be involved in the care also. This fragmentation of care can result in conflicting directions for care, overmedication or undermedication, and a confused client. **Continuity of care** is a bridge to quality care.

Community-based care becomes essential when clients are seen by several health care practitioners and move from one health care setting to another. Continuity allows for quality of care to be preserved in a changing health care delivery system. If all providers follow the basic principles of continuity of care, then the possibility of a detrimental impact from a decreased length of stay in the acute care setting, where care is coordinated, to a community setting, where care is provided through a variety of individuals, can be minimized. Continuity is the glue that holds community-based nursing care together and is one of the foundational concepts of this book. Continuity of care is discussed in Chapter 8.

## Collaborative Care

Closely related to continuity of care is collaborative care. Collaborative care among health care professionals is an essential part of holistic care because the primary goal of each practitioner should be to promote wellness and restore health. Regardless of the setting, the community-based nurse works with a variety of professionals as care for the client is assessed, planned, implemented, and evaluated.

The physician is responsible primarily for diagnosing the illness and initiating required medical or surgical treatment. Physicians have the authority to admit clients into a specific health care setting and to discharge them from that setting into another setting. The orders they write are followed by other professionals and the client, who report to the physician on outcomes. The pharmacist dispenses medications as directed by the physician.

Various therapists (physical, occupational, respiratory, speech) may be involved in the client's care, providing therapy in the acute care setting, a rehabilitation setting, a residential care setting, or the home. The client may visit the facility, or the therapist may visit the home.

A dietitian may be asked to adapt a specialized diet to a specific individual and family or to counsel and educate clients and their families. The social worker helps clients and families make decisions related to use of community resources, life-sustaining treatments, and long-term care. A chaplain or the client's spiritual advisor will also counsel the client and family and give spiritual support.

Although each professional is responsible for a specialized concern, each is also responsible for sharing information with others or for evaluating how care is proceeding. If one person in the chain fails to communicate, the bridge of continuity is weakened. Usually one person is designated as coordinator of these communications. In many cases this coordinator is the nurse. The nurse who coordinates collaborative care is discussed in Chapter 7.

## NURSING SKILLS AND COMPETENCIES

Although transitions have been made in health care in the past two decades, models of community-based care continue to develop. The Pew Health Professions Commission identified 21 competencies that health care professionals need in the 21st century. These competencies, listed in Box 1–2, emphasize community-based nursing care principles. Although these competencies apply to all health care professionals, the term "nurse" can be substituted in place of the term "practitioners" in the statements.

Nursing care in the acute care setting and the community differ greatly. Consequently, the nursing roles in each setting require different practice skills. Nursing roles differ in acute care, community-based health care, and home care. In the acute care setting, nurses spend the majority of their time in direct patient care and have little time for administrative, supervisory, or consultant roles.

The home care and community-based nurse spends almost three times as many hours as the acute care nurse in consultant roles (teacher, communicator). The community-based and home care nurses also spend five times as many hours in the administrator/manager role as the acute care nurse. In acute care, nurses spend 84% of their time doing direct client care; in community-based and home care nursing, only about 60% of time is spent on direct care.

The home care nurse spends more time in the supervision/management role than in the teaching or physical caregiver role. Home care incorporates critical aspects of both the hospital and community health nurse role. Nurses in home care

---

▶ **Box 1–2** Pew Commission : Twenty One Competencies ◀
for the 21st Century

1. Embrace a personal ethic of social responsibility and service.
2. Exhibit ethical behavior in all professional activities.
3. Provide evidence-based, clinically competent care.
4. Incorporate the multiple determinants of health in clinical care.
5. Apply knowledge of the new sciences.
6. Demonstrate critical thinking, reflection, and problem-solving skills.
7. Understand the role of primary care.
8. Rigorously practice preventive health care.
9. Integrate population-based care and services into practice.
10. Improve access to health care for those with unmet health needs.
11. Practice relationship-centered care with individuals and families.
12. Provide culturally sensitive care to a diverse society.
13. Partner with communities in health care decisions.
14. Use communication and information technology effectively and appropriately.
15. Work in interdisciplinary teams.
16. Ensure care that balances individual, professional, system, and societal needs.
17. Practice leadership.
18. Take responsibility for quality of care and health outcomes at all levels.
19. Contribute to continuous improvement of the health care system.
20. Advocate for public policy that promotes and protects the health of the public.
21. Continue to learn and help others learn.

———
Source: Bellack, J. P., & O'Neil, E. H. (2000). Recreating nursing practice for a new century: Recommendations and implications of the Pew Health Profession's Commission's final report. *Nursing and Healthcare Perspectives, 21*(1), 14–18.

---

express more job satisfaction than those working in acute care or community health (Simmons, Nelson, & Neal, 2001). Further, they are less likely to work weekends or nights.

Professional roles for the nurses in community-based care require competency in both knowledge and skills in communication, teaching, management, and direct physical caregiving (Box 1–3).

## Communication and Teaching

A competent nurse knows the principles and techniques of interpersonal communication and applies these in interactions with clients, caregivers, and other health care providers. In practice, the nurse identifies and interprets verbal and nonverbal communications. It is essential to recognize all recurring variables that influence the communication process. The nurse consistently and effectively uses

> ▶ **Box 1–3** Community-Based Nursing Competencies ◀

**Communication**

The nurse applies principles of interpersonal communication to interactions with clients, families, and other caregivers in all settings in the community.

**Teaching**

The nurse applies principles of teaching and learning to all learners, including the client, family member or caregiver, coworkers, and other care providers or community members.

**Management**

The nurse applies knowledge of leadership by performing the management functions of planning, organizing, coordinating, delegating, and evaluating care for a group of clients.

**Physical Caregiving**

The nurse applies knowledge of principles and procedures for providing safe and effective physical care.

interpersonal communication to establish, maintain, and terminate a therapeutic relationship. The interaction must effectively support the goals that are mutually established by the multidisciplinary team.

The nurse in the community-based setting must have a working knowledge of the principles of teaching and learning as they relate to the scope of practice. The nurse collects and interprets information to assess the learner's need to learn or readiness to learn. Individualized learning outcomes are developed and implemented in the teaching plan. Learning outcomes are evaluated, and modifications are made as indicated. Teaching is further developed in Chapter 6.

## Management

As a manager of care in the community, the nurse uses his or her leadership ability and carries out the management functions of planning, organizing, coordinating, delegating, and evaluating care for one client or a group of clients. This involves collecting and interpreting relevant data that leads to meeting priority needs of the client. The nurse assesses resources, capabilities of other providers, and the client or family's ability to provide ongoing care. This assessment and the established care plan goals provide the foundation used to develop a management plan geared toward the client's recovery.

The manager of care oversees the care of a group of clients, delegates nursing activities to coworkers, and assumes responsibility for care given under his or her direction. The manager may also work to maintain and improve the work environment by identifying opportunities for improvement and implementing change.

The nurse as manager is responsible for evaluation of every aspect of care. Evaluation of the client's ability to assess his or her own situation and condition and to plan and implement care is an essential component of the recovery process. The manager role extends not only to clients but also to other nursing personnel who are providing care under the direction and leadership of the registered nurse.

## Assessment and Physical Caregiving

The nurse must know the principles and procedures required for safe and effective physical care. Some of these procedures are ordered by the physician. The nurse either performs these procedures or observes the client or caregiver in performing the tasks. The community-based nurse performs less physical care than does the nurse in the acute care setting.

Assessment is key to quality nursing care in all settings. Because the nurse in the community often functions in a more autonomous role than the nurse in the acute care setting, sound assessment skills are even more essential. After systematically collecting and interpreting data related to the client's condition, the nurse initiates, continues, alters, or terminates physical nursing care. He or she identifies environmental variables in the home that may affect physical nursing care. Assessment also includes identification of the variables in the community that may influence physical nursing care.

The client, caregiver, and nurse set expected outcomes and outcome criteria and then develop a plan of care for providing the necessary physical care that will meet these goals. The plan is then implemented. The nurse removes hazards from the environment that threaten the safety of the client or others.

Effectiveness of the physical care, expected outcomes, and outcome criteria is evaluated, and modifications are made according to need. The nurse also evaluates the ability of other caregivers to provide adequate physical care for the client.

## Critical Thinking

Although thinking is a normal human skill, critical thinking is a skill that requires development. Critical thinking helps the nurse find options for solving client care problems. The home care nurse will find many problems to solve. He or she will need to identify signals that indicate an emergency situation or merely a need to call the physician. The nurse may have to think of adaptations that can be made with tools or facilities in the house or how to address situations that present a cultural or religious problem. The nurse may also help the client, caregiver, or family develop critical thinking skills to help them work through their own problems.

The critical thinking process is similar to the nursing process. There are many definitions of critical thinking, but the American Association of Colleges of Nursing (AACN) determined that an ideal critical thinker has the following abilities: questioning, analysis, synthesis, interpretation, inference, inductive and deductive reasoning, intuition, application, and creativity. Several models have been suggested for developing critical thinking skills (AACN, 1998). Box 1–4 will help the student or nurse to strengthen and build natural skills.

> ▶ **Box 1-4.**  Developing Self-Growth in Thinking Skills ◀

1. Make a list of your current thinking skills.
2. Keep a log (diary) of how you use thinking skills on a regular basis.
3. Share your log with a classmate. Learn from and applaud each other.
4. Read an article or book on thinking in nursing and discuss it with a classmate.
5. Draw a picture or write a paragraph that describes how you would like to enhance your thinking and the factors that hinder your thinking. Share it with a classmate.
6. Promise yourself always to consider at least three possible answers (hunches or conclusions) for every question.
7. Remind yourself that the path to responsible nursing care is along the path of critical thinking.
8. Give yourself a reward for your development of thinking skills.
9. Set goals for further development of your thinking skills.

Source: Craven, R. F., & Hirnle, C. J. (Eds.). (2000). *Fundamentals of nursing: Human health and function* (3rd ed., p. 135). Philadelphia: Lippincott Williams & Wilkins.

## Application of Nursing Process

Critical thinking is part of the nursing process. The nurse uses skillful thinking in knowing what assessments to make for each client and picking up on the cues of those assessments. Those assessments help the nurse determine the strengths and weaknesses of the client, family, and caregiver. Together they develop a problem statement, the nursing diagnosis. They plan expected outcomes and outcome criteria. Interventions are identified that are reasonable and acceptable to all parties. The person who will carry out those interventions is designated. The nurse may teach a procedure. The client may be able to do the procedure, but a caregiver may need to buy the supplies or help set up the equipment for the procedure each time it is used. Thinking is used in making evaluations. Many community-based nurses follow a managed care plan or are given physician's orders to follow. But the community-based nurse also uses the nursing process in therapeutic relationships with clients and caregivers. Nursing process is used in many of the chapters that follow.

## Documentation

Complete, accurate documentation is an essential element of nursing care in any setting but it is of particular importance in community-based settings. Creating a clear account of what the nurse saw and did not only provides a record of care but also creates a log of client progress. Unlike the acute care setting where several caregivers may be documenting care simultaneously, in some community settings such as the home, only the nurse may be documenting care.

Charting is used to determine eligibility for reimbursement for care provided. If services rendered by the nurse fall within the requirements of Medicaid,

Medicare, or other third-party payers, then the agency will be paid for the care rendered.

Charting is a legal document. In cases in which an agency and nurse are sued, charting of the incident in question will be used as the record of care provided and client response to that care. Litigation is often avoided or readily resolved if care is accurately and completely documented.

## Ethical–Legal Concerns

In community-based nursing, ethical dilemmas present challenges that differ from those in the acute care setting. There may be lack of formal institutional support, such as an ethics committee or ethics rounds in community-based care. In the acute setting, the nurse has 24-hour contact with the client and family, whereas care is intermittent and brief in the community setting. Problem identification and problem solving are troublesome when communication is fragmented over several weeks or months.

When care is provided in the home, respecting the client and family's desire for self-determination is foremost. This may limit the nurse's influence in the decision-making process. In contrast, the acute care setting is often thought of as "the turf" of the nursing and medical staff.

When family and nurse values collide, frustrating dilemmas may result. Some clients have limited resources and support systems. This may profoundly affect whether caregivers are accessible, available, and affordable. Interdisciplinary communication is difficult in community-based care; this fact may intensify difficulties with ethical issues.

The nurse may facilitate the discussion of ethical concerns as they arise, using an ethical framework and encouraging open dialogue between the client and appropriate family and friends. It is important to know one's own values. If conflicts arise when the nurse and family do not agree, the nurse may have to recommend that the family identify another party to facilitate discussions.

 **CONCLUSIONS**

Community-based nursing is not defined by a setting but by a philosophy of practice. Increasingly, health care is provided in community settings and not in acute care facilities. As a result, the client, family, friends, or neighbors provide care, rather than professional providers. The community-based nurse helps clients and families adapt to providing self-care.

Focusing on prevention, community-based nursing averts the initial occurrence of disease or injury and provides early identification and treatment or a comprehensive rehabilitation of a disease or injury. Continuity and collaborative care allow for quality care to be preserved in a changing health care delivery system. Community-based nurses use special skills and competencies to provide care within the context of the client's culture, family, and community.

# References and Bibliography

American Association of Colleges of Nursing. (1998). *Essentials of baccalaureate education and professional nursing practice.* Washington, DC: Author.

American Nurses Association, Community Health Nursing Division. (1999). *American Nurses Association standards of public health nursing practice.*

American Organization of Nurse Executives. (2000). The evolving role of the registered nurse. Chicago: Author.

Bellack, J., & O'Niel, E. (2000). Recreating nursing practice for a new century: Recommendations and implications of the Pew Health Commission's final report. *Nursing and Health Care Perspective, 21*(1), 14–18.

Buerhaus, P., Staiger, D., & Auerbach, D. (2000). Implications of an aging registered nurse workforce. *JAMA, 283*(22), 2948–2952.

Craven, R. C., & Hirnle, C. J. (2000). *Fundamentals of nursing: Human health and function* (3rd ed.). Philadelphia: Lippincott Williams & Wilkins.

Fawcett, J. (1984). *Analysis and evaluation of conceptual models of nursing.* Philadelphia: F.A. Davis.

Frachel, R. (1988). A new profession: The evolution of public health nursing. *Public Health Nursing, 51*(12), 84–91.

Health Resources and Services Administration. (2000). *The registered nurse population: Findings from the national sample survey of registered nurses.* Retrieved January 10, 2003, from http://www.hrsa_gov/newsroom

Health Resources and Services Adminstration. (2002). *Projected supply, demand, and shortages of registered nurses: 2000-2020.* Retrieved January 10, 2003, http://www.hrsa_gov/newsroom

Heller, B., Oros, M., & Durney-Crowley, J. (1999). *The future of nursing education: Ten trends to watch.* New York: National League for Nursing. Retrieved March 3, 2003, from http://www.nln.org

Hughes, K., & Marcantonio, R. (1992). Practice patterns among home health, public health, and hospital nurses. *Nursing and Health Care, 13*(10), 532–536.

Hunt, R. (1998). Community based nursing: Philosophy or setting. *American Journal of Nursing, 98*(10), 44–47.

Jitramontree, N. (2000). The impact of Medicare reimbursement changes on home health care: A nursing perspective. *Home Health Care Nurse, 18*(2), 116–121.

Josten, L. (1989). Wanted: Leaders for public health. *Nursing Outlook, 37,* 230–232.

Kalish, P., & Kalish, B. (1995). *The advance of American nursing* (3rd ed.). Philadelphia: Lippincott.

Leininger, M. (1970). *Nursing and anthropology: Two worlds to blend.* New York: Wiley.

Monteiro, L. (1991). Florence Nightingale on public health nursing. In B. Spradley (Ed.), *Readings in community health nursing.* Philadelphia: Lippincott.

National League for Nursing. (1997). *Final report: Commission on a workforce for a restructured health care system.* New York: Author. Available at http://www.nln.org/infrest3.htm

National League for Nursing. (2000a). *A vision for nursing education.* New York: Author. Available at http://www.nln.org/info-vision.htm

National League for Nursing, Council of Associate Degree Nursing Competencies Task Force. (2000b). *Educational competencies for graduates of associate degree nursing programs.* Boston: Jones & Bartlett Publisher.

Reed, F. C., & Wuyscik, M. A. (1998). Community health strategies: Teach what? Reflections on the transition from hospital teaching to teaching in the community. *Nurse Educator, 23*(3), 11–13.

Reverby, S. M. (1993). From Lillian Wald to Hillary Rodham Clinton: What will happen to public health nursing? [Editorial]. *American Journal of Public Health, 83,* 1662–1663.

Simmon, B. L., Nelson, D. I., Neal, L. J., (2001). A comparison of the positive and negative work attitudes of home health care and hospital nurses. *Health Care Management Review, 26*(3), 63–74.

U.S. Department of Health and Human Services. (2000). *Healthy people 2010: National health promotion and disease prevention objectives, full report, with commentary.* Washington, DC: U.S. Government Printing Office.

# LEARNING ACTIVITIES

## JOURNALING ACTIVITY 1-1

1. In your clinical journal, discuss a community with which you are familiar and describe what defines that community.
2. Identify some of the health needs of that community.
3. Where do members of this community receive health care?

## CLIENT CARE ACTIVITY 1-2

How can the nurse encourage self-care in the following client situations?

1. Jane is the 31-year-old mother of Jackie, a 4-month-old baby who has frequent apnea spells. Jane states, "I am afraid she will stop breathing at home. I can't figure out the monitor."
2. Stephan is a 60-year-old widower whose wife died 3 years ago. There is an increasing possibility that he will have to have his leg amputated below the knee as a result of a very large leg ulcer. Stephan has been hospitalized three times in the past 6 months because of uncontrolled diabetes. The last time, there were maggots in his leg ulcer.

## CLIENT CARE ACTIVITY 1-3

How can the nurse encourage disease prevention and health promotion in the following client situations?

1. Barb and Steve have a 10-month-old baby, Andy, who requires intermittent nursing care because of oxygen therapy and tracheotomy care. They have three other children, ages 2, 4, and 6. Andy has had three bouts of respiratory flu and two colds in the last 4 months. He has been hospitalized twice during that time. You are the home care nurse caring for Andy. You noticed on your last visit that Andy's brothers and sister kiss him, touch his trach tube, and cough on him. One of the children went in to use the bathroom and left the door open, and you noticed that he did not wash his hands afterwards. How do you use a preventative focus with Andy's home care?
2. Meg and Bob have a 3-year-old child, Mark, who has cerebral palsy. Meg provides 24-hour care for Mark with no assistance from anyone. You notice on your last home visit that Meg has lost weight, is not sleeping, and complains that she has no energy. You suspect that she may be suffering from depression. You recommend several counselors and respite care for Mark so Meg can get out occasionally. Meg states, "I come from a very large family. We never use a baby-sitter in our family." What do you do and say?

## PRACTICAL APPLICATION ACTIVITY 1-4

Describe an example from your clinical experience in which you believe continuity was interrupted.

- Indicate some things that could have been done to ensure continuity in these examples.
- Describe a time situation in which continuity was evident. What happened, and who and what made it happen?

## PRACTICAL APPLICATION 1-5

Contact your local or state department of health. You can either call them or visit their web site. What are the current issues facing your department of health? How are these issues related to nursing?

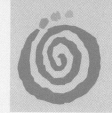

## CHAPTER 2

# Health Promotion and Disease Prevention

Roberta Hunt

## THE NURSE SPEAKS

When I went into nursing, I wanted to be a critical care nurse. I loved the idea of working with technology and having a lot of responsibility. Anatomy and physiology fascinated me, so critical care was a perfect fit for me. I worked for 5 years as a critical care nurse and really enjoyed it. The part about the job I liked the most turned out to be working with the families. When the families had questions, I was right there answering their questions. If a family member was feeling emotional and needed someone to listen, I actually enjoyed hearing their stories and trying to figure out how to be helpful. At the same time I was working in CCU, I was volunteering at the local senior citizens center, teaching classes on health topics that were identified by the clientele as being important to them. I began to make some home visits to some of the homebound seniors who had questions about their medications. I began to see the value of health promotion and disease prevention. Some of the people we saw in the CCU had conditions that could have been better managed at home, preventing an admission to the CCU. Some had diseases that could have been prevented. I also really enjoyed going to people's homes and taking care of them there. I looked into the home care agency in our hospital and learned that I could work one weekend a month as a home care nurse. I cut back on the CCU and began to gradually do more and more home care. That was 10 years ago, and I have never looked back. I love home care nursing.

— **Becky Carmondy, RN**
  Home Care Nurse

The U.S. health care system is the most expensive in the world, using 14% of the U.S. gross national product (GNP), at a cost of nearly $4,000 per person. The next most expensive health care system is in Canada, where 9% of the GNP is used for health care, at a per capita cost of $2,000. Most industrialized nations spend 8% to 10% of their GNP on health care. Every industrialized nation except the United States has a national health plan in place that covers all citizens (Anderson & Poullier, 1999).

Despite having the most expensive health care in the world, the United States lags behind other nations in key health indicators. The United States ranks 28th among nations in its infant mortality rate at 7.8/1,000 births. This average does not show the higher rates for certain minority groups. Life expectancy in the United States ranks behind Sweden, Germany, Italy, France, and Canada. Twenty-five percent of the nation's 1 1/2- to 3-year-old children are inadequately immunized against diphtheria, tetanus, pertussis, polio, measles, mumps, and rubella. Disadvantaged populations rank significantly worse than average in these and other health indicators (Federal Interagency Forum on Child and Family Statistics, 2002).

Nursing is a reflection of society's needs. Although a great deal of money is spent on health care in the United States, the level of health of U.S. citizens is disappointing. The consumer movement toward increased participation in wellness, weight loss, smoking cessation, and exercising has resulted in the preventive healthcare movement. Settings for practice have evolved naturally as nurses focus on health rather than illness. Nursing has taken on a new look as it assumes the role of health promotion and illness prevention.

This chapter begins with a discussion of health and its place on the health–illness continuum. The goals and priorities in the federal government's program—*Healthy People 2010*—are presented. A large part of the chapter is devoted to illustrating the difference between health promotion and disease prevention and the major strategies nurses will use to meet the goals of *Healthy People 2010,* with emphasis on the preventive focus. Levels of prevention and nursing roles are outlined. The chapter ends with a brief section on advocacy.

## HEALTH AND ILLNESS

Rather than focusing on curing illness and injury, community-based care focuses on promoting health and preventing illness. **Health** is defined by the World Health Organization (1986) as a "state of physical, mental and social well-being and not merely absence of disease or infirmity." This holistic philosophy differs greatly from that of the acute care setting.

Considering health—rather than illness—as the essence of care requires a shift in thinking. The **health–illness continuum** illustrates this model of care (Fig. 2–1). Health is conceptualized as a resource for everyday living. It is a positive idea that emphasizes social and personal resources and physical capabilities. Wellness is a lifestyle aimed at achieving physical, emotional, intellectual, spiritual, and environmental well-being. The use of wellness measures can increase stamina, energy, and self-esteem. These then enhance quality of life.

Improvement of health is not seen as an outcome of the amount and type of medical services or the size of the hospital. Treatment efficacy, rather than technology, drives care in this model. Here health is viewed as a function of collaborative efforts at the community level.

Care provided in acute care settings usually is directed at resolving immediate health problems. In the community, care focuses on maximizing individual potential for self-care, regardless of any illness or injury. The client assumes responsibility for health care decisions and care provision. Where health is the essence of care, the client's ability to function becomes the primary concern. The intent of care is not to "fix" with treatment but to enhance the quality of life and support actions that make the client's life as comfortable as possible.

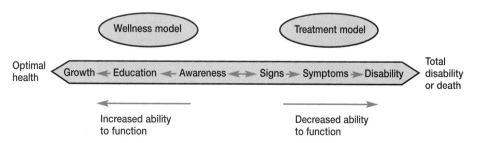

*Figure 2–1.* ▶ The health-illness continuum.

**Function** is defined by subjective and objective measurements. Both the client's abilities to perform activities of daily living (ADL) and the client's perception of how well he or she is functioning are considered. Clients may state that they are satisfied with their ability to care for themselves; however, objective data from laboratory reports, diagnostic tests, and caregivers' observations may show that this is not the case. On the other hand, clients may report that they are concerned about their ability to perform ADL, yet contrasting reports indicate that they are functioning quite well. The following Client Situation in Practice reflects this dichotomy.

## CLIENT SITUATIONS IN PRACTICE

### ▶ Perceptions of Health and Illness

Mary had a myocardial infarction 3 days ago. After two episodes of crushing chest pain, she reluctantly went to the emergency room. Laboratory values showed moderate heart damage. She, a 46-year-old single parent, is the sole provider for three adolescents. She is a physical therapist and works at an ambulatory clinic during the week and a nursing home on weekends. She says she feels fine and asks to go home so she can go back to work.

Mary's mother, Shirley, is extremely distraught about her daughter's condition and believes Mary is dying. Figure 2–2 illustrates the objective data versus Mary's subjective communication. The dissonance between subjective perceptions and objective data can interrupt and delay recovery.

A person's lifestyle is a dynamic process that involves needs, beliefs, and values. Choices in life therefore can be seen as opportunities for moving toward optimal health or wellness.

Wellness involves more than simply good physical self-care. It also requires using one's mind constructively, expressing one's emotions effectively, interacting constructively with others, and being concerned about one's physical and psychologic environment. Regardless of the setting for health care, wherever nurses practice, their concern is for the whole person, and they provide holistic care (Fig. 2–3).

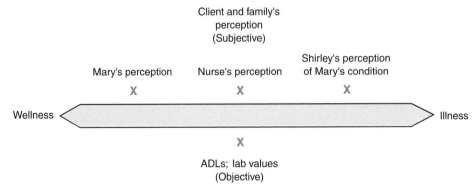

*Figure 2–2.* ▶ Subjective perceptions of health and function may differ from each other and from objective data.

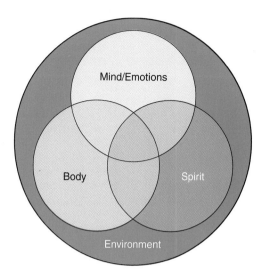

**Figure 2–3.** ▶ Schematic representation of holism. The system is greater than and different from the sum of the parts. Wherever the setting, the nurse's concern is for the whole person.

 ## HEALTHY PEOPLE 2010

*Healthy People 2010* offers a simple but powerful idea: Provide the information and knowledge about how to improve health in a format that enables diverse groups to combine their efforts and work as a team. It is a road map to better health for all, which can be used by many different people, communities, professional organizations, and groups whose concern is a particular population group or particular threat to health (U.S. Department of Health and Human Services [DHHS], 2000). Publication of this vision was the result of a national consortium of health care professionals, citizens, and private and public agencies from across the United States.

*Healthy People 2010* states that its purpose is to commit the nation to the attainment of two broad goals:

1. To eliminate health disparities
2. To increase quality and years of healthy life

Measurable targets or objectives to be achieved are organized into 28 priority areas (Box 2–1).

### Eliminate Health Disparity

The first goal of *Healthy People 2010* is to eliminate health disparities. These include differences in health and access to health care services by gender, age, race or ethnicity, education or income, disability, geographic location, or sexual orientation. For example, men have a life expectancy that is 6 years less than women. Information about the biologic and genetic characteristics of African Americans, Hispanics, Native Americans, Alaska Natives, Asians, Native Hawaiians, and Pacific Islanders does not explain the health disparities experienced by these groups compared with the white, non-Hispanic population in the United States. See Box 2–2 for a summary of health disparity in the United States.

## HEALTHY PEOPLE 2010

**BOX 2-1   Focus Areas**

1. Access to quality health services
2. Arthritis, osteoporosis, and chronic back conditions
3. Cancer
4. Chronic kidney disease
5. Diabetes
6. Disability and secondary conditions
7. Education and community-based programs
8. Environmental health
9. Family planning
10. Food safety
11. Health communication
12. Heart disease and stroke
13. Human immunodeficiency virus (HIV)
14. Immunization and infectious diseases
15. Injury and violence prevention
16. Maternal, infant, and child health
17. Medical product safety
18. Mental health
19. Nutrition and obesity
20. Occupational safety and health
21. Oral health
22. Physical activity and fitness
23. Public health infrastructure
24. Respiratory diseases
25. Sexually transmitted diseases
26. Substance abuse
27. Tobacco use
28. Vision and hearing

It is believed that these disparities are a result of the complex interaction among genetic variations, environmental factors, and specific health behaviors. Inequalities in income and education underlie many health disparities, with income and education often serving as a proxy measure for each other. In general, population groups that suffer the worst health status are also those that have the highest poverty rates and the least education. Poverty is more prevalent in populations of color (Fig. 2-4).

Disparities in health care can be eliminated through continued commitment to understanding why disparities exist. Effective strategies to eliminate and overcome disparities need to be identified. Nurses have a role in working more closely with communities to ensure that relevant research findings are implemented quickly. There is a need to evaluate transcultural competence (discussed in Chapter 3) as it relates to health care disparities. Last of all, capacity for health services research among minority institutions and minority investigators is lacking. Nurses have a role in seeing that these deficiencies are addressed (Agency for Healthcare Research and Quality, 2002).

▶ **Box 2-2** Racial and Ethnic Disparities in Health Care ◀

The overall health of Americans has improved in the last few decades, but all Americans have not shared equally in these improvements. Among nonelderly adults, for example, 17% of Hispanic and 16% of Black Americans report they are in only fair or poor health, as compared with 10% of White Americans. One may ask: In people who receive health care, how much do differences in race and ethnicity contribute to disparities in that health care?

Primary care is central to the health care system in the United States. Research shows that having a source of care raises the chance that people receive adequate preventive care and other health services. Data from the Agency for Healthcare Research and Quality (AHRQ) Medical Expenditure Panel Survey shows that about 30% of Hispanic and 20% of Black Americans lack a usual source of health care, compared with less than 16% of White Americans. Further, Hispanic children are nearly three times as likely as non-Hispanic children to have no usual source of health care.

Race and ethnicity influence a patient's chance of receiving many specific procedures and treatments. Of nine hospital procedures investigated in one AHRQ study, five were significantly less common among African-American clients than among White patients; three of those five were also less common among Hispanics, and two were less common among Asian Americans. Other AHRQ research revealed additional disparities in client care for various conditions and care settings. Researchers in Boston examined the quality of care provided to hospital clients with congestive heart failure or pneumonia. The quality of care was measured by physician adherence to standards of care as well as by physician review. Although there was no difference in quality of care for those clients from poor communities compared with other clients, African-American clients received a lower quality of care than white clients.

Source: Agency for Health Care and Quality Research (2002). Addressing racial and ethnic disparities in health care fact sheet. Retrieved December 12, 2002, from http://www.ahcpr.gov/research/disparit.htm

Nurses can help reduce health disparities by (1) educating themselves regarding issues of disparity, (2) identifying vulnerable populations in their communities, and (3) advocating for vulnerable populations. Suggestions for advocacy activities for nurses include the following:

▶ Empowering each client and family member they care for who experiences disparities in health care
▶ Discussing disparities in their communities with colleagues
▶ Writing about disparities for hospital, clinic, or professional organization newsletters
▶ Writing letters to, or calling and making an appointment to speak to, local or state politicians to describe evidence of health disparities that they encounter

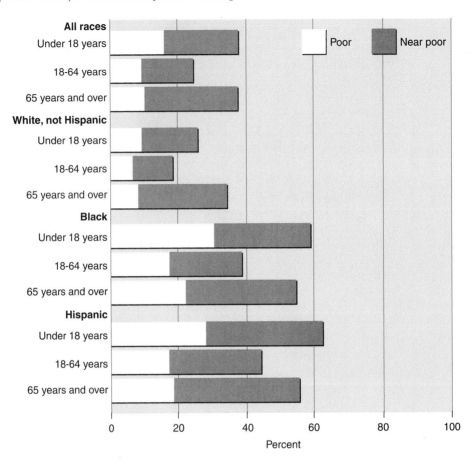

NOTES: Poor is defined as family income less than 100 percent of the poverty level and near poor as 100-199 percent of the poverty level. See Data Table for date points graphed and additional notes.

SOURCE: U.S. Census Bureau, Current Population Survey

***Figure 2–4.*** ▶ Low income population by age, race, and Hispanic origin: United States, 2000. Note: Poor is defined as family income less than 100% of the poverty level and near poor as 100% to 199% of the poverty level. Source: U. S. Census Bureau, Current Population Survey.

## Increase the Quality and Years of Healthy Life

The fact that individual health is closely linked to community health was discussed in Chapter 1. Likewise, community health is affected by the collective behaviors, attitudes, and beliefs of everyone who lives in the community. The underlying premise of *Healthy People 2010* is that the health of the individual is almost inseparable from the health of the larger community. One way to increase the quality and years of healthy life for communities is to follow the recommendations of *Healthy People 2010*. This road map for improving health is based on the concepts of health promotion, disease prevention, and health protection.

 ## HEALTH PROMOTION VERSUS DISEASE PREVENTION

Sometimes people confuse health promotion and disease prevention. It is easy to do so because some approaches and interventions are the same or overlap. **Health promotion** strategies relate to individual lifestyle, which has a powerful influence over one's long-term health. Educational and community-based programs, such as smoking cessation programs, are designed to address lifestyle. **Disease prevention services** include counseling, screening, immunization, and chemoprophylactic interventions for individuals in clinical settings. Health promotion activities are used to make a person who already feels well feel better, and disease prevention activities are used to make a person who feels well prevent possible future illness. For example, Jill jogs every morning before work. She enjoys jogging, finding that it stimulates her for the day's activities and makes her feel good. Jill jogs to promote wellness, so Jill is participating in a health promotion activity. On the other hand, Nancy jogs because her physician has told her to do so. She is overweight and has a family history of heart problems. Her physician tells her she needs exercise to help prevent future cardiovascular problems. Nancy jogs to prevent illness, so Nancy is participating in a disease prevention activity.

Health protection strategies relate to environmental or regulatory measures that confer protection on large population groups. Rather than the individual focus of health promotion, health protection involves a communitywide focus.

 ## THE PREVENTION FOCUS

The prevention focus is a key concept of community-based nursing. Prevention is conceptualized on three levels: primary prevention, secondary prevention, and tertiary prevention. An overview of these levels of prevention appears in Table 2–1. Different preventive strategies are found at each level of prevention. These strategies fall into a continuum of essential activities that prevent disease or injury, prolong life, and promote health. The following services are categorized as preventive strategies: counseling, screening, immunization, and chemoprophylactic interventions for clients in clinical settings.

Health protection and health promotion activities conducted by nurses in community-based settings usually occur at the primary level, although they may occur at secondary and tertiary levels also.

Some of the preventive activities listed in Table 2–1 are further developed in Table 2–2 which shows the goals of these selected activities.

**TABLE 2-1** • Levels of Disease Prevention and Examples of Activities

| Level | Description | Activities[a] |
|---|---|---|
| Primary | Prevention of the initial occurrence of disease or injury | Immunization, family planning, retirement planning, well-child care, smoking cessation, hygiene teaching, fluoride supplements, fitness classes, alcohol and drug prevention, seat belts and child seat car restraints, environmental protection |
| Secondary | Early identification of disease or disability with prompt intervention to prevent or limit disability | Physical assessments, hypertension screening, developmental screening, breast and testicular self-examinations, hearing and vision screening, mammography, pregnancy testing |
| Tertiary | Assistance (after disease or disability has occurred) to halt further disease progress and to meet one's potential and maximize quality of life despite illness or injury | Teaching and counseling regarding lifestyle changes such as diet and exercise, stress management and home management after diagnosis of chronic illness, support groups, support for caretaker, Meals On Wheels for homebound, physical therapy after stroke or accident, mental health counseling for rape victims |

[a]Some prevention activities listed above overlap into health promotion or health protection.

**TABLE 2-2** • Activities at Each Level of Prevention

| Level | Activities | Goal of the Activity |
|---|---|---|
| Primary | Immunization clinics | Prevention of communicable diseases such as polio, pertussis, rubella |
| | Smoking cessation | Prevention of lung and heart disease, cancer |
| | Tobacco chewing prevention | Prevention of cancer of the mouth, tongue, and throat |
| | Sex education with emphasis on condom use | Prevention of acquired immunodeficiency syndrome (AIDS) and other sexually transmitted diseases (STDs) |
| Secondary | Programs to teach and motivate men to do self-exam for testicular masses | Early identification and treatment of testicular cancer |
| | Blood pressure screening | Early identification and treatment of hypertension to prevent strokes and heart disease |
| | Programs to teach and motivate women to do breast self-exams | Early identification and treatment of breast cancer |
| Tertiary | Counseling, low-sodium diet, exercise for management of hypertension | Minimize the effects of hypertension |
| | Exercises and speech therapy after a cerebrovascular accident | Restore function and limit disability |

There are numerous reasons for adopting preventive steps; cost benefit is one. For example, the direct and indirect costs of infectious diseases are significant. Every hospital-acquired infection adds an average of $2,100 to a hospital or home care bill. Bloodstream infections result in an average of $3,517 in additional hospital charges per infected individual because the client's stay averages an additional 7 days (DHHS, 2000). These costs are realized in every setting where health care is provided. A typical case of Lyme disease diagnosed in the early stages incurs about $174 in direct medical treatment costs. Delayed diagnosis and treatment can result in complications that cost from $2,228 to $6,724 per client in direct medical costs in the first year alone.

As researchers develop more technology and treatment choices, these costs (and, therefore, potential cost savings) increase. The lifetime costs of health care associated with HIV, in light of recent advances in diagnostics and therapeutics, have grown from $55,000 to $155,000 or more per person (DHHS, 2000). These costs mean that HIV prevention efforts may be even more cost effective, providing cost savings to society.

In addition to being cost effective, appropriate prevention interventions result in enhanced client satisfaction and faster recovery. Historically, the major portions of primary and tertiary prevention services have been delivered from community-based settings. This is still appropriate in the current health care system.

## Primary Prevention

**Primary prevention** is commonly defined as prevention of the initial occurrence of disease or injury. Primary prevention activities include immunizations, family planning services, classes to prepare people for retirement, and counseling and education on injury prevention. These are categorized as primary prevention because they prevent the initial occurrence of a disease or injury. Table 2–1 lists examples of specific primary prevention activities.

Also included in primary prevention are health promotion and health protection activities. Health promotion focuses on activities related to lifestyle choices in a social context for individuals who are already essentially healthy. Examples of health promotion include exercise and nutrition classes and prevention programs for alcohol and other drug abuse. Smoking cessation programs are often targeted at healthy individuals, offering them a lifestyle choice.

Prevention is also accomplished through health protection. Health protection focuses on activities related to environmental or regulatory measures that provide protection for large population groups. This category would include activities directed at preventing unintentional injuries through motor vehicle accidents, occupational safety and health, environmental health, and food and drug safety. Other examples of health protection include seat-belt and child car seat restraint laws and laws prohibiting smoking in public places. Implementation of child car seat restraint laws has prevented a significant number of deaths and disabilities among children in the United States over the past 20 years. It has been effective as a health protection activity. Environmental protection and pollution control are other primary levels of prevention that are also health protection factors.

## Secondary Prevention

The intent of **secondary prevention** is the early identification and treatment of disease or injury to limit disability. Identification of health needs, health problems, and clients at risk is the inherent component of secondary prevention. Activities of secondary prevention include screening programs for blood pressure, breast cancer, scoliosis, hearing, and vision. Intervention does not prevent scoliosis, but it does provide early identification and subsequent treatment of a condition that already exists in school-age children. Likewise, mammography does not prevent breast cancer, but it provides an opportunity for early identification and treatment. Typically, screening efforts should address conditions that cause significant morbidity and mortality in the target age group. Table 2–1 lists other examples of specific secondary prevention activities.

## Tertiary Prevention

**Tertiary prevention** maximizes recovery after an injury or illness. Most care provided in acute care facilities, clinics, and skilled nursing facilities focuses on tertiary care. Rehabilitation is the major focus in this level of prevention. Rehabilitation activities assist clients to reach their maximum potential despite the presence of chronic conditions. Teaching a client who has had a hip replacement how to create a safe home environment that prevents falls is an example of tertiary prevention.

Shelters for battered women and counseling and therapy for abused children are further examples of tertiary prevention. Other examples are listed in Table 2–1.

 **NURSING COMPETENCIES AND SKILLS AND LEVELS OF PREVENTION**

Despite an increasing emphasis on disease prevention and health promotion, and despite ample evidence demonstrating the effectiveness of preventive services, such services are underutilized (Amonkar, Madhavan, Rosenbluth, & Simon, 1999). This emphasis has generated numerous opportunities for nurses to participate in health promotion and disease prevention activities in all levels of prevention (Dixon, 1999). Now that you understand the levels of prevention, this section discusses the role of the nurse at each level of prevention in two types of community-based care: the ambulatory and home care settings. Typically, the prominent nursing competencies in these settings are those of communicator and teacher. Competencies as manager and physical care provider also are essential in the home setting. This can be true of ambulatory care as well, depending on the setting.

The role responsibilities for each level of prevention differ in each setting. Levels of prevention and the role of the nurse in community-based care may be affected by the particular position and the educational preparation of the nurse. Table 2–3 illustrates this relationship. Table 2–1 provides additional examples of preventive strategies in community-based settings.

## Primary Prevention

### Ambulatory Health Care

Nurses communicate information about primary prevention in the ambulatory setting. For example, a nurse may provide information on the importance of infant seats, child restraints, and helmets to all the mothers at a well-child clinic. School nurses may communicate with families through written flyers sent home with the children. Subjects may include the communicability and the methods of transmission of high-risk diseases, as well as prevention for conditions such as chickenpox, influenza, and head lice. Parents of preschool children can obtain vital information

**TABLE 2–3** • Educational Preparation Needed to Provide Community-Based Nursing at Three Levels of Prevention

| Client Served | Levels of Prevention | | |
| --- | --- | --- | --- |
| | Primary[a] | Secondary[b] | Tertiary[c] |
| **Individual client** | Sexuality; teaching about using condoms | Counseling and HIV testing | Nutrition teaching to the client with AIDS to maximize health |
| | Family planning | Early prenatal care | Support groups for parents of low-birth-weight infants |
| | Dietary teaching and exercise programs to assist clients with obesity | Screening for early identification of diabetes | Teaching to a newly diagnosed diabetic about diet and how to administer insulin |
| **Family** | Education about infection control in the home of a family member on a ventilator there | Tuberculosis screening for a family at risk | Teaching to a family caregiver about how to follow sterile procedure for a dressing change |
| **Group** | Prenatal classes for pregnant adolescents | Vision screening for first graders | Support groups for children with asthma |
| | Sexuality teaching about AIDS and other STDs | Hearing screening at a senior center | Swim therapy for physically disabled |
| **Communities** | Fluoride water supplementation | Organized screening programs such as health fairs | Shelter or relocation provision for victims of natural disasters |
| | Environmental cleanup of paint and other substances containing lead | Lead screening of children in a community | Development of programs to assist children with developmental delays caused by lead exposure |

Key: [a]Associate Degree Nurse; [b]Baccalaureate Nurse; [c]Master of Science in Public Health

and clarification from school nurses about when, where, and why their children can receive periodic checkups and immunizations.

Teaching in clinics, schools, and occupational settings may be directed to individuals or groups. Topics cover a wide range and include such things as immunizations, family planning, and prenatal care. At adult clinics, nurses can provide current information to clients about health promotion, diet, exercise, stress management, and weight reduction. Women of childbearing age may attend classes on family planning and prenatal teaching, an essential primary prevention strategy. In the occupational setting, nurses may provide information about injury prevention, repetitive motion injuries, and sensory losses secondary to job tasks. They disseminate information about shift work, offer strategies to avoid sleep disturbances, and provide information about the importance of health promotion activities such as exercise. Many companies provide recreational programs and physical activities at work or in the community through their occupational health programs.

The manager of care in these settings applies knowledge about the principles of leadership by performing management functions for a group of clients. This includes managing all aspects of care and involves communication, teaching, and physical care.

The physical caregiver role in the clinic, school, occupational health setting, and home is usually provided at the tertiary level of prevention. Evaluation of the physical care provided to a client, however, is a function of the manager of care and may take place in all of the previously discussed settings. The manager evaluates the teaching, physical care, and communication skills of the home health aide, for instance, or the care manager teaches a licensed practical nurse in the clinic and school.

### Home Health Care

Clients in the home frequently require episodic care for acute health care conditions. Opportunities for primary prevention are limited. Home care nurses communicate information to the client and family regarding primary prevention strategies because in community-based care, the nurse considers the client in the context of the family. The nurse influences the family's health behaviors in many areas that are not directly related to the client's condition. For example, if the client's spouse asks about immunizations for their children, the nurse has the opportunity to teach about the immunization schedule and where to get affordable care.

## Secondary Prevention

### Ambulatory Health Care

Secondary prevention can involve alerting clients about the time frames for health screening (eg, mammography, Pap smears, glaucoma screening, breast examinations, lipid levels). The clinic nurse may see clients who are at risk for certain conditions, alert them to their risk, and provide information about community services that may be able to assist them.

Preschool screening, vision and hearing testing, and scoliosis screening are secondary prevention strategies provided in the school. In addition, school nurses teach secondary prevention by educating parents about the screening programs available for their children.

Often the workplace is the site where screening is done for hypertension, hearing loss, exposure to hazardous substances, and breast cancer. The nurse disperses information about the services and provides educational programs.

Client need determines in which setting information may be presented. For example, as a manager of care in the clinic, the nurse may not have the opportunity to assess the family caregiver's abilities in assisting a client with insulin injections. However, the nurse in the home can better assess how well the family can assist and support the client. The nurse, as the manager of care in the home, may decide that the family caregiver needs additional teaching to administer the insulin because he or she could not accurately draw up the insulin during an early morning nursing visit.

### Home Health Care

Care in the home usually involves short visits. Thus, opportunities for communicating secondary prevention information are limited. However, home health care nurses do inform the client and family about services in the community that may help them with the client's care, early identification and treatment of conditions related to the client's diagnosis, and general health promotion and disease prevention.

## Tertiary Prevention

### Ambulatory Health Care

Clinic nurses often give their clients information about community resources. Parents of children with a chronic disease, for instance, may receive a list of organizations that provide emotional support, respite care, and information and referral. Clients with chronic conditions benefit from teaching that is directed at successful rehabilitation and prevention of related complications. Physical care in the clinic may include changing a dressing, wrapping a sprained ankle, and giving an intravenous infusion.

Through the schools, parents can learn about community services available for children with chronic conditions. In some states, children with disabilities are mainstreamed into the public schools. These children and their families need tertiary prevention education. In all states, children with less severe chronic conditions attend school and benefit from health care instructions.

Some schools provide a significant amount of physical caregiving through school-based clinics. Services may include physical examinations, routine screenings, venipuncture for laboratory studies, family planning, and even prenatal care. Nurses may also provide direct nursing care to some children on an ongoing basis (eg, children on a mechanical ventilator or children with conditions that result in frequent urinary catheterization). The school nurse also dispenses prescription medications and provides first aid in emergencies.

In the occupational setting, physical care is primarily first aid. The nurse may tell personnel with chronic conditions or recent acute conditions about the opportunities and advantages of returning to work. Return-to-work programs assist personnel with chronic injuries or illnesses and illustrate the tertiary prevention approach of maximizing individual potential for health through teaching.

### Home Health Care

A primary role of home health care nurses is to provide health instruction to clients and family members. Because home health care clients generally require only episodic care and usually have a chronic condition, most teaching is directed toward tertiary prevention. Teaching may focus on rehabilitation or restoration for those with a recent stroke, head injury, fractured hip, diagnosis of a chronic condition, or surgery.

Physical care provided in the home is usually at the tertiary level of prevention. To receive payment for services, most home health care has a physical care component such as completing dressing changes while teaching and implementing good infection control techniques with the client and the family.

Although the client is the main concern, a holistic nursing style means that nurses also provide care for family and other support persons. Chapter 13 covers this topic in more detail.

## ADVOCACY

An advocate is a person who pleads or defends the cause of another. Advocates work to change the system by revealing injustices and inadequacies. **Advocacy** involves teaching, changing the system, guiding others, serving as a role model, collaborating with professionals, encouraging prevention activities, and exploring and communicating about community resources. Steps in advocacy, listed in Box 2–3 represent power that is inherent in knowledge. The expertise and competence of nurses can also be used in supporting the needs and views of their clients and their clients' families. Nurses can be advocates for clients who feel they have been excluded from participation in health care decisions or who have little trust in the health care system or political representatives.

▶ **Box 2–3** Steps of Advocacy ◀

**Understanding and Knowledge of Self—Personally and Professionally**
- Knowing oneself: awareness of personal goals and how these goals may affect relationships with clients
- Realistic self-concept: awareness of one's own limitations and abilities that will affect what one can and cannot support
- Self-knowledge about values clarification: awareness of one's biases and prejudices, morals, and ethical values. This gives one a good knowledge and understanding of personal views of what is fair and acceptable and how that may affect one's approach to a relationship with the client.

**Knowledge of Treatment and Intervention Options**
- Development of knowledge base of procedures and actions
- Awareness of rationale for specific therapies

**Knowledge of Health Care System**
- Awareness of how systems relate to each other, the client, and the community
- Awareness of the relationship of outside influences, such as politics and economics, to oneself.

**Knowledge of How to Put Advocacy into Action**
- Assessment—contextual approach
  What does the client believe is the most important problem?
  What support or resources does the client already have in place?
  What does the client know or not know (eg, health services, treatment options)?
  In what areas does the client feel a need for personal control to be established in his or her life?
- Planning—mobilization of resources, consultations, collaboration with other disciplines
- Implementation—education, empowerment of client (The nurse assists the client in asserting control over the variables affecting the client's life. The nurse must be a role model for assertiveness to make this important step effective.)

Community-based nurses who have rapport with their clients know the problems their clients face: the mother who lacks child care, the older adult who lacks transportation, the school child who is afraid to use the rest rooms in the school, the adolescent who is afraid of the violence on the street, the wife who faces abuse from her husband, the poor who struggle to make ends meet. One nurse characterized her home visits as mutual disclosure: "It's all about listening to each other." Together the client and the nurse have power and use it to improve the client's health status.

Who is better situated as an advocate for the individual and families than the community-based nurse who knows clients' needs and has a knowledgeable understanding of local services?

 ## CONCLUSIONS

Settings for nursing practice have evolved as a reflection of society's need to focus on health rather than illness. State and local health departments are using *Healthy People 2010* as a framework to put disease prevention into action. The prevention focus is a key concept of community-based nursing. Different preventive strategies are found at three levels of prevention. Advocacy is another form of community-based nursing in which the nurse supports the needs and views of the people he or she serves. The nurse and client working together have power.

### References and Bibliography

Agency for Health Care and Quality Research. (2002). *Addressing racial and ethnic disparities in health care fact sheet.* Retrieved December 12, 2002, from http://www.ahcpr.gov/research/disparit.htm

Amonkar, M., Madhavan, S., Rosenbluth, S., & Simon, K. (1999). Barriers and facilitators to providing common preventive screening services in managed care settings. *Journal of Community Health, 24*(3), 229–247.

Anderson, G. F., & Poullier, J. P. (1999). Health spending, access, and outcomes: Trends in industrialized countries. *Health Affairs, 18*(3), 178–192.

Dixon, E. (1999). Community health nursing practice and the Roy Adaptation Model. *Public Health Nursing, 16*(4), 290–300.

Federal Interagency Forum on Child and Family Statistics. (2002). *American's children: Key national indicators of well being,* 2002. Washington, DC: U.S. Government Printing Office.

U.S. Department of Health and Human Services. (2000). *Healthy people 2010* (Conference edition, Vols. 1–2). Washington, DC: Author.

U.S. Department of Health and Human Services. (2002). *Fact sheet on national healthcare disparities report: Update on current status.* Retrieved January 13, 2003, from www.ahrq.gov

World Health Organization. (1986). Twelve yardsticks for health. New York: WHD.

## LEARNING ACTIVITIES

### JOURNALING 2-1

1. In your clinical journal, identify issues you have observed in your clinical experiences that relate to health rather than to illness.
2. Discuss how this differs from what you previously thought of as health.
3. How does this observation affect your impression of the role of the nurse in the community?

4. In your clinical journal, identify issues you have observed in your clinical experiences that relate to *Healthy People 2010* goals.
5. What can you do as a nurse to affect these health issues?

### CLIENT CARE 2-2

1. Primary nursing roles and levels of prevention determine the primary nursing role(s) and level of prevention for each of the following clients.
   - **Jack.** Jack is a 43-year-old man with a colostomy. He has evidence of early skin breakdown around the stoma site despite the fact that he has followed the established protocol. The clinic nurse notes the problem at Jack's first visit to the clinic after his surgery. She teaches him about a new product that may interrupt the skin breakdown.
     a. Determine the primary nursing role.
     b. Identify the level of prevention the nurse is using.
   - **Stephen.** Stephen is a 12-year-old boy with a neurologic condition that requires self-catheterization every 2 hours. He has had three bladder infections in the past 2 months. The school nurse has taught Stephen about the infectious cycle and the importance of hand washing and has watched Stephen self-catheterize in an attempt to identify the reason for the frequent infections.
     a. Determine the primary nursing role.
     b. Identify the level of prevention the nurse is using.

### PRACTICAL APPLICATION 2-3

You have been asked to start a support and education group for people in your community who have had strokes.

1. Describe how you will decide who in the community should participate in the group. Then assume you have identified those who will be attending your group and write objectives for them.
2. Discuss how the components of community-based nursing apply to these problems:
   a. Self-care
   b. Preventive care
   c. Care within the context of the community
   d. Continuity of care
   e. Collaborative care
3. Identify levels of prevention on which you will focus. Determine if there are levels you will not include.
4. State for your group two likely basic or physical needs at each level of prevention.
5. List two goals for the basic or physical needs you have chosen in number 4.
6. State for your group two likely psychosocial needs at each level of prevention.
7. List for group members two objectives for the psychosocial needs at each level of prevention.

### PRACTICAL APPLICATION 2-4

1. You work in an emergency department. An older woman and her husband enter. The woman is loud and combative, and her blood alcohol level is well above normal.
   a. Identify the level of prevention on which you will focus.
   b. Determine if any level of prevention will not be included at all.
   c. List the reasons for focusing on tertiary prevention in home health care.

# CHAPTER **3**

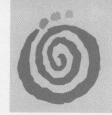

# Cultural Care

Paula Swiggum

## THE NURSING STUDENT SPEAKS

Although I had been having experiences with those from other cultures all of my life, my first true immersion into the lives of another culture occurred when I volunteered to help children who had recently come to America from Somalia. I became involved with helping them to both read and speak better English, as well as how to count money and tell time. Most importantly, we were just friends trying to help them assimilate into a culture so very different from their own.

Before my first day "on the job" I went through my text and reviewed the Somali culture, trying to increase my knowledge so that I would know just how to act. The more I thought about it, the more nervous I became. How was I going to remember everything? How was I going to communicate with a child who looks and speaks so differently from myself?

In nursing class you learn so many things, but it was through this experience that I learned perhaps my most important lesson. Although not as profound as Einstein's theory of relativity, it is a lesson that I hold close to my heart. In watching these children play, it occurred to me how similar we all are. Many times we get so focused on the differences that lie between us, that we forget that we are all human, with many of the same basic needs. Sometimes we just have different means to our ends. We all need to be loved, nurtured, and cared for; we all desire and strive to achieve that sense of wellness, wholeness, and belonging. It is in keeping these principles close to heart that I have been able to provide the best cross-cultural care to all of my clients. Respecting our differences and embracing our similarities are what's important.

— **Stephanie Larson**
   Nursing Student
   Gustavus Adolphus College

The increasing diversity of people in the United States is becoming more evident each day. One needs only to walk the streets of urban areas and farming communities to notice the changing face of America. Recent immigrants have come from the far reaches of the world, primarily Southeast Asia, East Africa, and Latin American countries. Thirty million could be added to the population between 1990 and 2030, according to the U.S. Census Bureau (1998), further increasing the U.S. population diversity (Andrews & Boyle, 2003). New groups bring with them a variety of languages, customs, modes of dress, and other cultural practices. Nurses in the 21st century are challenged to provide care to persons whose customs are unfamiliar. Because culture influences health and well-being in a myriad of ways, the professional nurse must understand what that means for each client encountered.

Nurses have always been concerned with the whole person, their physical, emotional, psychologic, spiritual, social, and developmental dimensions. With the increasing numbers of immigrants coming to the United States, especially in the last 30 years, the new challenge is to understand the cultural dimension. Culture incorporates not only customs, but also beliefs, values, and attitudes shared by a group of people and passed down through generations.

*Healthy People 2010* (U.S. Department of Health and Human Services [DHHS], 2000) calls for the elimination of disparity among groups in access to quality health care services and an increase in community-based programs that are culturally and linguistically appropriate. It states, "The U.S. population is composed of many diverse groups. Evidence indicates a persistent disparity in the health status of racially and culturally diverse populations as compared with the health status of the overall U.S. population." Information about the disparity of health outcomes for minority groups is essential for nurses who plan and carry out nursing interventions in community settings. For example, the infant mortality rate among Alaskan Natives, Native Americans, and African Americans is double that of Whites. The death rate for heart disease is 40% higher for African Americans than for Whites. The knowledge of these and other disparities noted in *Healthy People 2010* can lead community-based nurses to learn about diverse cultural factors that must be taken into account to improve health status within cultural groups (Andrews & Boyle, 2003). Transcultural nursing knowledge is essential to attain the goals of understanding and improving health, as outlined in the document.

This chapter will discuss transcultural nursing and its historical beginnings. In addition, key concepts will be explored related to cultural care, cultural awareness, and culturally appropriate nursing competencies involving assessment and intervention. Because there is such a multitude of cultural groups and practices, nurses cannot have knowledge of each and every one. Therefore, a culturally sensitive approach will be discussed, one that incorporates how to discover important cultural beliefs affecting health and wellness and the available resources.

 ## HISTORICAL PERSPECTIVES

Discussions of cultural competence in nursing are not new. In fact, the field of transcultural nursing had its roots in the early 1900s, when public health nurses cared for immigrants from Europe who came from a wide range of cultural backgrounds and had diverse health care practices. In the late 1940s, Dr. Madeleine Leininger held the belief that "care is the essence of nursing, and the central, dominant and unifying focus of nursing" (Leininger & McFarland, 2002, p. 73). She then began to see the importance of nursing care that was based on the client's culture, that is, their unique values, beliefs, practices, and **lifeways** passed down from one generation to the next. The idea that culture and care are inextricably linked led her to study other cultures, and she became the first nurse to obtain a PhD in anthropology. **Transcultural nursing** (a term coined by Leininger) is a body of knowledge and practice for caring for persons from other cultures.

Since those early days, the theory of cultural care diversity and universality was developed by Dr. Leininger to "generate substantive knowledge for the discipline of nursing" (Leininger, 2002). The world was on a fast track to multiculturalism, and nurses did not have the knowledge to provide care that was culturally appropriate. Having this knowledge is a moral and ethical obligation for nurses as they strive to provide the best care possible to all their clients. Community nurses have been among the nurses most interested in this field because they work directly with individuals and families in their own settings and see the need firsthand.

Although the first large groups of immigrants came to America primarily from Europe in the early 1900s, the recent wave of immigrants to the United States has come from all over the world, including Latin America, Asia, Africa, and other areas. Figure 3–1 depicts the country of origin for immigrants from 1850 to 2000. Today, both urban and rural communities have significant numbers of members whose country of origin is not the United States. The Native American population has significant numbers who live off the reservation and contribute to the multicultural makeup in cities and towns.

Many nurse leaders and educators have embraced the need for culture specific care, and various approaches to gaining this knowledge have been developed. Dr. Josepha Campinha-Bacote, a Cape Verde native who now lives and works in the United States, developed one such model. Her model involves the components of cultural awareness, cultural knowledge, cultural skill, and cultural encounter (Campinha-Bacote, 2002). It will be used here as a framework to help nurses learn the concepts necessary to gain cultural competence working within the community setting.

 ## CULTURAL AWARENESS

Before nurses can intervene appropriately with clients from another culture, they must first understand their own, that is, have a self-awareness of their own cultural background, influences, and biases. Only with this **cultural awareness** can they appreciate and be sensitive to the values, beliefs, lifeways, practices, and problem-solving methods of a client's culture.

One exercise that can be illuminating for nurses is to respond to a "cultural tree" in which one's own cultural heritage is evaluated in terms of the various components that make up a culture. Figure 3–2 depicts the components of a cultural tree. By considering specific examples and anecdotes about family traditions and beliefs, one becomes aware of beliefs and practices that are highly influenced by one's cultural background. There can be amazing diversity, even within a group that outwardly appears very much alike.

This new awareness of one's own cultural influences helps the nurse avoid attitudes that can be detrimental to the nurse–client relationship. **Cultural blindness** occurs when the nurse does not recognize his or her own beliefs and practices, nor the beliefs and practices of others. **Ethnocentrism** refers to the idea that one's own ways are the only way or the best way to behave, believe, or do things. For example, a dominant cultural value in the United States is planning for the future. Calendars are kept religiously, goals are set, events are planned weeks and months in advance, and money is saved for retirement. In other cultures, value is placed on the present, and there is a belief that life is preordained, so there is no point in planning or trying to change the future. Future-oriented individuals may feel that this is the only correct way to live and may be disdainful of those with another time orientation. This is ethnocentrism.

Another concept in mainstream American culture that is taken for granted as normal is the concept of time. Americans live by the clock, make time, waste time, kill time, want to know what time, and worry about enough time. In many cultures, one's daily activities take place as the need arises without regard to a prescribed time of day. For members of these cultures, "being on time" for an appointment may have a range of several hours. The community nurse must be aware of these views and accommodate them accordingly.

Percent distribution. For 1960-90, resident population. For 2000, civilian noninstitutional population plus Armed Forces living off post or with their families on post.

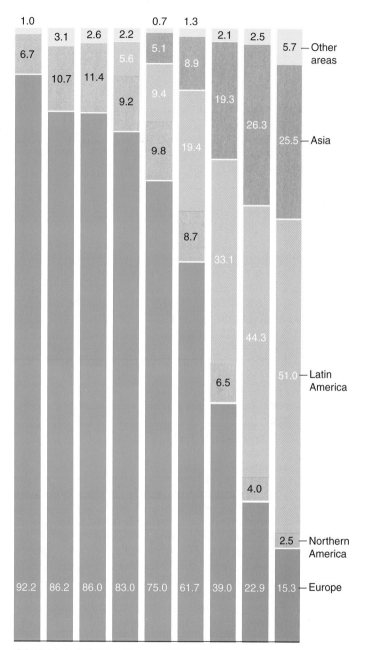

**Figure 3–1.** ▶ Foreign-born population by region of birth: selected years 1850 to 2000. Source: U.S. Census Bureau Web Site.

*SOURCE: U.S. Census Bureau, 2001, Table 2 and 1-1.*

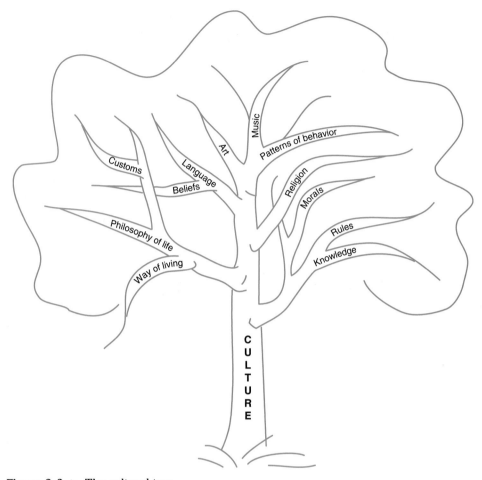

***Figure 3–2.*** ▶ The cultural tree.

The reliance on self is another dominant cultural value in the United States. There are more than 100 words in the English language that begin with the word "self." In many languages there is no translation for the word "self." Individual needs are secondary to the needs of the group. This has strong implications for the concept of self-care. Mainstream American culture places high value on taking care of one's self. People are reluctant to have someone do for them what they think they can do for themselves. This is not so for all cultures.

## CLIENT SITUATIONS IN PRACTICE

### ▶ The Meaning of Self-Care

Maria, a Mexican woman, gave birth 2 days ago. For a period of time called "la quarentena" or "la dieta," specific rules apply regarding the postpartum woman's activity and diet (Andrews & Boyle, 2003). During this time, she is not to do any

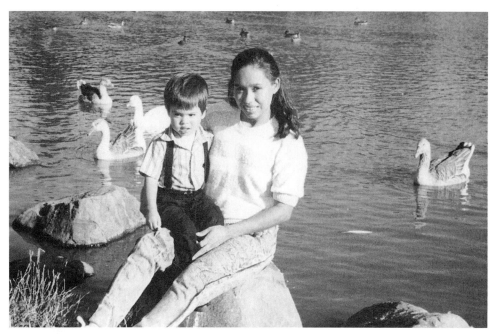

***Figure 3–3.*** ▶ Family relationships and childcare are strongly influenced by cultural traditions.

heavy lifting, exercise, or housework. Family and community members take over the chores of the household, including child care and meal preparation (Fig. 3-3) Jane, a community nurse visiting during this postpartum period, is aware of this cultural practice and provides teaching according to her client's values, which are different than the more active approach to a mother's recovery from childbirth practiced in her own culture.

Because nurses working in the community are frequently visiting postpartum mothers and their newborns, it is essential that they understand how strongly culture influences postpartum self-care and how much that may vary from Western practices.

The way that health decisions are made is culturally based. These decisions are private and individual for some, while others wouldn't think of making a treatment decision without first consulting their extended families.

## CLIENT SITUATIONS IN PRACTICE

### ▶ Client's Right to Know

In the Pakistani culture, the individual's autonomy is secondary to the family's responsibility for health care decisions. Abby is the nurse assigned to a Pakistani woman who has metastatic liver cancer in a home care setting. She would be obligated not to divulge the serious nature of the client's terminal illness. Pakistanis believe that this prevents distress and allows the client to die in peace (Andrews & Boyle, 2003).

Some people come from backgrounds where stoicism is the norm and pain is not expressed, while others have the view that openly verbalizing pain is expected.

## CLIENT SITUATIONS IN PRACTICE

### ▶ Pain Expression

Eva, a community-based nurse, is caring for a Vietnamese client. She knows this culture idealizes stoicism that may suppress the verbalization of pain in disease states where the nurse would expect pain to be expressed. This awareness leads Eva to make a physician referral before her client's disease is in an advanced stage (Lasch, 2000).

In each example, cultural self-awareness is essential to help the nurse recognize and value the right of others to follow their cultural beliefs and practices. Awareness of one's own cultural values opens the nurse's mind to the possibility that the client's values, beliefs, and practices may vary in ways that are very different from his or her own, which can significantly impact the provision of care.

The effective nurse will recognize other cultural beliefs and practices as valid and accommodate the client's ways in providing care. The nurse should ask, "How will knowing these things about my client influence my care?"

 ## CULTURAL KNOWLEDGE

Once nurses are more sensitive and aware of their own cultures and biases, they are ready to discover the culture and lifeways of the community within which they work. **Cultural knowledge** encompasses the familiarity of the worldview, beliefs, practices, and problem-solving strategies of groups that are ethnically or culturally diverse (Campinha-Bacote, 2002).

Community-based nursing practice requires that the nurse have cultural knowledge of the community. This knowledge allows the nurse to use a preventive approach and facilitate self-care according to the client's particular culture. Collaboration and continuity are also enhanced when the nurse knows the cultural community in which he or she is working with the client. Having cultural knowledge about the community will influence what is seen, leading to a more thorough and appropriate assessment and intervention.

Lack of cultural knowledge stands in the way of cultural competence. Nurses can have wonderful intentions and be sensitive and caring, but if there is a lack of specific knowledge about the client's culture, then mistakes are bound to be made.

## CLIENT SITUATIONS IN PRACTICE

### ▶ The Use of Touch

John, a community health nurse, is visiting a family in the Hmong community of St. Paul. As he walks in the door, a young boy is standing there, and John reaches out to touch his head in greeting and as an expression of caring. Lacking cultural knowledge of the Hmong, the nurse is unaware of a strong taboo against touching the head, which is considered the most sacred part of the body, where the brain is, and thinking processes take place. This unintentional affront compromises the nurse's ability to provide care to the family.

## CLIENT SITUATIONS IN PRACTICE

### ▶ Postpartum Care

Concesca is a new immigrant to the United States from Guatemala. She takes her 2-week-old infant in for a checkup. As the umbilical cord has dried and is ready to fall off, the physician plucks it away and tosses it into the trash as Concesca looks on in horror. In her culture, the umbilical cord is precious and is saved in a special place by the mother.

The physician wasn't being cruel, but he was ignorant of cultural knowledge related to postpartum practices in Guatemalan culture. A simple question asked by the doctor or nurse such as, "What cultural practices are important to you in the care of your newborn?" would have alleviated the trauma to this young woman.

## Generic and Professional Knowledge

Dr. Madeleine Leininger uses the terms "emic" and "etic" to describe types of care (Leininger & McFarland, 2002). **Emic** refers to the local or insider's views and values about a phenomenon. **Etic** refers to the professional or outsider's views and values about a phenomenon. The community-based nurse uses both these types of care knowledge and verifies with the client and family those areas that are meaningful and acceptable to them. Discovering how generic (emic) and professional (etic) systems are alike or different assists the nurse in providing culturally congruent care to individuals or groups.

In Mexican–American culture, there are several levels of healers within the curanderismo folklore system. At one level is a curandero, or folk healer, who is believed to have God-given gifts of healing. This folk healer may treat those with a wide range of physical and psychologic problems, ranging from back pain and gastrointestinal distress to irritability or fatigue. After a diagnosis is made, the curandero may use treatments such as massage, diet, rest, indigenous herbs, prayers, magic, or supernatural rituals (Andrews & Boyle, 2003). The nurse working in a Mexican—American community should know about the levels of folk healers used by her clients and inquire as to the consultation and treatment already rendered.

Using this emic understanding of the client's beliefs about health issues, the community nurse can coordinate that care with professional (etic) care that would be acceptable to the client. If massage or a specific diet treatment has been successful, then those interventions can be incorporated into a plan of care. When cultural practices are acknowledged and respected by the professional nurse, clients are more willing to incorporate Western medicine that may augment and enhance the response to treatment.

## Components of Cultural Assessment

Six phenomena related to a cultural assessment are discussed in this section (Box 3-1).

## ASSSESSMENT TOOLS

### Box 3–1  Six Phenomena of Cultural Assessment

- *Communication.* A continuous process by which one person may affect another through written or oral language, gestures, facial expressions, body language, space, or other symbols.
- *Space.* The area around a person's body that includes the individual, body, surrounding environment, and objects within that environment.
- *Social organization.* The family and other groups within a society that dictate culturally accepted role behaviors of different members of the society and rules for behavior. Behaviors are prescribed for significant life events, such as birth, death, childbearing, child rearing, and illness.
- *Time.* The meaning and influence of time from a cultural perspective. Time orientation refers to an individual's focus on the past, the present, or the future. Most cultures combine all three time orientations, but one orientation is more likely to dominate.
- *Environmental control.* The ability or perceived ability of an individual or persons from a particular cultural group to plan activities that control nature, such as illness causation and treatment.
- *Biologic variations.* The biologic differences among racial and ethnic groups. It can include physical characteristics, such as skin color; physiologic variations, such as lactose intolerance, or susceptibility to specific disease processes.

Giger, J. N., & Davidhizar, R. E. (1991). *Transcultural nursing: Assessment and intervention.* St. Louis. Mosby–Year Book.

### Communication

Because the community-based nurse spends much of his or her time teaching and communicating roles, knowledge of communication styles and meanings is essential. Verbal and nonverbal behavior, space between persons talking, family member roles, eye contact, salutations, and intergender communication patterns vary significantly among cultures. For example, lack of eye contact to Western cultures is seen as impolite and may indicate indifference or no interest. In Native American and Southeast Asian cultures, on the other hand, lack of eye contact is a gesture of respect. In conversations, European Americans tend to answer quickly, often before the person speaking has finished; however, Native Americans use silence before answering to carefully absorb what the other has said and to formulate their own response. A nurse working within this community must be aware of this and allow time for these interactions.

In many Eastern cultures, agreeing by nodding or saying "yes" is considered polite, whether or not the individual really agrees or understands what has been asked. To a Hmong person, saying, "yes" to a medical explanation may simply mean that the person is politely listening, not that they have agreed to or even understood what was said. The Hmong appear passively obedient to protect their own dignity by not appearing ignorant and also to protect the doctor's dignity by acting deferential (Fadiman, 1997).

## CLIENT SITUATIONS IN PRACTICE

### ▶ Client Teaching

Nicole is a nurse teaching about medication regimens and wound care in a community setting. Being familiar with the cultural beliefs of her clients, she uses other means of ensuring understanding rather than simply asking, "Do you understand?" She expects return demonstrations or verbal explanations back to her, helping to ensure that her teaching is effective. For example, Nicole may say, "To be sure that your mother will get her medication in the best way to help her, tell me the times you will give her this pill." Or she may say, "Give me some examples of the kinds of foods that you can prepare for your father so that he will minimize the amount of grease in his diet." A respectful and caring approach is a universal dimension of care.

### *Space and Physical Contact*

The concept of space is another important dimension of cultural knowledge. How close people stand by each other in conversation, overt expressions of affection or caring with touch, and rules relating to personal space and privacy vary greatly among cultures. For example, in Italian and Mexican cultures, physical presence and touching is valued and expected. Family members of both genders embrace, kiss, and link arms when walking. In Middle Eastern cultures, close face-to-face conversations where one can almost feel the breath of the other person is the norm, whereas in the United States, the normal space for conversation between persons is an arm's length. In Muslim cultures, it is inappropriate for males and females to even shake hands before marriage. It would be highly improper and distressing for a female Somalian client to be assessed by a male nurse.

## CLIENT SITUATIONS IN PRACTICE

### ▶ Physical Contact

An Iranian child of the Muslim faith is brought in to the local clinic by his parents. The office nurse refrains from shaking hands with the child's father when greeting him. This ensures a feeling of being respected for the father, and a trusting relationship is fostered.

The professional nurse learns about these cultural traditions and beliefs by reading, observing, and asking questions. When in doubt, it is always appropriate to ask, "In your culture, what is considered proper relating to touching and physical space?"

### *Time*

The Western orientation to time and its value was discussed previously. Because the concept of time has such different meanings in various cultures, it is important for the nurse to know of this dimension within the cultural group receiving care. Implications for making appointments, follow-up care, and proper medication administration need to be considered. For example, a physician may prescribe a medication to be taken three times a day with meals. Three meals a day is the norm for most Americans, but this is not so in all other cultures. The nurse should find out when the family has a meal and how much time there is between meals to determine how to explain the regimen within this client's normal patterns of eating.

When scheduling a home visit, 2:00 PM is an exact time to a nurse accustomed to Western orientation to time, but it may mean "sometime in the afternoon" to a person who doesn't share that value of exactness to clock time. Clarifying with the client and family what is meant by a designation of an appointment time saves frustration for both parties.

Another aspect of time is that of past, present, or future orientation. As described already, traditional American culture is future oriented. Calendars and plans for the future are a part of everyday American life. In contrast, Native-American cultures tend to be past oriented, with a focus on ancestors and traditions. African-American culture tends to focus on the present, with an emphasis on "now" and day-to-day activities. Persons without a future orientation need a different approach when discussing preventive care. The nurse may involve the client by saying, "Because of the strong tendency toward developing diabetes that exists in your family, in what ways can we work together to help you avoid this disease in the future?"

### Social Organization

The community-based nurse must understand the family patterns of the groups within the community being served. "The family is the basic unit of society. Cultural values can determine communication within the family group, the norm for family size, and the roles of specific family members" (Kozier, Erb, Blais, & Wilkinson, 2000, p. 209). Nurses should consider, learn about, and assess for these things:

What is the definition of family in this cultural group; does it include primarily the nuclear family, or is the extended family considered the basic unit?

Are there gender or age roles that affect the choice of whom the nurse should address when entering the home or in consultation about a client's health?

What are the traditional roles within the family that affect caregiving?

What value is placed on children and the elderly, and how does that affect health care decision making within the family?

What is the status of females within the culture, and how does that affect the acceptability of a health care provider?

What is the expected family involvement in health care decisions, and who is the primary decision maker within the family?

How is information regarding the health of a family member shared with others in the community?

What role does religion play in health care practices and decision making within the culture and the family unit?

*Biologic Variations*

To perform a thorough assessment and provide culturally congruent care, the community-based nurse who knows biologic variations specific to his or her clients will be most effective. Although some biologic variations are obvious (eg, skin color, hair texture, facial features, stature, and body markings), others require knowledge based on medical information and research. For example, Africans and African-American persons have a much higher incidence of sickle cell disease than other groups. Much of the world's population (many Asians, Africans, Hispanics, and Native Americans) is lactose intolerant, or unable to digest milk sugars. To provide health teaching related to a diet that includes milk and milk products to people in these groups is ethnocentric. Native Americans have a high incidence of diabetes mellitus. Health assessment by community-based nurses working with this population should include screening for high blood-sugar levels and culturally appropriate preventative teaching.

The action, absorption, excretion, and dose parameters of many pharmacologic agents also vary among ethnic groups. Genetic differences, structural variation in binding receptor sites, and environmental conditions may affect the drug action in different groups of people. Blood pressure medications, analgesics, and psychotropic drug doses may be significantly different depending on the ethnic group requiring the medication (Andrews & Boyle, 2003). Adult doses for many medications are not determined by weight as for pediatric doses; instead, body mass should be considered for groups of small stature, such as people of Japanese and Korean descent. The nurse should also ask about herbal remedies that the client might be taking that could affect the action or metabolism of certain medications. Table 3–1 lists some common diseases and their effect on different populations.

*Environmental Control*

There are three predominant views on the relationship between the environment and health: magicoreligious, biomedical, and humoral. The magicoreligious view sees illness as a having a supernatural force; that is, malevolent or evil spirits cause disease, or illness is a punishment from God. People from Hispanic and Caribbean cultures may have this health belief system. Because the belief is that a supernatural influence (rather than organic) caused the health problem, people with this perspective will look for a supernatural counterforce to rid them of the problem. People with this belief will seek a voodoo priestess or spiritualist who has the powers to remove "spells" from a variety of sources. Although Western medicine has classified voodoo illness as a psychiatric disorder, nurses who practice cultural care will understand this view of illness and intervene accordingly.

In the biomedical view, disease and illness are believed to be caused by microorganisms or a malfunction of the body. People with this health view look to medicines, medical treatment, or surgery to cure their illness.

The humoral health belief looks for a balance or harmony with nature (Kozier et al., 2000). Many Eastern cultures ascribe to the theory of yin and yang being opposite forces that must be kept in balance. Imbalance results in illness or disease. The hot and cold theory of many Latino and Asian cultures is similar. "Central to humoral theory is the belief that the healthy body is characterized by evenly distributed warmth and that illness results when the body is attacked by an increase of either hot or cold" (Andrews & Boyle, 2003, pp. 52–53).

**TABLE 3–1 • Biocultural Aspects of Disease**

| Disease | Remarks |
| --- | --- |
| Alcoholism | Native Americans have double the rate of Whites; lower tolerance to alcohol among Chinese and Japanese Americans |
| Anemia | High incidence among Vietnamese due to presence of infestations among immigrants and low-iron diets; low hemoglobin and malnutrition found among 18.2% of Native Americans, 32.7% of Blacks, 14.6% of Hispanics, and 10.4% of White children under 5 years of age |
| Arthritis | Increased incidence among Native Americans<br>Blackfoot 1.4%<br>Pima 1.8%<br>Chippewa 6.8% |
| Asthma | Six times greater for Native American infants < 1 year; same as general population for Native Americans ages 1–44 years |
| Bronchitis | Six times greater for Native American infants < 1 year; same as general population for Native Americans ages 1–44 years |
| Cancer | Nasopharyngeal: High among Chinese Americans and Native Americans<br>Breast: Black women 11/2 times more likely than White<br>Esophageal: No. 2 cause of death for Black males ages 35–54 years<br>*Incidence:*<br>White males 3.5/100,000<br>Black males 13.3/100,000<br>Liver: Highest among all ethnic groups are Filipino Hawaiians<br>Stomach: Black males twice as likely as White males; low among Filipinos<br>Cervical: 120% higher in Black females than in White females<br>Uterine: 53% lower in Black females than White females<br>Prostate: Black males have highest incidence of all groups<br>Most prevalent cancer among Native Americans: biliary, nasopharyngeal, testicular, cervical, renal, and thyroid (females) cancer<br>Lung cancer among Navajo uranium miners 85 times higher than among White miners<br>Most prevalent cancer among Japanese Americans: esophageal, stomach, liver, and biliary cancer<br>Among Chinese Americans, there is a higher incidence of nasopharyngeal and liver cancer than among the general population |
| Cholecystitis | *Incidence:*<br>Whites 0.3%<br>Puerto Ricans 2.1%<br>Native Americans 2.2%<br>Chinese 2.6% |
| Colitis | High incidence among Japanese Americans |
| Diabetes mellitus | Three times as prevalent among Filipino Americans as Whites; higher among Hispanics than Blacks or Whites<br>Death rate is 3–4 times as high among Native Americans ages 25–34 years, especially those in the West such as Utes, Pimas, and Papagos<br>*Complications:*<br>Amputations: Twice as high among Native Americans versus general U.S. population<br>Renal failure: 20 times as high as general U.S. population, with tribal variation (eg, Utes have a 43-times higher incidence) |
| G6PD | Present among 30% of Black males |

*(continued)*

**TABLE 3–1 • Biocultural Aspects of Disease** *(Continued)*

| Disease | Remarks |
|---|---|
| Influenza | Increased death rate among Native Americans ages 45+ |
| Ischemic heart disease | Responsible for 32% of heart-related causes of death among Native Americans; Blacks have higher mortality rates than all other groups |
| Lactose intolerance | Present among 66% of Hispanic women; increased incidence among Blacks and Chinese |
| Myocardial infarction | Leading cause of heart disease in Native Americans, accounting for 43% of death from heart disease; low incidence among Japanese Americans |
| Otitis media | 7.9% incidence among school-age Navajo children versus 0.5% in Whites; up to $\frac{1}{3}$ of Eskimo children < 2 years; increased incidence among bottle-fed Native Americans and Eskimo infants |
| Pneumonia | Increased death rate among Native Americans ages 45 + |
| Psoriasis | Affects 2–5% of Whites, but < 1% of Blacks; high among Japanese Americans |
| Renal disease | Lower incidence among Japanese Americans |
| Sickle cell anemia | Increased incidence among Blacks |
| Trachoma | Increased incidence among Native Americans and Eskimo children (3–8 times greater than general population) |
| Tuberculosis | Increased incidence among Native Americans<br>Apache    2.0%<br>Sioux    3.2%<br>Navajo    4.6% |
| Ulcers | Decreased incidence among Japanese Americans |

Based on data reported in Overfield, T. (1995). *Biologic variation in health and illness: Race, age, and sex differences.* New York: CRC Press; Office of Minority Health. (1995). *Cancer in minority communities. Closing the gap.* Washington, DC: U.S. Government Printing Office; and Andrews, M., & Boyle J. (1999). *Transcultural concepts in nursing care* (pp. 46–47). Philadelphia: Lippincott Williams & Wilkins.

## CLIENT SITUATIONS IN PRACTICE

### ▶ Humoral Health Theory

To the Chinese, childbirth is seen as an experience in which the body loses heat balance that must be restored. Mrs. Yiu, a postpartum Chinese woman, will refuse ice water and will accept only foods that are seen has "warm," such as chicken and rice. Bathing would contribute to the loss of body warmth and would be refused for a period of time after childbirth. The nurse visiting this client in a community setting would be sensitive to these practices and provide care accordingly.

Many variations exist among cultural groups as to how health care is managed and decisions are made. It is important to also keep in mind that individual families may have their own roles, beliefs, and practices that differ from the larger cultural group. This may reflect the degree to which the family has been acculturated to Western cultural patterns and beliefs, or it may be a regional or familial variation. Professional nurses who desire to provide effective care that is culturally congruent to the beliefs of the client are aware of the potential for variations and know what questions to ask. While it is helpful to have a holding knowledge (i.e., knowledge of a group learned from transcultural nursing texts, literature, and previous encounters) of cultural groups, the nurse must always verify with each client which beliefs and practices are personally relevant to him or her. In this way, cultural sensitivity and respect are conveyed even when the nurse is not well versed in the lifeways of a particular group.

### Acculturation and Assimilation

Two other concepts are important for nurses to keep in mind as they learn about the culture of particular groups. Individuals within a group may adhere to the traditional culture to varying degrees; this variation may result from acculturation or assimilation.

As new groups enter a different society, **acculturation** may occur as they learn the ways to exist in a new culture. This may include learning to drive, going to school, negotiating public transportation, getting a job, and interacting in an environment unlike that of the home country. As these activities become more comfortable, individuals become more acculturated to the dominant society, yet they may retain much of their own cultural traditions within their communities. For example, a young Somalian girl may continue to wear her traditional Muslim attire (hijab) and retain the tradition of gender roles while going to an American high school and getting a job at a fast-food restaurant on weekends.

**Assimilation** takes place when individuals or groups identify more strongly with the dominant culture in values, activities, and daily living. This usually occurs over longer periods of time, sometimes generations. These assimilations are important for the nurse to keep in mind as there may be a wide variation in how cultural traditions are carried out, even within the same family. The parents may have emigrated from another country, but the children have been raised surrounded by the dominant culture and have, therefore, assimilated more aspects of the dominant culture.

## CULTURAL SKILL

Campinha-Bacote describes **cultural skill** as the ability to collect relevant cultural data regarding the client's health history. Up to this point we have discussed the need for nurses to examine their own cultural traditions, beliefs, values, and practices to increase awareness of how influential their culture is on their view of the world and to open their mind to the valid variations in worldviews of varying cultures. This helps to avoid cultural blindness, cultural imposition, and ethnocentrism. It is then the nurse's responsibility to learn as much as possible about the ethnic or cultural groups encountered in the community where the nursing care is being delivered. A holding knowledge of the emic or folk care practices along with the etic or professional care practices gives the community nurse a basis from which to individualize care that is culturally sensitive to the client as an individual or as a family. Practices within cultural groups or families may vary significantly from general descriptions; therefore, knowing the questions to ask for culturally specific care is essential to avoid stereotyping. Having cultural skill is essential to that process.

Leininger defines a **culturologic assessment** as a "systematic identification and documentation of culture care, beliefs, meanings, values, symbols and practices of individuals or groups with a holistic perspective" (Leininger & McFarland, 2002, p. 117). Community-based nurses focus on preventive care. These nurses assess the health risks of a particular group and consider cultural practices and beliefs to plan teaching and activities to prevent disease or health risks (primary prevention). Using culturally based knowledge of generic or folk health care practices in the group, community-based nurses then incorporate their **etic** and **emic care** knowledge to diagnose and treat threats to health and wellness (secondary prevention). Tertiary prevention in the community seeks to rehabilitate or prevent recurrence of health problems. Through a skillful culturologic assessment, the community nurse has listened to the clients' perception of the health problem and compared it to his or her own perception, explaining and acknowledging the similarities and differences. Involving members of the community, the nurse then negotiates a treatment plan that will be seen as beneficial to the community.

Numerous models for culturologic assessment have been developed by various authors in the field of transcultural nursing (Andrews & Boyle, 2003; Giger & Davidhizer, 2002; Leininger, 2002; Heineken & McCoy, 2000). Each organizes assessment data in a different manner, and individual nurses will determine which model works best within their scope of practice and the community served. A cross-cultural assessment tool (Box 3-2) can be useful with any client (Heineken & McCoy, 2000). The questions are open ended and provide the opportunity for the client to describe his or her perception of the health problem. For example, in response to the second question, "How would you describe this problem you have?", the parents of a Hmong child with epilepsy might respond, "The spirit catches you and you fall down" (Fadiman, 1997).

The culturologic assessment gives the nurse good information with cultural implications to use as a basis for planning teaching and treatment plans. All clients have a right to have their values, beliefs, and practices considered, respected, and incorporated into the plan of care. (Heineken & McCoy, 2000).

---

## ASSSESSMENT TOOLS

### Box 3-2   Heineken and McCoy's Cross-Cultural Assessment Tool

- If the patient is an immigrant, ask: How is this kind of illness treated in your country?
- How would you describe this problem you have? Or is there someone else I should talk to?
- What does this sickness do to you?
- How long have you had the problem? Why has the problem happened to you?
- Why do you think the problem began when it did?
- What do you think is wrong, out of balance, or causing the problem?
- What has been done so far?
- What do you think will help your problem clear up? What should be done?
- What does the family think should be done?
- Apart from me (us), who else do you think can help you get better?
- How serious do you think this situation/problem is?

Heineken, J. & McCoy, N. (2000). Establishing a bond with clients of different cultures. *Home Healthcare Nurse, 18*(1), 45–51.

## CULTURAL ENCOUNTER

The **cultural encounter** is the opportunity for the nurse to engage in direct contact with the members of cultural communities. Through frequent contact with numerous members of a cultural group, the nurse keeps in mind that variations will exist within the community and stereotypical expectations are to be avoided. Trust builds over time between the caregiving nurse and members of the community, and it is essential to the well-being of both.

Using knowledge of etic and emic care practices and having completed a culturologic assessment, the nurse now uses the skills and competencies necessary to effect healthful outcomes for the clients in the community. Leininger has identified three modalities that "guide nursing judgments, decisions or actions so as to provide cultural congruent care that is beneficial, satisfying and meaningful to people nurses serve" (Leininger & McFarland, 2002, p. 43). These three modalities are defined in Table 3–2.

### Cultural Care Preservation

The first of the modalities is cultural care preservation and/or maintenance. After careful assessment and observation, the nurse identifies those cultural care practices that are helpful to the client. The nurse then assists, supports, facilitates, or enables the client and family to preserve those actions or behaviors. For example, in the Amish community, the extended family, neighborhood, and church expect to assist and care for members within the community. The nurse working in this community encourages and supports ways to enlist the help of the extended community and facilitates ways to let the care needs be known (Fisher, 2002).

**TABLE 3–2** • Leininger's Guidelines for Providing Culturally Congruent Care

| Modality | Definition |
| --- | --- |
| Cultural care preservation and/or maintenance | Refers to those assistive, supporting, facilitative, or enabling professional actions and decisions that help people of a particular culture to retain and/or preserve relevant care values so that they can maintain their well-being, recover from illness, or face handicaps and/or death |
| Cultural care accommodation or negotiation | Refers to those assistive, supporting, facilitative, or enabling creative professional actions and decisions that help people of a designated culture (or subculture) adapt to or negotiate with others for a beneficial or satisfying health outcome with professional care providers |
| Cultural care repatterning or restructuring | Refers to those assistive, supporting, facilitative, or enabling professional actions and decisions that help a client reorder, change, or greatly modify lifeways for new, different, and beneficial health care patterns while respecting the client's cultural values and beliefs and still providing beneficial or healthier lifeways than before the changes were coestablished with the client(s) |

Leininger, M. N. & McFarland, M. (2002). *Transcultural Concepts, theories, research, practice* (p. 84) New York: McGraw-Hill.

## Cultural Care Accommodation

The second mode of cultural care accommodation or negotiation refers to those nursing actions and decisions that assist or enable the client and family to continue with practices that are meaningful to them but may be altered due to circumstances. For example, the nurse in the community may be setting up a referral for a client to be seen in a clinic for follow-up care. The client is Muslim and must adhere to the practice of praying five times a day. The nurse will negotiate with the client as to times of day that would provide enough time between prayers for an appointment or assist in helping the client find a place within or near the clinic where these prayers may be said.

In another example, the community-based nurse is doing a follow-up visit to a Jewish child recently diagnosed with type 1 diabetes. Knowing the Jewish restriction of pork products, the nurse might intervene to ask the physician to prescribe a nonporcine insulin product.

In addition to assisting the client in carrying out his or her religious practices, the respect and care shown by the nurse toward these clients enhances trust and feelings of caring support.

## Cultural Care Repatterning

The third way in which nurses make decisions or intervene is cultural care repatterning or restructuring. When the nurse assesses the client, family, and community and finds practices that may be detrimental to health and well-being, he or she will work with the client to change behaviors that are harmful.

### CLIENT SITUATIONS IN PRACTICE

#### ▶ Dietary Repatterning

Joan is working within the Navajo community, where members observe the practice of eating bread fried in fat as a staple in the diet. Knowing that this much fat soaked into the bread is detrimental to a community at risk for heart disease, Joan works with the Navajo women to explore ways to decrease the amount of fat in servings of fry bread. Together they may decide that placing the fry bread vertically or on paper towels before serving may decrease the amount of fat as it drips off before eating. Because the nurse works with the client(s) to diminish risks to health, the changes are more likely to take effect.

Box 3-3 presents research that led nurses to provide culturally competent care using three modes of action in an ambulatory care setting. Note how knowing the culture and learning the emic care can lead to simple but important nursing actions and decisions that will be perceived by the clients as cultural care.

Whether the nurse is validating and supporting helpful existing practices, helping clients to negotiate ways to maintain their health care practices, or working to identify and change harmful behaviors, it is essential that he or she work with the community as a partner. Because optimum health care for all clients is the goal of nursing, these three modes of nursing actions and decisions, in close cooperation with the clients, can be enormously beneficial and satisfying to both the community and the nurse.

## ASSESSMENT TOOLS

### Box 3–3   Research Related to Community-Based Nursing Care

## Research Informs Practice

The purpose of this study was to examine the cultural beliefs and practices of Puerto Rican families that influence feeding practices and affect the nutritional status of infants and young children. The goal of the study was to outline strategies that would enable nurses to provide culturally congruent care for this population. Resulting cultural care modalities are listed below.

### Cultural Care Modalities for the Puerto Rican Client in an Ambulatory Care Setting

#### CULTURAL CARE PRESERVATION MODALITIES

Reinforce family caring values of nurturance and succorance.

Respect and understand use of religious symbols and protective care symbols.

Touch the infant or child and say "God bless you" if complimenting the child.

Treat the family with respect, use professional demeanor, maintain eye contact.

Promote continuity of care.

#### CULTURAL CARE ACCOMMODATION MODALITIES

Use the Spanish language to include the grandmother; reinforce intergenerational caregiving.

Promote *respeto* (respect) and *confianza* (confidence, trust) by accommodation (or deference) to family and community values.

Encourage introduction of traditional, healthy foods—rice, beans, and eggs—at the appropriate time, linking their use with green vegetables and meat.

Encourage the generic folk practice of *Ponche* as needed, with additional health considerations.

Develop a comprehensive bilingual feeding assessment guide to improve anticipatory guidance.

#### CULTURAL CARE REPATTERNING MODALITIES

Include grandmother and kin in a collaborative participatory approach to feeding.

Emphasize the cultural ideology and beliefs. Explain how a new approach will contribute to a big, healthy baby.

Anticipatory guidance about overfeeding formula should begin at 2–4 weeks.

*(continued)*

## ASSESSMENT TOOLS

**Box 3–3   Research Related to Community-Based Nursing Care**
*(Continued)*

Anticipatory guidance about not adding solids to the bottle should be given at
4–8 weeks before the practice is initiated. Stress the ease of feeding solids by
mouth at 4–6 months of age.
Develop Spanish-language pamphlets linking emic and etic feeding practices.
Provide nutrition and cooking demonstration classes with a cultural theme, linking emic and etic foods for mothers, fathers, and grandmothers.
Advertise classes on Spanish-speaking radio and TV stations.
Develop a nutritional outreach program including bilingual Puerto Rican mothers who are interested in nutrition and health.

Higgins, B. (2000). Puerto Rican cultural beliefs: Influence on infant feeding practices in western
New York. *Journal of Transcultural Nursing, 11*(1), 19–30.

## CLIENT SITUATIONS IN PRACTICE

### ▶ Planning for a Cultural Encounter

Sarah is a home health care nurse assigned to visit Ahmed and her 2-week-old
newborn son. This Somalian family consists of Ahmed, her husband, 3-year-old
daughter, and the new baby. The family has been in the United States for 4
months, after spending a year in a refugee camp in Kenya. Both Mohammed and
Ahmed were residents of Mogadishu before the civil war and were from middle-
class traditional Somalian families. Both speak English, although not fluently. Prenatal history indicates the baby was born by C-section after a reported uneventful
pregnancy, notable only for the fact that Ahmed's first prenatal visit with a physician was 1 week prior to the child's birth. She experienced false labor and was
brought to the physician's office by her neighbor.

   Sarah is preparing to visit Ahmed and her new baby for the first time. What are
some considerations she should think about prior to her visit?

   *Sarah should consider the traditional Somali practice of female circumcision and
her own cultural beliefs related to that practice. She cannot assume Ahmed is circumcised or to what degree, but the decision to have a C-section may have been a result
of this possibility (although circumcised women can give birth vaginally as well).*

   Sarah knows that most Somalians are Muslims. Where can she find out some
basic beliefs and practices of those who practice Islam?

   *Sarah can review current literature and transcultural-nursing books as well as
access information on-line related to Muslim religious practices. She notes that
99% of Somalians are Sunni Muslims. She knows this will be an important question
to ask as culture and religion are highly intertwined in Somalia.*

What basic cultural practices are important for Sarah to know prior to visiting this Somalian family?

*Gender roles are quite specifically defined in traditional Somali culture. Sarah will know that she must not offer to shake hands with Mohammed, as physical contact with a woman other than a close family member is forbidden. She will also know that female modesty is a high priority when assessing Ahmed's incision.*

Sarah plans to discuss family planning. What is important for her to know in providing culturally sensitive care?

*In the Muslim religion, children are seen as gifts from Allah, and many children are considered a blessing. Preventing conception is not acceptable, but the concept of family "spacing" to preserve the mother's health and provide adequate time for weaning the youngest child is an appropriate approach to take (Lawrence & Rozmus, 2001; Callister, 2002).*

As in any cultural encounter, Sarah must proceed slowly, know some basic cultural practices and beliefs she is likely to encounter, verify the degree to which the client is acculturated, and establish a climate of trust using cultural sensitivity and respect.

 ## CONCLUSIONS

All nurses, regardless of their own cultural background, are obligated to learn what is important to their clients. "Health and illness states are strongly influenced and often primarily determined by the cultural background of the individual" (Leininger, 1970, p. 22). Cultural awareness of one's own background, beliefs, values, and practices opens the nurse's mind to value and support the diversity of others. Cultural knowledge learned from books, formal coursework, and discussions with community members gives the nurse a background or framework in which to understand the cultural health care beliefs of a group. This information can then be validated or altered based on individual interactions. Cultural skill is the ability to conduct a culturologic assessment that will guide nursing actions and decisions. In the cultural encounter, the nurse reinforces, negotiates, or assists clients to repattern care practices for optimum health care.

An attitude of sensitivity, acceptance, and sincere desire to work with culturally diverse clients results in continuity and collaborative care and promotes a trusting relationship with the client. Nurses in the community setting must establish a bond based on trust with the home health care client to provide excellent care and do so cost effectively (Heineken & McCoy, 2000). Using knowledge of the generic or emic care practices of the cultural community and integrating these with professional or etic knowledge, the nurse assists in self-care by encouraging existing healthy behaviors and establishing preventive measures that are culturally congruent and acceptable in creating a healthy future for each community served.

# What's on the Web

Center for Cross-Cultural Health
**Internet address:**
*http://www.crosshealth.com*
This Minneapolis-based organization offers excellent information and resources for culturally competent medical and nursing care.

Ethnomed
**Internet address:** *http://www.ethnomed.org*
This Web site, through the University of Washington, offers excellent information on a wide range of cultures.

Transcultural Nursing Society
**Internet address:** *http://www.tcns.org*
This is an excellent Web site, with links to other resources, information about membership in the Transcultural Nursing Society, and transcultural nursing workshops, courses, and certifications. The site also provides an on-line index for all articles published in the *Journal of Transcultural Nursing* since 1989.

## References and Bibliography

Andrews, M., & Boyle, J. (1998). *Transcultural concepts in nursing care*. Philadelphia: Lippincott Williams & Wilkins.

Andrews, M., & Boyle, J. (2003). *Transcultural concepts in nursing care*. Philadelphia: Lippincott Williams & Wilkins.

Callister, L. C. (2001). Culturally competent care of women and newborns: Knowledge, attitude and skills. *Journal of Obstetric, Gynecologic and Neonatal Nursing, 30*(2), 9–15.

Callister, L. C. (2002). Toward evidence based practice. Culture care conflicts among Asian-Islamic immigrant women in United States hospitals. *American Journal of Maternal Child Nursing, 27*(3), 194.

Campinha-Bacote, J. (2002). The process of cultural competence in the delivery of healthcare services: A model of care. *Journal of Transcultural Nursing, 13*(3), 181–184.

Fadiman, A. (1997). *The spirit catches you and you fall down*. New York: Noonday Press.

Giger, J. N., & Davidhizar, R. E. (2002). The Giger and Davidhizar transcultural assessment model. *Journal of Transcultural Nursing, 13*(3), 185–188.

Heineken, J., & McCoy, N. (2000). Establishing a bond with clients of different cultures. *Home Healthcare Nurse, 18*(1), 45–51.

Higgins, B. (2000). Puerto Rican cultural beliefs: Influence on infant feeding practices in western New York. *Journal of Transcultural Nursing, 11*(1), 19–30.

Kozier, E., Erb, G., Blais, K., & Wilkinson, J. (2000). *Fundamentals of nursing, concepts, processes and practice*. Redwood City, CA: Addison Wesley.

Lasch, K. E. (2000). Culture, pain and culturally sensitive pain care. *Pain Management in Nursing 1*(3)(Suppl. 1), 16–22.

Lawrence, P., & Rozmus, C. (2001). Culturally sensitive care of the Muslim patient. *Journal of Transcultural Nursing, 12*(3), 228–233.

Leininger, M. M. (1970). *Nursing and anthropology: Two worlds to blend*. Columbus, OH: Greyden Press.

Leininger, M. M. (2002). Culture Care Theory: a major contribution to advance transcultural nursing and practice. *Journal of Transcultural Nursing 13*(3), 189–192.

Leininger, M. M., & McFarland, M. (2002). *Transcultural nursing concepts, theories, research, practice*. New York: McGraw-Hill.

Overfield, T. (1995). *Biologic variation in health and illness. Race, age, and sex differences.* New York: CRC Press; office of Minority Health (August 1995).

Stewart, E. C. and Bennett, M. J. (1991). *American cultural patterns: In a cross-cultural perspective* (revised edition). Yarmouth, Maine: Intercultural Press.

U.S. Census Bureau (1998).

U.S. Department of Health and Human Services. (2000). *Healthy people 2010: National health promotion and disease prevention objectives, full report, with commentary.* Washington, DC: U.S. Government Printing Office.

# LEARNING ACTIVITIES

## LEARNING ACTIVITY 3–1

Using the cultural tree in Figure 3–2, write the ways in which your family of origin or your cultural background influence each area depicted on a branch. Discuss your findings with another student.

1. In what areas was culture a strong influence?
2. In what areas has acculturation or assimilation influenced your beliefs and preferences compared to what your grandparent may have answered?
3. What similarities and differences did you note in comparing your tree to another student's responses?
4. By participating in this activity, what awareness did you gain that may be helpful to you in caring for clients from other cultures?

## LEARNING ACTIVITY 3–2

Make a list of various ethnic and minority or cultural groups (e.g., Native Americans, Asians, the elderly, Latinos, WASPs [White, Anglo–Saxon, Protestants], Jews) and write a stereotype you have or have heard about each group.

1. How does knowing these stereotypes exist make you more sensitive to clients about potential barriers in daily living and access to health care?
2. In what way can nurses break through stereotypes to deliver the best possible care?

## LEARNING ACTIVITY 3–3

Read the following list of American cultural values and reflect on how these values may vary significantly from those of other cultural groups.

### AMERICAN CULTURAL VALUES

Doing: value of activity, ie, keeping busy
Problem solvers: conceive of more than one course of action
Achievement: personal, visible, measurable, materialistic
Choices: effects are preferably measurable, visible, materialistic

Practical: adjust to immediate situations without much thought for long-term effects
Exploration of values: "oughtness," "should"
Self-centered
Equality and fairness
Majority rule
Decision makers are responsible for subsequent action, rational order to the world; cause and effect, world and nature are controllable
Separation of work from play
Hard work ethic
Time is money
Temporal orientation: toward the future, can improve on the present with effort and optimism; action and hard work = goal achievement (positive)
Training and education very important
Source of motivation lies in individual, not society
Need feedback: sensitive to praise/blame; need to be liked
Competitive: individual and ascriptive (team, country, etc.)
Failure is the result of lack of will and effort of the individual
Individualism vs. individuality
Limits role of authority: to providing services, protecting rights of individuals, inducing cooperation and adjudicating differences
Equality of opportunity
Social equality
Don't like obligations socially
Competition within cooperation
Cooperation to get things done more important than social relationship of doers
Physical comfort and health
Private property and free enterprise
(Excerpted from Stewart, 1991)

Follow these instructions in your clinical journal:

1. Describe several of the values that are part of your everyday way of living.
2. How do those values influence how you see other cultural ways that differ?
3. Knowing that significant value orientation differences may exist between you and your clients in the community, describe accommodations you might make to provide culturally sensitive care within that setting.

## LEARNING ACTIVITY 3–4

Using a cultural assessment guide referenced in the chapter, conduct a cultural assessment on a client from a cultural group that differs from your own. What specific information did you learn that would guide your nursing actions related to (1) cultural preservation, (2) cultural accommodation, and (3) cultural repatterning?

## LEARNING ACTIVITY 3–5

Keep a journal of your nursing encounters with persons from cultures different than your own. Discuss how prepared you felt in each interaction and what cultural beliefs, values, or lifeways you discovered in each encounter. How did that knowledge affect the care you provided?

# Family Care

Roberta Hunt

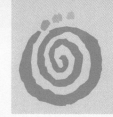

## KEY TERMS

| | |
|---|---|
| affective interventions | family structure |
| behavioral interventions | family systems theory |
| cognitive interventions | functional assessment |
| developmental assessment | genogram |
| family developmental tasks | healthy family functioning |
| family functions | role conflict |
| family health | structural family assessment |
| family role | |

## CHAPTER TOPICS

- **Significance of Family Care**
- **Nursing Competencies and Skills in Family Care**
- **Conclusions**

**THE NURSE SPEAKS**

For many years, the nursing students at our college had the opportunity to see patients in a pediatric primary care clinic. To meet the needs of working parents, this clinic was open during the week from 5:00 to 9:00 PM. One evening, one of my students completed the initial assessment with Ty, a 3-year-old boy. Ty was accompanied by his mother and father and two younger siblings.

Ty had a history of frequent otitis media and was being seen that evening for ear drainage, ear pain, and a low-grade fever. Ty was accustomed to the routine and allowed the student to do the initial assessment as he sat on his mother's lap.

The pediatrician did her evaluation and diagnosed otitis media of the right ear. Because the pediatrician was familiar with the family, she asked if they had kept the referral appointment she had made for Ty to see an ear, nose, and throat (ENT) specialist the month before. The mother, who spoke very little English, shook her head no.

After leaving the room, the pediatrician voiced her concern with us because she noted hearing impairment as a result of the otitis media. Next, she wrote a prescription for an oral antibiotic, which was filled at the clinic, and found a sample bottle of oral analgesic. The nursing student and I went back to see the family and to review the home care instructions. I encouraged the student to have the mother and father administer the first dose of antibiotic and analgesic before the family left the clinic. The student questioned why she would need to observe this as Ty had a long history of otitis media. I again encouraged her to observe the mother and father administer the medications. The student asked the parents to administer the first dose of medications while at the clinic. The parents agreed, so Ty's mother washed her hands, read each medication bottle, and precisely measured the exact amount to be administered. Next, Ty's mother placed him across her lap and attempted to administer the oral antibiotic into his right ear. In utter surprise, the nursing student stopped the mother before she was able to place the medication into Ty's ear. The student politely explained how the medications worked and the need to administer both medications orally. At this point, a staff person who could serve as an interpreter was able to visit with the family, and it was discovered that the parents had routinely given the oral medications into whichever ear was affected.

Through the assistance of the interpreter, the student reviewed the home care instructions with the parents. The parents verbalized their understanding of the route of administration, and each medication was correctly administered by the mother before leaving the clinic. The parents agreed to a follow-up by a community health nurse and the ENT specialist.

We all learned an important lesson that evening in the midst of a very busy pediatric clinic—that is, the value of making time for discharge teaching along with a return demonstration, especially when administering medications to children.

— **Susan O'Conner-Von, DNSc, RNC**
Assistant Professor, School of Nursing
University of Minnesota
Minneapolis, Minnesota

Not only is the family the basic social unit in American society, but also it is the most influential and dynamic unit. It has been the primary focus of nursing care in the community since the establishment of public health nursing in the late 19th century. The family performs a variety of key functions and has a central role in promoting and maintaining the health of its members.

Understanding family structure, roles, and functions is paramount in providing comprehensive nursing care. Knowledge of **healthy family functioning** allows the nurse to identify unhealthy functioning and take appropriate actions. In the current health care climate, the nurse must be cognizant of the needs, feelings, problems, and views of the family when providing care to the individual client.

Numerous models depict the relationship between nursing care and the family. These models reflect three ways to consider the family as it relates to nursing care.

*Care of the individual in the context of the family.* This point of view considers the family as it relates to the recovery of the individual client. Consequently, the client is the focus, and the context is the family.

*The family's impact on the recovery of the client.* In this model, the influences that family structure, function, development stage, and interpersonal interactions have on the recovery of the client are considered.

*Improvement of the family's collective health.* This method focuses on the family as the unit of service. In this model, the nurse assesses the family, determines the family's health problems or diagnoses, and develops goals with the family that are intended to improve its collective health.

This chapter discusses all three models by which nursing care is provided to families. However, **family health** will be considered primarily in the context of the impact of the family on the health of the individual who has been identified as the client. Nursing process skills will focus on the health of the family as it relates to the health recovery of the individual client.

## SIGNIFICANCE OF FAMILY CARE

Regardless of which method is used, it is evident the family and individual are closely interrelated. The individual's health affects the family, and the family's health affects the client.

### Concepts

Definitions of family have evolved over the past several decades. Definitions usually include family structure, roles, and function. The definition currently accepted by most health care professions is that of a social group whose members share common values and interact with each other over time. Usually, but not always, they live together. In this text, we will use this definition but also consider those whom the client has identified as family or significant others.

#### Family Structure

Traditionally, the family has been defined as the nuclear family, or a family with a mother, father, and two or more children. The characteristics of the "typical" family in the United States have changed markedly over the past 20 years. During that time, the typical family has evolved to the point where the traditional nuclear family—mother, father, and 2.2 children—no longer represents the majority of the population. Many different family structures exist. Table 4–1 lists the various **family structures** and their components; Figure 4–1 depicts different family structures.

In 1970, 85% of all children under age 18 were living with two parents; in 1993, only 71% were, and in 2001, 69% of all children were living with two parents. The proportion of children living with only one parent almost doubled between 1970 and 2001, rising from 12% to 22%. For White children, 78% were living with two parents in 2001; however, only 38% of African-American children and 65% of Hispanic children lived with both parents (Federal Interagency Forum on Child and Family Statistics, 2002).

Marked differences in income are apparent among the different family structures. Children in married-couple families are much less likely to be living in poverty than children living only with their mother. In 2000, 8% of children in married-couple families were living in poverty, compared with 40% in female-householder families. The contrast by family structure is especially pronounced among certain racial and ethnic groups. For example, in 2000, 8% of African-American children in married-couple families lived in poverty, compared with 49% of African-American children in female-householder families. Twenty-one percent of Hispanic children in married-couple families lived in poverty, compared with 48% in female-householder families. Most children in poverty are White and not Hispanic. However, the proportion of African-American or Hispanic children in poverty is much higher than the proportion of White, non-Hispanic children. Children under 18 continue to represent a large segment of the poor populations (40%) although they make up only about 25% of the total population. To complicate matters, in 2001, 13% of all children had no health insurance (Federal Interagency Forum on Children and Family Statistics, 2002). These statistics are important because the level of health and the quality of health care are affected by poverty. Those living in poverty, and consequently receiving poor health care, represent a large number of families in the United States.

### Family Roles

A **family role** is an expected set of behaviors associated with a particular family position. Roles can be formal or informal. Formal roles are recognized by expectations associated with the roles, such as wife, husband, mother, father, or child. Examples of formal roles include breadwinner, housekeeper, child caretaker, financial manager, or cook. Informal roles are those that are casually acquired within a

**TABLE 4–1 • Family Structures**

| Structure | Participants |
| --- | --- |
| Nuclear family | Married couple with children |
| | Unmarried couple, heterosexual or same sex with children |
| Nuclear dyad | Couple, married or unmarried; heterosexual or same sex |
| Single-parent family | One adult with children (separated, divorced, widowed, or never married) |
| Single adult | One adult |
| Multigenerational family | Any combination of the first four family structures |
| Kin network | Two or more reciprocal households (related by birth or marriage) |

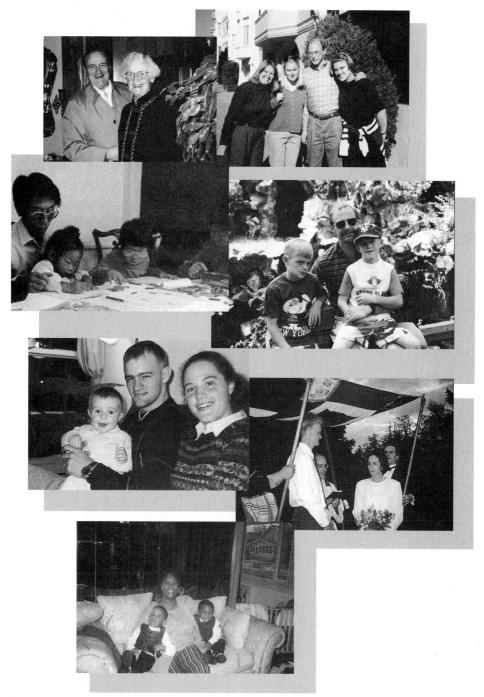

***Figure 4–1.*** ▶ Various family structures.

family. An example of an informal role would be the family member who plans the social schedule or who takes out the garbage.

**Role conflict** may occur when the demands of one role conflict with or contradict another. This may also occur when one family member's expectations conflict with another's expectations. Role overload occurs when an individual is confronted with too many role responsibilities at one time. For instance, when a woman with children returns to school, she may have difficulty managing the roles of cook, driver, housekeeper, wife, and child care provider while keeping up with her schoolwork. The new role of student competes with the prior roles, and role overload occurs.

Illness or hospitalization of a family member causes role conflict or overload for all family members. Flexibility with family roles becomes particularly important during crises. Hospitalization and illness often require shifts in family roles and responsibilities. If one family member is ill, other family members may have to assume certain roles temporarily or permanently. In some situations, this may mean that a child assumes a parental role if one of the parents becomes ill or is hospitalized. During illness, various family members' ability to take on different roles facilitates the family's adaptation or return to homeostasis. Role flexibility also allows the family to provide support to the family member who is recovering from an illness or injury. Similarly, role flexibility in a family may allow the ill family member to be more comfortable with giving up roles, thus facilitating recovery.

### Family Functions

**Family functions** are defined as outcomes, or consequences, of family structure. They are the reason families exist. Functions are divided into several categories: affective, socialization, reproductive, economic, and health care, as shown in Figure 4–2.

The affective function of the family is defined as the family's ability to meet the psychologic needs of family members. These needs include affection and understanding. This is considered by some as the most vital function of families.

Socialization or social placement is the second function. Socialization is the process of learning to adapt to life in a family and a community. This involves helping children adapt to the norms of the community and become productive members of society. This socialization process is built into all cultures. Specific functions include a variety of day-to-day family and social experiences that prepare children to assume adult roles. These may include learning the norms of dress and hygiene and preparing and eating food.

The third function, reproductive, is procreation. It may be thought of as the family's provision of recruits for society to ensure the continuity of the intergenerational family and society.

Economic functions encompass the allocation of adequate resources for family members. This entails the provision of sufficient income to provide for basic necessities. It also includes the allocation of these resources to all family members, especially those unable to provide for themselves.

Providing for health care and the physical necessities is the final family function. Physical care is the provision of material necessities, such as food, clothing, and shelter. Family health care includes health and lifestyle practices, such as nutrition, chemical use and abuse, recreation, and exercise and sleep practices.

Family functions can also be viewed in relation to Maslow's hierarchy of needs. Maslow's theory is directionally based and presents the concept that the needs at the bottom of the model must be met before the next level can be addressed (Fig.

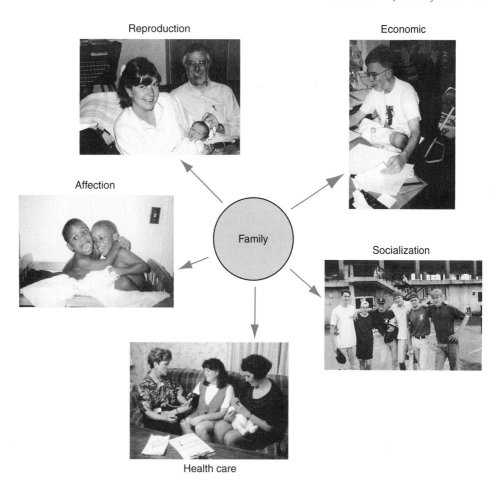

Reproduction

Economic

Affection

Family

Socialization

Health care

***Figure 4–2.*** ▶ Basic family functions.

4–3). According to Maslow, the family must first meet physiologic needs (eg, food, fluids, shelter, sleep) before members can consider any other opportunities in life.

Safety needs include both physiologic and psychologic safety of family members. The infant experiences safety when held securely in the arms of the parent. The young child experiences safety in the family when the environment is sufficiently structured to protect the child from harm. Adolescents feel safe in an environment that allows freedom and provides responsibility and structure.

Physiologic and psychologic safety remains important to adults. Physical safety includes living in a safe community. Increasingly, urban neighborhoods are more and more violent, resulting in residents feeling unsafe. Psychologic safety evolves from living a relatively structured life with some definite social expectations of one's self and those around us.

Another family function is meeting love-and-belonging needs. We all need meaningful relationships with other people. In classic research by Spitz (1945), two groups of infants and children were studied. Both groups received excellent physical care, but the second group received little demonstrative affection. Members

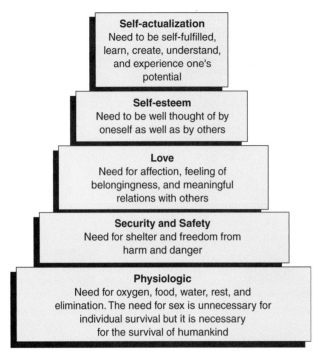

*Figure 4–3.* ▶ Maslow's hierarchy of needs. According to Maslow, basic physiologic needs must be met before the person can move on to higher-level needs. Adapted from Maslow, A. H. (1954). *Motivation and personality.* New York: Harper & Row.

of the first group were talked to, held, and caressed. There was a higher mortality rate as well as impaired development among the infants and children of the second group who received no physical affection. This demonstrates the vital importance of meeting the love-and-belonging need.

Fulfillment of esteem needs is also a family function. Self-esteem comes from feeling that we are valued by those around us. The family introduces the child to self-esteem. Family members may assist one another to feel good about themselves through acceptance and approval.

Self-actualization is being "true to oneself," to fulfill one's potential. Self-actualization is not what one chooses to do in life, but how one feels about that choice. To joyfully do in life what one wants and is suited to do is self-actualization.

### Family Systems Theory

The identification of the family as the unit of care is an emerging trend in family systems theory. **Family systems theory** defines family as a collection of people who are integrated, interacting, and interdependent. The actions of one member influence the actions of other members. The family system has a boundary; people recognize the family members. This boundary is selectively permeable according to the family's wishes, so items such as material goods, people, and information are allowed in or out according to the perceived needs of the system. Families with closed boundaries in one area may, for instance, be reluctant to use community resources.

After a crisis or during a transition from one developmental stage to another, the family system may experience disequilibrium. This imbalance causes a large amount of energy to be expended by individual family members in an attempt to cope with the discomfort. The family will attempt to return to the previous state of equilibrium. A nurse who is knowledgeable about family systems theory can facilitate healthy functioning.

The nurse considers the actions of family members as they apply to the health of the individual client. Family boundaries can be assessed to determine the likelihood that the family will use needed services. Similarly, disequilibrium of the family system as it pertains to the client can also be assessed.

## Family Health

### The Health–Illness Continuum

The family's structure, roles, ability to fulfill family functions, culture, and developmental tasks all affect the way the family functions. When a family member is ill, adaptation depends on each of these areas. An individual's place on the wellness–illness continuum affects all members of the family and all interactions within the family.

Family structure also affects the health recovery of an individual. In a family with two adult members, recovery may be different from that in a family headed by one adult. Certainly, when an individual lives alone, there is a greater need to tap extended family and friends for support and assistance than when the family has other adult members.

Family roles have an impact on the health recovery of the individual, and the health of the individual affects family roles. It is difficult to fulfill the usual functions of the family during times of stress or illness. When a family member is hospitalized, it may be difficult to fulfill the family's basic physical necessities and care. Examples include the inability to provide meals, maintain a regular bedtime, or wash laundry.

### Family Needs During Illness

Health care professionals are placing increased emphasis on the needs and roles of the family during a loved one's critical illness. Studies show that although nurses are often in the best position to meet families' needs, their needs are not always met (Holden, Harrison, & Johnson, 2002). The standards for comprehensive and effective family care by the Association for the Care of Children's Health focus on the immediate emotional and practical needs of the family in crisis. These recommendations may be adapted to all family care:

▶ Recognizing that the family is the primary constant in the client's life, which requires nurse and family collaboration
▶ Sharing information
▶ Providing support
▶ Recognizing family strengths
▶ Respecting different methods of family coping (Tomlinson, Thomlinson, Peden-McAlpine, & Kirschbaum, 2002)

Families require similar assistance from nursing staff during the course of a lifelong chronic condition. Taanila, Jarvelin, and Kokkonen (1998) found from a 10-year study that families need quality information and advice at the time of diagnosis, as well as ongoing communication concerning both emotional and factual issues. This research showed a relationship between the quality of information given to families and their feelings of insecurity and helplessness.

## TABLE 4–2 • Family Needs During Stages of Illness

| Stage Priority | Family Needs | Education Needs | Role of the Nurse | Psychosocial Issues |
|---|---|---|---|---|
| **Prediagnosis** | Information<br>Relief from anxiety<br>To be with and<br>  helpful to the client<br>Support and personal<br>  needs | | Counselor<br>Educator | Presurgery fear |
| **Diagnosis** | Relief from anxiety<br>Information<br>To be with and<br>  helpful to the client<br>Support and personal<br>  needs | Complications<br>Postdischarge<br>  care | Support system<br>Educator<br>Assessor of family<br>  systems | Diminished support of<br>  friends<br>Empathy |
| **Treatment** | Relief from anxiety | Treatment op-<br>  tions and<br>  outcomes | Support for com-<br>  fort measures<br>Resource person<br>Support for personal<br>  needs<br>Support for emotions | Decreased work hours<br>Limited time with family<br>Socialization at hospital<br>Peer support<br>Community support<br>Changes, jealousy<br>Cause of disease<br>Isolation<br>Special treatment<br>Health fears<br>Overprotection<br>Empathy |
| **End of life** | Relief from anxiety<br>To be with and<br>  helpful to the client<br>Support | Terminal care<br>  planning | Support for<br>  emotions | Confrontation of<br>  possible death<br>Maturational lag<br>Spirituality<br>Social support<br>Need to help similar<br>  families<br>Long-term outcome<br>Preparation<br>Continued counseling |

Adapted from Marino, L., & Kooser, J. (1986). *The psychosocial care of clients and their families: Periods of high risk.* In L. Marino (Ed.), *Current nursing* (pp. 53–56). St. Louis: Mosby.

Adapted from Freeman, K., O'Dell, C., & Meola, C. (2000). Issues in families of children with brain tumors. *Oncology Nursing Forum, 27*(5), 843–848.

In addition to these needs, families experience stages or landmarks when a family member is ill (Freeman, O'Dell, & Meola, 2000; Marino & Kooser, 1986). As with any stage theory, these landmarks are not rigid pathways but, rather, fluid progressions. These stages could apply to chronic, acute, or terminal illnesses. Family needs during illness vary according to these stages and the family roles and relations to the person experiencing illness. Table 4–2 outlines these needs.

In the first stage, the prediagnostic period, signs and symptoms of the disease appear. The client and family often perceive this stage as a threat. There may be concern about the future, along with misconceptions and misinformation that compound existing fears. The nurse's role is that of counselor and educator.

In the second stage, a diagnosis is made. The client and family may experience a variety of responses—from denial and anger to guilt—as they attempt to cope with the diagnosis. During this stage, the role of the nurse requires that the nurse educate, assess the family system, and assist the family in identifying and garnering their support system. They may have education needs in the areas of complications and postdischarge care if they are hospitalized.

The third stage, the treatment period, may be characterized by optimism, despair, anger, dependency, feelings of powerlessness, and fear of recurrence or long-term impairment. This is the stage of the "long, hard pull," which may last for months, but more often for years. Frequently, the nurse's role during the treatment period involves providing physical comfort measures, assisting with contacting and referring to resources, and giving positive feedback and encouragement.

The last stage is the end of life. Both terminal and chronic illnesses apply in this final stage. The client may have feelings of hopelessness and fear of abandonment; the family feels guilt, relief, or a profound sense of loss. The nurse provides support during this grieving process.

 ## NURSING COMPETENCIES AND SKILLS IN FAMILY CARE

Nurses are in a unique position among health care professionals in their close proximity to clients. As nursing has moved away from a task orientation, it has adopted a more holistic view of clients as individuals with a life beyond their illness. The next step is to address the needs of families whose lives have been irrevocably changed by the illness of one member (Whyte & Robb, 1999). Providing nursing care to families is a logical development of the holistic approach to care of the client. It could become a cornerstone of nursing practice (Whyte & Donaldson, 1999).

The essential considerations when caring for individuals in the context of their families are as follows:

- ▶ One part of the family cannot be understood in isolation from the rest of the system.
- ▶ A family's structure and organization cannot be understood in isolation from the rest of the system.
- ▶ Communication patterns between family members are essential in the functioning of the family (Whyte & Robb, 1999).

Nurses need to be competent in using the nursing process as they work with clients and family members.

### Family Assessment

The intent of the assessment process as it applies to the client in community-based nursing is to determine the nursing needs and intervene for the client. Initially a nurse collects information about the family to treat the client. Family interviewing, rather than family therapy, is an appropriate technique for intervention.

## ASSESSMENT TOOLS

### Box 4-1   Family Assessment Guide

**Family Members**

| Member | Birth Date | Sex | Marital Status | Education |
|--------|-----------|-----|----------------|-----------|
| | | | | |
| | | | | |
| | | | | |
| | | | | |
| | | | | |

**Genogram**

**Stage of Illness**

In what stage of illness is this family? (See Table 4-2.)

_____

_____

What are this family's priority needs?

_____

_____

What is the role of the nurse in this stage?

_____

_____

_____

*(continued)*

## ASSESSMENT TOOLS

**Box 4-1   Family Assessment Guide** *(Continued)*

**Development Assessment**

What is this family's developmental stage?

_____

Is the family meeting the tasks of its stage?

_____

_____

_____

Does, or will, the client's health problem interrupt the family's ability to meet the developmental tasks? If yes, how does it interrupt it?

_____

_____

_____

State nursing interventions to assist family members in meeting their developmental tasks.

_____

_____

_____

**Functional Assessment**

Does the family meet the individual's need for affection, love, and understanding?

_____

_____

_____

Does the family meet the individual's need for physical necessities and care?

_____

_____

_____

_____

*(continued)*

**ASSESSMENT TOOLS**

**Box 4-1   Family Assessment Guide** *(Continued)*

Does the family have the economic resources necessary to provide for the basic needs of the family?

_____

_____

_____

Is the family meeting the function of reproduction as defined by the family?

_____

Is the family meeting the family function of socialization? Is the family fulfilling the function to socialize children to become productive members of society?

_____

_____

_____

Does the family attempt to actively cope with problems?

_____

_____

_____

_____

**Assessment of Presence of Characteristics of a Healthy Family**

Is communication between members open, direct, and honest, and are feelings and needs shared?

_____

_____

_____

Do family members express self-worth with integrity, responsibility, compassion, and love to and for one another?

_____

_____

_____

*(continued)*

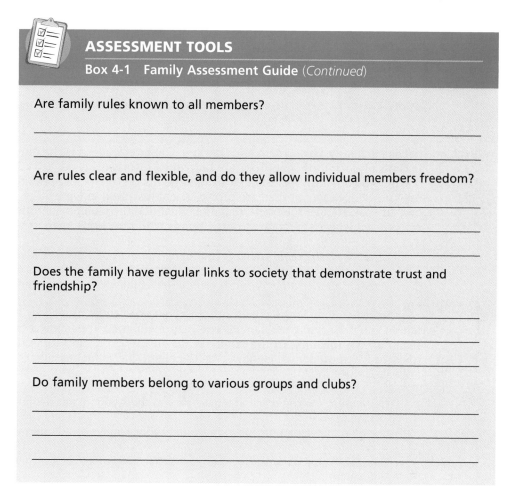

**ASSESSMENT TOOLS**

**Box 4-1   Family Assessment Guide** (Continued)

Are family rules known to all members?

_____

_____

Are rules clear and flexible, and do they allow individual members freedom?

_____

_____

_____

Does the family have regular links to society that demonstrate trust and friendship?

_____

_____

_____

Do family members belong to various groups and clubs?

_____

_____

_____

### The Family Interview

The principles used in an effective interview with a client apply to a family interview. Effective communication is essential in the first step of establishing a trusting relationship. The interview might start with an informal conversation so all participants are put at ease. It is helpful to have all the family members present during this interview. It is also beneficial to encourage them all to participate.

Numerous family assessment tools are available. A short family assessment form is shown in Box 4–1. Many agencies have a standard form that they use for all family interviews.

The assessment may determine if a family's response is adaptive or maladaptive. This permits the nurse to identify problem areas and the need for additional assessment and referral. For example, after a family interview, the nurse may share with the family concerns expressed by one member about family communication. The nurse may then suggest that the family explore this with a social worker, public health nurse, physician, clergy member, or counselor. A finding in assessment by the community-based nurse is the family's need for further assessment by a professional, such as a family therapist or social worker with special ex-

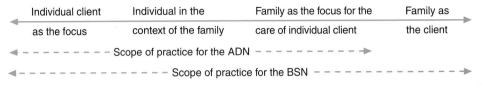

**Figure 4–4.** ▶ Focus of nursing care for individuals and families.

pertise in family assessment and therapy. The intervention is the nurse's action to initiate a referral to an appropriate individual or organization.

The type of family assessment used depends on the focus of the treatment and the knowledge level of the care provider, as illustrated in Figure 4–4. Family members are asked questions regarding the client and the client's condition. The client is assessed within the context of the family with questions such as the following:

> *Question to the client:* What is your understanding of a diabetic diet?
> ▶ *Question to the mother:* What is your understanding of your son Jon's diabetes?
> *Question to the father:* What is your understanding of your son Jon's diabetes?

When the family is the client, other realms need to be assessed. These include family functions such as financial role responsibilities, the family's emotional system, and the meaning to the family of the health event and its outcome. Consequently, when the family is viewed as the client, individual members of the family are asked questions:

> *Question to the client:* What impact do you think your illness has had on your family?
> ▶ *Question to the parents:* How do you feel your family has adjusted to your son's illness?
> *Question to the parents:* How has your son's illness affected your family's finances?

The first step in assessing the family as the client is to determine the family's impact on the recovery of the client. This is appropriate especially when the family's functioning is clearly impeding the recovery. Figure 4–5 illustrates the levels that are necessary in a comprehensive family assessment.

Overall, the intent of evaluating the family is to analyze the client's potential for recovery and self-care, given the familial conditions. To facilitate the client's return to the highest level of wellness, the circumstances in which the client lives must be considered.

### Models of Family Assessment
#### DEVELOPMENTAL ASSESSMENT

The health of a family's functioning may be evaluated by a family **developmental assessment** considering normal **family developmental tasks.** As individuals have development stages that they must go through to move to the next stage of development, so do families. Duvall (1977) developed a commonly used theory of development stages of family life as it relates to nursing care. According to Duvall, there are predictable stages within the life cycle of every family; each stage includes distinct family developmental tasks (Table 4–3). Stages of the family life

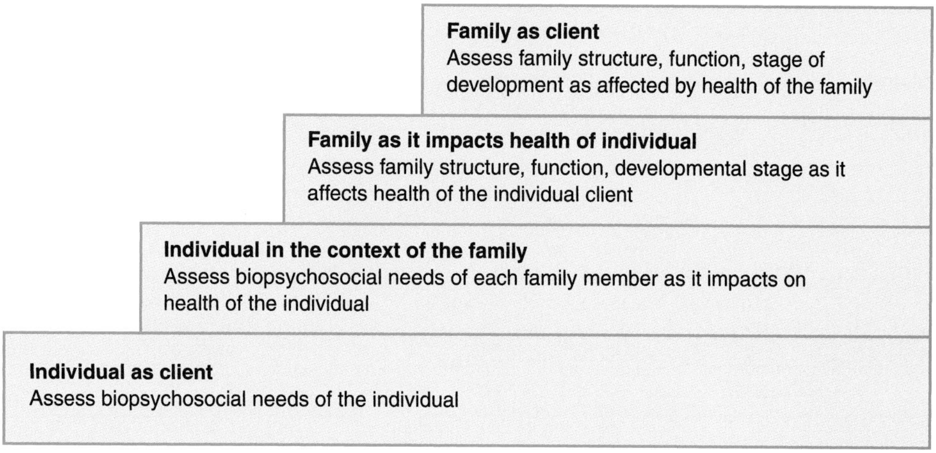

**Family as client**
Assess family structure, function, stage of development as affected by health of the family

**Family as it impacts health of individual**
Assess family structure, function, developmental stage as it affects health of the individual client

**Individual in the context of the family**
Assess biopsychosocial needs of each family member as it impacts on health of the individual

**Individual as client**
Assess biopsychosocial needs of the individual

***Figure 4–5.*** ▶ Levels necessary to assess in a comprehensive family assessment.

cycle follow no rigid pattern. The family enters each stage with the birth of the first child or according to the age of the oldest child in the family. This model can be used as a guide to assessment by following these steps:

1. Determine the family's developmental stage. This can be done by determining the age of the oldest child in the family and correlating it with the level in Table 4–3.
2. Consider the family members' health problems in the context of the tasks in their developmental stage. Is it likely that the health condition will interrupt the family's developmental tasks?
3. Determine if family members are meeting the tasks at their levels of development.
4. Identify the nursing interventions that would assist the family in meeting these developmental tasks.

Because of the wide variety of family structures, not all families fit neatly into this family stage theory. For individuals who do not marry, remain childless, divorce, remarry to form a blended family, or are in same-sex unions, the stages are viewed differently. In families in which the stages of the family life cycle are disrupted, the emotional processes and issues relating to transition and development also differ from those set out in Duvall's stages.

Disruption of the family cycle because of a divorce causes additional steps to be taken to restabilize the family for further development. Family life cycle stages for divorced or disrupted families are compared with healthy families in Figure 4–6. In the postdivorce phase, the single custodial parent experiences a different emotional process and transition than does the noncustodial parent. The developmental issues differ as well (Table 4–4).

Families with remarriage may experience emotional transitions or developmental issues as well (Table 4–5). Emotional transitions include attaining an adequate emotional separation from the previous marriage and accepting and dealing with fears about forming a new family. In addition, when beginning a blended family, members must find the time and patience necessary to permit

**TABLE 4–3** • Stages of the Family Life Cycle

| Stage | Scope of the Stage | Family Developmental Tasks |
|---|---|---|
| Married couple | Couple makes commitment to one another | Establishing a mutually satisfying marriage<br>Fitting into the kin network |
| Childbearing | Oldest child is infant through 30 mo | Adjusting to infants and encouraging their development<br>Establishing a satisfying family life for both child and parent |
| Preschool | Oldest child is 2½–6 y | Adapting to the needs of preschool children in growth-producing ways<br>Coping with lack of privacy and energy |
| School age | Oldest child is 7–12 y | Fitting into age-appropriate community activities<br>Encouraging the children's achievement |
| Teenage | Oldest child is 13–20 y | Balancing freedom with responsibility as teens mature and emancipate<br>Establishing outside interests and career |
| Launching | First child leaves home to last child leaving home | Assisting young adults to work, attend school or military, with marriage, with appropriate rituals |
| Middle-aged parents | Empty nest to retirement | Rebuilding marital bond<br>Cultivating kin ties with younger and older family |
| Aging family | Retirement to moving out of family home | Coping with loss and living alone<br>Adapting to retirement and aging |

Adapted from Allender, J. A., & Spradley, B. W. (2001). *Community health nursing: Concepts and practice* (5th ed., p. 440). Philadelphia: Lippincott Williams & Wilkins.

another emotional adjustment. Resolving the feelings of attachment to a previous spouse and accepting the new family model require transitions by individuals. Developmental issues are also seen in each phase of the new marriage.

Family developmental tasks involve meeting the basic family functions discussed earlier in this chapter. The needs of the individual family members, family developmental tasks, and family functions must mesh.

Meeting these needs is not necessarily easy in families. The conflict that often occurs in families with adolescents illustrates this point. Typically, adolescents are attempting to break away from parents and spend more time with friends than family. Yet, parents may wish for the adolescent to participate as more of an adult in family activities. This conflict may be compounded, for instance, when family members need adequate rest to provide health care to a family member, but the adolescent's need is to stay out late and get support and approval from peers.

### STRUCTURAL FAMILY ASSESSMENT

**Structural family assessment** considers the family's composition. A structural assessment defines the immediate family members, their names, ages, and the relationship among those who live together. A **genogram** is constructed to clarify the relationship and information about each member of the family. Symbols often used for the genogram are shown in Figure 4–7.

Genograms can be helpful to nurses in many settings. An inpatient nurse can quickly sketch a genogram and identify family members; this helps to define

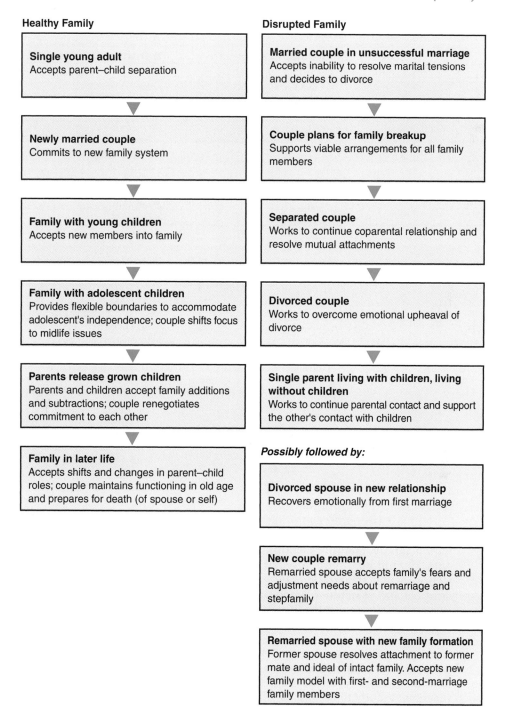

**Healthy Family**

> **Single young adult**
> Accepts parent–child separation

▼

> **Newly married couple**
> Commits to new family system

▼

> **Family with young children**
> Accepts new members into family

▼

> **Family with adolescent children**
> Provides flexible boundaries to accommodate adolescent's independence; couple shifts focus to midlife issues

▼

> **Parents release grown children**
> Parents and children accept family additions and subtractions; couple renegotiates commitment to each other

▼

> **Family in later life**
> Accepts shifts and changes in parent–child roles; couple maintains functioning in old age and prepares for death (of spouse or self)

**Disrupted Family**

> **Married couple in unsuccessful marriage**
> Accepts inability to resolve marital tensions and decides to divorce

▼

> **Couple plans for family breakup**
> Supports viable arrangements for all family members

▼

> **Separated couple**
> Works to continue coparental relationship and resolve mutual attachments

▼

> **Divorced couple**
> Works to overcome emotional upheaval of divorce

▼

> **Single parent living with children, living without children**
> Works to continue parental contact and support the other's contact with children

*Possibly followed by:*

> **Divorced spouse in new relationship**
> Recovers emotionally from first marriage

▼

> **New couple remarry**
> Remarried spouse accepts family's fears and adjustment needs about remarriage and stepfamily

▼

> **Remarried spouse with new family formation**
> Former spouse resolves attachment to former mate and ideal of intact family. Accepts new family model with first- and second-marriage family members

***Figure 4–6.*** ▶ Comparison of healthy family life cycle stages to disrupted family stages. Liebermann, A. (1990). *Community and home health nursing.* Springhouse, PA: Springhouse Corporation.

**TABLE 4–4** • When Families Divorce

| Phase | Emotional Responses | Transitional Issues |
|---|---|---|
| 1. Stressors leading to marital differences | Reveal the fact that the marriage has major problems | Accept the fact that the marriage has major problems |
| 2. Decision to divorce | Accept the inability to resolve marital differences | Accept one's own contribution to the failed marriage |
| 3. Planning the dissolution of the family system | Negotiate viable arrangements for all members within the system | Cooperate on custody, visitation, and financial issues<br>Inform and deal with extended family members and friends |
| 4. Separation | Mourn loss of intact family<br>Work on resolving attachment to spouse | Develop coparental arrangements/relationships<br>Restructure living arrangements<br>Adapt to living apart<br>Realign relationship with extended family and friends<br>Begin to rebuild own social network |
| 5. Divorce | Continue working on emotional recovery by overcoming hurt, anger, or guilt | Give up fantasies of reunion<br>Stay connected with extended families<br>Rebuild and strengthen own social network |
| 6. Postdivorce | Separate feelings about ex-spouse from parenting role<br>Prepare self for possibility of changes in custody as children get older; be open to their needs<br>Risk developing a new intimate relationship | Make flexible and generous visitation arrangements for children and noncustodial parent and extended family members<br>Deal with possibilities of changing custody arrangements as children get older<br>Deal with children's reaction to parents' establishing relationships with new partners |

Allender, J. A., & Spradley, B. W. (2001). *Community health nursing: Concepts and practice* (5th ed., p. 442). Philadelphia: Lippincott Williams & Wilkins.

which family members should be involved in the collaboration of planning care, including being present at care conferences with professional staff. Genograms may also be used in discharge planning by identifying the need for support and assistance when the client returns home. Genograms may help the home care nurse clarify the dynamics of the family in relation to the recovery of the client.

### FUNCTIONAL ASSESSMENT

Six family functions must be considered during **functional assessment:** affective, health care and physical necessities, economics, reproduction, socialization and placement, and family coping.

Through interviews, the nurse collects information about the family members' perceptions of how well the family is fulfilling basic functions. To assess family functions, the nurse may ask questions from each of the following categories.

**TABLE 4–5** • Remarriage and Blending Families

| Phases | Emotional Responses | Developmental Issues |
|---|---|---|
| 1. Meeting new people | Allowing for the possibility of developing a new intimate relationship | Dealing with children's and ex-family members' reactions to a parent dating |
| 2. Entering a new relationship | Completing an "emotional recovery" from past divorce and loss of marriage<br>Accepting one's fears about developing a new relationship<br>Working on feeling good about what the future may bring<br>Discovering what you want from a new relationship<br>Working on openness in a new relationship | |
| 3. Planning a new marriage | Accepting one's fears about the ambiguity and complexity of entering a new relationship such as the following:<br>New roles and responsibilities<br>Boundaries: space, time, and authority<br>Affective issues: guilt, loyalty, conflicts, unresolvable past hurts | Recommitting to marriage and forming a new family unit<br>Dealing with stepchildren as custodial or noncustodial parent<br>Planning for maintenance of coparental relationships with ex-spouses<br>Planning to help children deal with fears, loyalty conflicts, and membership in two systems<br>Realigning relationships with ex-family to include new spouse and children<br>Restructuring family boundaries to allow for new spouse or stepparent |
| 4. Remarriage and blending of families | Forming a final resolution of attachment to previous spouse<br>Accepting of new family unit with different boundaries | Realigning relationships to allow intermingling of systems<br>Expanding relationships to include all new family members<br>Sharing family memories and histories to enrich members' lives |

Allender, J. A., & Spradley, B. W. (2001). *Community health nursing: Concepts and practice* (5th ed., p. 442). Philadelphia: Lippincott Williams & Wilkins.

> ▶ Is the family meeting the individual's need for affection, love, and understanding?
> Is the family meeting the individual's need for physical care?
> Does the family have the economic resources required to provide for basic needs of the family?
> Is the family meeting the function of reproduction, as defined by the family?
> Is the family meeting the family function of socialization? Is the family fulfilling the function of socialization of its children for them to become productive members of society?
> Does the family attempt to actively cope with problems?

### Using Characteristics of a Healthy Family for Assessment

The characteristics of a healthy family can be used as the baseline for family assessment. Family health depends on the ability of family members to share and to understand the feelings, needs, and behavior patterns of each individual (Satir, 1972). Healthy families demonstrate the following characteristics:

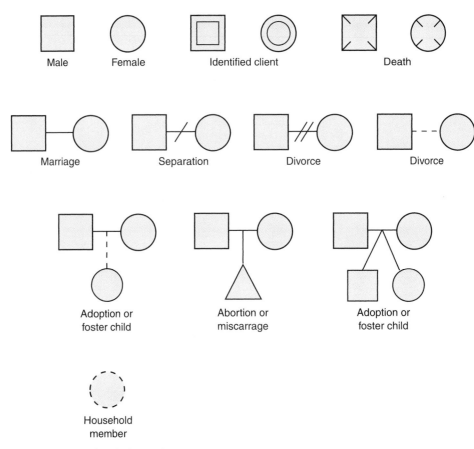

*Figure 4–7.* ▶ Symbols used in genograms.

▶ There is a facilitative process of interaction among family members.
▶ The family enhances the development of its individual members.
▶ Role relationships are structured effectively.
▶ The family actively attempts to cope with problems.
▶ The family has a healthy home environment and lifestyle.
▶ The family establishes regular links with the broader community.

In addition, interactions in a healthy family display the following qualities:

▶ Communication among members is open, direct, and honest, with shared feelings.
▶ Family members express self-worth with integrity, responsibility, compassion, and love to, and for, one another.
▶ All members know the family rules. Rules are clear and flexible and allow individual members their freedom.
▶ The family has regular links with society, which demonstrate trust and friendship.
▶ Family members belong to various groups and clubs.

## Nursing Diagnosis: Identifying Family Needs

After the family interview and assessment are completed and analyzed, the nurse can identify family strengths and needs. Again, the primary focus in community-based nursing is the care of the client. Assessment and identification of the needs of the family are focused on the family's effect on the care and recovery of the client.

The process of identifying the needs of the family follows the same steps as those used for the client. By comparing the collected data about the family with defining characteristics of the North American Nursing Diagnosis Association (NANDA) diagnosis, the nurse can arrive at the appropriate diagnosis for the client in the context of the family.

Maslow's model (Figure 4-3) is valuable in individualizing and prioritizing care for individuals in the context of the family. Again, food and shelter, the most basic family needs, must be met first. When these needs are met, the priority of care can shift to safety and then up the hierarchy of needs. The priorities of the family can change as the circumstances of the family change.

## Planning: Expected Outcomes

The process of planning care for families is similar to planning for an individual's care. The primary goal is to define expected outcomes in relation to the recovery of the client. The family may benefit from these established expected outcomes; however, the primary intent is to enhance the recovery of the client.

Mutual goal setting in which the client and the family are included is the corner-stone of effective planning in relation to families. Examples of outcomes for family interventions are listed in Box 4–2. It is essential that family members be a part of the planning process because, ultimately, it is the family members who are the primary caregivers and implement the plan of care. The process of goal setting has a positive effect on the health care provider's interactions with families. Mutual goal setting also has a positive effect on family interactions and compliance and accountability with the plan of care. Like individual clients, family members tend to resist being told what to do; they are much more likely to work toward goals they have chosen and support.

## Nursing Interventions

Nursing interventions fall into three levels of family functioning: cognitive, affective, and behavioral. **Cognitive interventions** involve the act of knowing, perceiving, or understanding. An example is teaching a client or family member about the exchange system for a diabetic diet. **Affective interventions** have to do with feelings, attitudes, and values. Helping family members to understand their fears about a loved one's diagnosis of diabetes is an illustration of an affective intervention. **Behavioral interventions** are those that have to do with skills and behaviors. Teaching clients about giving themselves insulin injections and beginning a group exercise program for newly diagnosed diabetic clients are examples of behavioral interventions. Like other steps of the nursing process, interventions must be directed primarily toward the health recovery of the client.

Nursing interventions provide specific directions and a consistent, individualized approach to the client's care. They are written as instructions for others to follow. Obviously, interventions in community-based care require the active involvement of the client and the family to determine the appropriate interventions. The client or family will often be responsible for implementing the interventions at home. As with goal setting, the client and family are more likely to comply with the plan of care if

▶ **Box 4–2**    Examples of Outcomes for Commonly ◀
Used Nursing Diagnoses

Decisional Conflict: The client or family will state advantages and disadvantages of choice by _____ (date).

Anticipatory Grieving: The client and/or family will express grief by _____
(date).

Dysfunctional Grieving: The client and/or family will share grief with significant others by _____ (date).

Parental Role Conflict: The parents will demonstrate control over decision
making regarding the child and collaborate with health professionals in
making decisions about the health/illness care of the child by _____
(date).

Social Isolation: The client and/or family will state the reasons for feelings
of isolation by _____ (date).

Altered Parenting: The parent will demonstrate increased attachment behaviors such as holding infant close, smiling and talking to the infant,
seeking eye contact with infant, and holding the infant by _____ (date).

Risk for Violence: The client or family member will experience control of
behavior with assistance from others by _____ (date). The client
and/or family will identify factors that contribute to violence by _____
(date).

Ineffective Disabling Family Coping: The client and/or family will discuss
the physical assault by _____ (date). The client and/or family will identify factors that contribute to violence by _____ (date).

Impaired Adjustment: The client and/or family member will identify the
temporary and long-term demands of the situation by _____ (date).

Relocation Stress Syndrome: The client and/or family member will identify
the most difficult aspect of relocation by _____ (date).

_____
Adapted from Carpenito, L. (2002). *Nursing diagnosis: Application to clinical practice* (9th ed.).
Philadelphia: Lippincott Williams & Wilkins.

they are active participants in the planning of interventions. Examples of expected
outcomes and nursing interventions appear in Table 4–6.

The Internet is an excellent resource for researching appropriate nursing interventions for families. For example, the Bright Futures for Families Web site
(http://www.brightfutures.org), supported by the Maternal and Child Health Bureau
of the U.S. Department of Health and Human Services, offers tools to prepare families
for health supervision to make them full participants in the process, to demonstrate
the value of health supervision, and to teach families what to expect from health professionals.

Nursing interventions for families may include strategies in primary, secondary,
and tertiary prevention. Primary prevention encompasses nursing interventions
that obviate the initial occurrence of a disease. When attempting to implement interventions for individual clients, it is often necessary to involve family members

**TABLE 4–6** • Examples of Expected Outcomes and Nursing Interventions for Commonly Used Nursing Diagnoses for Family Intervention

| Nursing Diagnosis | Expected Outcome | Nursing Intervention |
|---|---|---|
| Ineffective Management of Therapeutic Regimen | Client and family will describe disease process, causes, and factors contributing to symptoms and regimen for disease or symptom control by _____ (date). | Promote learning by providing information to client or family regarding strategies to enhance symptom control. |
| Effective Management of Therapeutic Regimen | Client and a family member will state a desire to manage the treatment of illness and prevention of sequelae by _____ (date). | Discuss possible changes in client's condition that may affect illness and usual management. |
| Health-Seeking Behavior | Client and family will state the benefits of abstinence from tobacco use by _____ (date). | Promote learning by providing written information regarding the benefits of abstinence from tobacco. |
| Impaired Home Maintenance Management | Client and family members will identify factors that restrict self-care and home management by _____ (date). | Provide referral sources that the family agrees are appropriate to assist with household tasks. |
| Knowledge Deficit | Client and family members will demonstrate aseptic technique when using a heparin lock by _____ (date). | Demonstrate and provide written information by _____ (date) about aseptic technique when using a heparin lock. |

Adapted from Carpenito, L. (2002). *Nursing diagnosis: Application to clinical practice* (9th ed.). Philadelphia: Lippincott Williams & Wilkins.

because they are affected as well. An example is family planning. In some cultures, partners make decisions together about birth control and the spacing of children. In other cultures, the female or male partner decides independently of the other about family planning.

## CLIENT SITUATIONS IN PRACTICE

### ▶ Intervention at the Primary Prevention Level

Pam is a nurse working in a clinic whose clients are primarily from Southeast Asia. When she first began teaching female clients about family planning, Pam did not include the husband or significant other. Over time, she discovered that the use of birth control, for many of her clients, was decided by the male partner. By involving the male partner in planning (choosing a method of birth control and teaching the couple about its use), the couples were more likely to comply.

Secondary prevention is early detection and treatment of a condition. In some families, lack of information may be a barrier to seeking services related to secondary prevention.

## CLIENT SITUATIONS IN PRACTICE

### ▶ Intervention at the Secondary Prevention Level

Tom is a nurse working in a day care center for older adults. One of the clients who comes to day care, Irene, is having problems with her eyesight and comes from a family with a history of glaucoma. Tom has been encouraging her to have her eyes tested. Although Irene has severe arthritis, she is alert and cognitively intact. Irene tells Tom that she does not want to ask her son to take her to anymore clinic visits. The son is unaware of his mother's vision problems. Tom learns that only by involving another family member (Irene's son) will the secondary prevention strategy (vision screening) occur.

Tertiary prevention is seeking treatment and rehabilitation for maximizing recovery. In some situations, the family is compliant with nursing care but is not aware of resources in the community that may support the client's care.

## CLIENT SITUATIONS IN PRACTICE

### ▶ Intervention at the Tertiary Prevention Level

Kristi is a staff nurse working on a medical–surgical unit in a hospital. Her situation illustrates tertiary prevention. Kristi is in charge of Barb's discharge planning. Barb has had a fusion of three cervical vertebrae and will be discharged from the hospital in 4 days. She lives alone; however, her daughter (the mother of five children) lives an hour's drive from Barb's home. After discharge, Barb will need assistance with activities of daily living for at least 2 weeks at home, will not be permitted to drive for 6 weeks, and will receive physical therapy four times a week starting 2 weeks after discharge. Kristi, Barb, and Barb's daughter sit down together to plan for the care and assistance Barb will need at home. They also discuss the community services that may be able to transport Barb to physical therapy until she is permitted to drive.

## Evaluation

Evaluation has a profound effect on the quality of care in community-based nursing. It is a joint effort among the nurse, family, and other caregivers. As is true in an acute care setting, evaluation leads to more assessment or refinement of the goals set out in the care plan and results in the identification of additional diagnoses, expected outcomes, or interventions.

The following questions for reflection may be useful during evaluation of the family care plan:

What additional data are required to evaluate progress?

Did the nursing diagnosis focus on the most important problem for this family as it relates to the potential for the client to do self-care?

What other nursing problems apply to this family and client?

Were the diagnosis, expected outcomes, and interventions realistic and appropriate for this client and family?

Were the family strengths considered when the expected outcomes and interventions were defined? If not, how could these strengths be used to enhance the outcome?

Are the nurse, client, and family satisfied with the outcome? If not, what would provide satisfaction?

The nursing process continues in an ongoing, circular, and dynamic manner. Information gained from asking the above questions is used to define a new problem and identify new or additional expected outcomes and interventions as the ongoing process of providing care and evaluating its effect continues.

## Documentation

Complete and accurate information is an essential element of nursing care of the client or family. Creating a clear account of what the nurse saw and did related to the family's care provides a record of that care. This includes documentation of the client and family's strengths and needs. Charting is used to determine eligibility for care needed and for reimbursement for care provided.

## CLIENT SITUATIONS IN PRACTICE

### ▶ The Family and Nursing Process

Jane, a home health care nurse, is assigned to care for Becky, a 30-year-old homemaker who is the mother of three preschool children (Joe, age 4, Kevin, age 2, and Michael, age 2 months). Becky has been diagnosed with liver cancer. Jack, Becky's husband, is a 32-year-old accountant with his own accounting firm. Jack's parents are in good health and live in another city. Ila, Becky's mother, lives in the same neighborhood as Jack and Becky. Becky's father died 10 years ago, and Ila remarried Stephen last year. Ila has severe arthritis. Becky also has a sister and brother who both live out of state.

As Becky's home care nurse, Jane completes a family assessment during the first visit. She begins the family interview by getting acquainted with all of the family members. Joe shows her the new toy his grandmother sent for his birthday; Kevin is very shy and sits in Becky's lap during the home visit. Jack holds the baby. Jane hopes to be able to identify how much support the family will be able to provide to Becky from this family assessment. She is also interested in identifying any problem areas where intervention is needed. The completed family assessment is shown in Box 4–3.

### Identification of the Nursing Diagnosis

Jane reviews her family assessment as well as Becky and Jack's responses. She identifies these family strengths:

The family and a large number of supportive friends are willing to assist with care of the children and the home.

A strong marital bond between Becky and her husband is apparent; they show mutual support and love.

The family has a stable financial status.

(*Client Situation continues on page 104*)

## ASSESSMENT TOOLS

### Box 4–3 Family Assessment

### Family members

| Member | Birth Date | Sex | Marital Status | Education |
|--------|-----------|-----|----------------|-----------|
| Becky | 7/15/76 | F | Married | College grad |
| Jack | 11/10/74 | M | Married | College grad |
| Joe | 9/18/02 | M | | |
| Kevin | 2/15/04 | M | | |
| Michael | 2/22/06 | M | | |

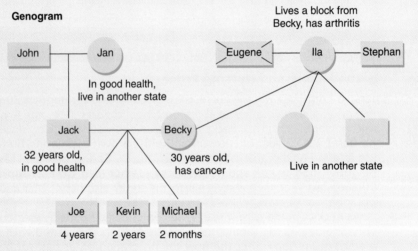

Genogram

John — Jan
In good health, live in another state

Lives a block from Becky, has arthritis

Eugene — Ila — Stephan

Jack
32 years old, in good health

Becky
30 years old, has cancer

Live in another state

Joe
4 years

Kevin
2 years

Michael
2 months

### Stage of Illness

In what stage of illness is this family? (See Table 4-2.)

*Diagnosis stage*

What are this family's priority needs?

*Relief from anxiety information, to be with and helpful to the client, and support for*

*personal needs*

What is the role of the nurse in this stage?

*Emotional support, educator, assessor of family*

*(continued)*

**ASSESSMENT TOOLS**

Box 4–3 **Family Assessment** (*Continued*)

## Developmental Assessment

What is this family's developmental stage?

*Preschool age stage*

Is the family meeting the tasks of its stage?

*No, the added energy depletion of Becky's illness has caused profound exhaustion for all members of the family*

Does, or will, the client's health problem interrupt the family's ability to meet the developmental tasks? If yes, how does it interrupt it?

*Becky's illness has interrupted the family's ability to meet the developmental tasks. Becky and Jack state they are "unable to keep up with the demands of the kids, the baby, and rigors of daily living."*

State nursing interventions to assist family members in meeting their developmental tasks.

1. Identify specific parental roles that Becky and Jack want to retain.
2. Identify parental responsibilities that they are willing to give up to someone else.
3. Identify possible support persons who could assist more with child care.
4. Determine other household tasks that can be assumed by family members or community services.

## Functional Assessment

Does the family meet the individual's need for affection, love, and understanding?

*Both Becky and Jack continue to be very affectionate and loving to each other and their children. This is evident in the way they interact with each other and with the children, hold the children, explain things to them, and comfort them. The children are in turn affectionate to Becky. Becky states, "My sister has provided me with a lot of emotional support."*

(continued)

## ASSESSMENT TOOLS

### Box 4–3 Family Assessment *(Continued)*

**Does the family meet the individual's need for physical necessities and care?**

*Jack is able to continue working, and he still has the opportunity to take some time off if necessary. Becky is unable to fulfill her prior role responsibilities of homemaker, which included cooking, cleaning, marketing, and most of the child care. Becky states that she is "exhausted and able to participate only in a limited manner in the care of the children and the work of running the household." Becky states, "I want to be able to bathe the kids and read them their bedtime story. I also want to continue to give Michael his bottles." Note disorderly surroundings with the children's toys, dirty clothes, and dirty dishes scattered in all of the rooms. The children are cranky, and the baby cries most of the visit.*

**Does the family have the economic resources necessary to provide for the basic needs of the family?**

*Jack states, "My job is very secure. I have been lucky that I have a job which allows me to provide so well for my family. I have a lot of vacation time saved up because we were going to take a big family vacation next summer."*

**Is the family meeting the function of reproduction as defined by the family?**

*Yes*

**Is the family meeting the family function of socialization? Is the family fulfilling the function to socialize children to become productive members of society?**

*Becky states, "It is very hard to provide guidance and discipline for Joe because I am so tired. He wears me down. Maybe he should be in day care a few days a week. There is a day care at our church, which is only a few blocks away."*

**Does the family attempt to actively cope with problems?**

*Becky says, "Jack does not want to talk about the future and what the doctor has said about my prognosis. He believes that I will be better by summer. He has been so angry since the diagnosis." Jack says, "I believe that Becky will be better by summer. She has the best doctor in the Midwest, and people survive from cancer all the time."*

*(continued)*

## ASSESSMENT TOOLS

### Box 4–3 Family Assessment (*Continued*)

### Assessment of Presence of Characteristics of a Healthy Family

**Is communication between members open, direct, and honest, and are feelings and needs shared?**

*Becky says, "It is hard for Jack to share his feelings with me. I think he talks to his dad but not to me. Sometimes his dad tells me what he has said. It's hard for me to tell him what I really think because it seems like then I am giving up." Jack says, "I have a close relationship with my dad. It is so hard for me to talk to Becky about my fears because I want to be upbeat and hopeful; I don't want her to have to comfort me."*

**Do family members express self-worth with integrity, responsibility, compassion, and love to and for one another?**

*Both Becky and Jack express love and concern for each other. They are so concerned about each other that Becky states, "Our concern for each other gets in the way of open communication."*

**Are family rules known to all members?**

*Becky and Jack describe the family in precisely the same way—"Becky is responsible for the care of the children and the home and Jack is the bread winner."*

**Are rules clear and flexible, and do they allow individual members freedom?**

*Both state that before Joe was born, Becky worked full time and the home maintenance was shared. Becky says that since she became ill, Jack has assumed many of the responsibilities at home. Becky states, "He is working too hard and is exhausted. We need help!"*

**Does the family have regular links to society that demonstrate trust and friendship?**

*During the home visit, three neighbors came over with food, and two people called. There were many plants, cards, and flower arrangements in the house. Becky stated, "Our friends have been wonderful. They have offered to take the kids, brought food, and visited."*

**Do family members belong to various groups and clubs?**

*The family is active in a church, and Jack is involved in an environmental group. Becky has many friends in the neighborhood.*

She identifies these family needs:

There is difficulty managing the home and child care of three preschool children. This was evident when Becky stated she needed help managing the family's daily needs. Jane also observed that the house was very disorganized.

There is the potential for ineffective family coping. This was evident when Becky and Jack were unable to be honest and open when discussing Becky's illness and prognosis.

Becky has difficulty in performing her role of child caretaker because of her disabling illness.

### Setting Priorities

To identify the priority of family needs, Jane uses Maslow's hierarchy of needs. Recognizing that the family and client must have their basic needs addressed first, she concentrates on the family's difficulty in managing the home and the child care.

As a result, Jane believes that this is Becky and Jack's priority problem:

Impaired Home Maintenance Management related to Becky's complex care regimen as evidenced by a disorderly home environment and Becky's statement, "I can only care for the kids a few minutes at a time. We need help."

### Planning

At the second home visit, Jane, Becky, and Jack discuss the family assessment. Jane shares her conclusion about their primary problem. She asks Becky and Jack for their impressions, and they agree that the major concern is the care of the home and the children. Becky adds, "I am concerned about being able to continue to provide care for the kids. I'm also worried about Jack and me having time together and being able to talk."

The three decide to address the problems about home management and save the discussion about communication for the third visit. Jane suggests that if some of the issues regarding care of the home and family are addressed, Becky may have more energy for the children.

### Expected Outcomes

Jane, Becky, and her husband define the following outcomes that address impaired home maintenance. The goal is to accomplish them by the third visit.

1. Becky and Jack will identify home maintenance tasks that need to be done daily and weekly.
2. Becky and Jack will compile a list of family members and friends who are able and willing to assist with these tasks.
3. Becky and Jack will match the list of tasks with the list of people and contact them within the next 3 days.
4. Becky will call Jane with the list of tasks that their family and friends can do.
5. Jack will contact the list of community agencies that Jane gave him to see what assistance they can provide.

### Nursing Implementation

Jane lists the specific nursing interventions she has identified for the plan of care:

1. Jane will assist the family in determining a realistic plan for both health care and home maintenance.

2. Jane will identify resources in the community that can assist with the tasks that the family and friends cannot do. She will contact Jack and give him the list of resources and telephone numbers.
3. Jane will schedule periodic home visits to evaluate the effectiveness of the plan and identify any changes that occur in Becky's condition that may need intervention.

### Evaluation

At the third home visit, Jane, Becky, and Jack evaluate the plan to date. The first four outcomes were met; however, Jack did not contact the community agencies. He will contact them next week. Jane and the family agree on the plan and the method for evaluating the plan. Jane also reviews the list of community resources with Becky and Jack. They all agree on which one to contact. They agree to discuss Becky's concern about caring for her children at the next visit.

## CONCLUSIONS

The family is the basic social unit of American society and has long been the primary focus of nursing care in the community. Understanding family structure, roles, and functions is essential in providing comprehensive nursing care both in the acute care and community-based setting. Knowledge of healthy family functioning permits the nurse to identify unhealthy functioning and take appropriate action, including referrals to community resources. Often, families with an ill family member are in crisis and require nursing intervention or referrals.

Today, more than ever, the nurse must be cognizant of the needs, feelings, problems, and views of the family when providing care for the individual client. Community-based nursing requires the nurse to provide care in the context of the client's family to enhance self-care. This is accomplished by assessing the client in the context of the family.

To provide continuous care with a preventive focus, the nurse must consider the family's ability and needs. The care of the client in the context of the family is enhanced by following the principles of community-based care.

# What's on the Web

Bright Futures for Families Web site
**Internet address**:
*http://www.brightfutures.org*

This Web site is supported by the Maternal and Child Health Bureau of the U.S. Department of Health and Human Services.

## References and Bibliography

Allender, J. A., & Spradley, B. W. (2001). *Community health nursing: Concepts and practice* (5th ed.). Philadelphia: Lippincott Williams & Wilkins.

Carpenito, L. (2002). *Nursing diagnosis: Application to clinical practice* (9th ed.). Philadelphia: Lippincott Williams & Wilkins.

Duvall, E. M. (1977). *Marriage and family development* (5th ed.). Philadelphia: Lippincott.

Duvall, E. M., & Miller, B. (1985). *Marriage and family development* (6th ed.). New York: Harper & Row.

Federal Interagency Forum on Children and Family Statistics. (2002). *American's children: Key national indicators of well-being, 2002.* Washington, DC: U.S. Government Printing Office.

Freeman, K., O'Dell, C., & Meola, C. (2000). Issues in families of children with brain tumors. *Oncology Nursing Forum, 27*(5), 843–848.

Holden, J., Harrison, L., & Johnson, M. (2002). Families, nurses and intensive care patients: A review of the literature. *Journal of Clinical Nursing, 11*(2), 140–148.

Marino, L., & Kooser, J. (1986). The psychosocial care of cancer clients and their families: Periods of high risk. In L. Marino (Ed.), *Cancer nursing* (pp. 53–66). St. Louis: Mosby.

Maslow, A. H. (1954). *Motivation and personality.* New York: Harper & Row.

Satir, V. (1972). *People making.* Palo Alto, CA: Science and Behavioral Books.

Spitz, R. (1945). Hospitalization: Inquiry into genesis of psychiatric conditions in early childhood. *Psychoanalytic Study of the Child, 1.*

Taanila, A., Jarvelin, M., & Kokkonen, J., (1998). Parental guidance and counseling by doctors and nursing staff: Parents' view of initial information and advice for families with disabled children. *Journal of Clinical Nursing, 7*(6), 505–511.

Tomlinson, P., Thomlinson, E., Peden-McAlpine, C., & Kirschbaum, M. (2002). Clinical innovation for promoting family care in paediatric intensive care: Demonstration, role modeling and reflective practice. *Journal of Advanced Nursing, 38*(2), 161–170.

Whyte, D., & Donaldson, J. (1999). All in the family: Activating family support can dramatically improve care. *Nursing Times, 95*(32), 47–48.

Whyte, D., & Robb, Y. (1999). Families under stress: How nurses can help. *Nursing Times, 95*(30), 50–52.

# LEARNING ACTIVITIES

### LEARNING ACTIVITY 4–1

You are working in a chemical dependency day treatment unit for adolescents. Your primary client is Chris, a 16-year-old boy, admitted yesterday. His father, Michael, and his stepmother, Joanna, brought in Chris after a family fight. Michael says that Chris' grades in school have been on a downhill slide since his sophomore year began 6 months ago. Both parents have noticed that Chris' behavior has changed. He is spending more time in his room; his appearance has become disheveled; and he is increasingly more listless, fatigued, hostile, and erratic. Michael describes his son as a cheerful, focused boy—until this year.

Chris has a 13-year-old brother, and both boys live for a week with their mother, Lori, and a week with their father, Michael, and his second wife, Joanna. Lori and Michael have been divorced for 4 years. Michael and his new wife have a 1-year-old daughter. Lori visited Chris this morning. While at the treatment center, she mentions that she is suing Michael for money he owes her. After lunch, you are visiting with Michael, and he relates to you that two of Lori's brothers are lawyers, and the family is always suing someone for something. Last year, he says, Lori claimed that she had lupus and collected disability payments until the insurance company discovered it was a phony claim.

During the initial family conference, Lori blames Michael for Chris's problems, maintaining that Michael has suffered from depression over the past years. Michael talks about his feelings: that the ongoing battle between him and Lori is stressful for their children. He wants the conflict to end.

1. Construct a genogram for this family.
2. Identify which stage of illness this family is experiencing. List data that led you to this conclusion.
3. Describe additional information you will need to plan care.
4. Identify the developmental stage of each member of the family. Explain how you will use this information.
5. Identify the developmental stage of each family. Explain how you will use this information when planning care for Chris.
6. Detect which family functions are not being met.
7. Develop outcomes you hope to see with this family.
8. Propose referrals you could initiate.

## LEARNING ACTIVITY 4–2

Complete a family assessment on the family of a client you are caring for in clinical who has a nontraditional family structure. Use the family assessment tool in the text of this chapter (Box 4.1) to collect basic information on the family. After you have completed the family assessment, respond to the following questions.

1. Identity the family problem or need that may interfere with the client's recovery.
2. Identity the family problem or need that may interfere with the client's ability to maximize his or her functioning within the limitations of his or her health condition.
3. Identify the family strengths that will enhance the client's recovery.
4. What client or family expected outcomes do you hope to see based on the family's needs stated in the first question?
5. List nursing interventions that will help you, the client, and the family achieve the outcomes you have identified.
6. Describe ways you will evaluate your nursing plan for the family.

## LEARNING ACTIVITY 4–3

Identify three agencies in your community that provide health services for families. Using the form in the Instructor's Manual for Chapter 2, group project No. 2, analyze the agency you have selected.

## LEARNING ACTIVITY 4–4

Locate a local, state, or federal program that assists families. Call the state or county department of health in your community for suggestions or the public health or public health nursing division. Common federal programs are Headstart; the Women, Infants, and Children (WIC) Program; and immunization programs. These all have Web sites and are administered through county or state agencies. What are the goals of the program you contacted? Do you think the program creates benefits for families? What are the benefits? (This can be a program in your own community, such as an after-school program for children or a federal program like Headstart.)

**LEARNING ACTIVITY 4–5**

1. In your clinical journal, create a genogram of your family showing three generations.
   - What patterns do you see regarding health issues as you analyze your own genogram?
   - Determine which developmental stage your family is in by using Table 4–3 or Table 4–5. Examine whether your family members are meeting the developmental tasks of the stage. If not, analyze which is preventing this from occurring.
   - What was the most important thing you learned from doing this activity?
2. In your clinical journal, discuss a situation you have observed or served as the caregiver in which the family enhanced or interrupted the client's self-care or return to maximum functioning. What was the family doing to influence the client's health? What else could they have done? Use theory from this chapter to support your ideas.
   - What did you do (or would you have done) as a nurse to facilitate family involvement in this situation? What did you learn from this experience? What would you do differently next time? Use a theory from this chapter to support your ideas.

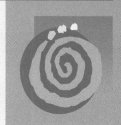

# SKILLS FOR COMMUNITY-BASED NURSING PRACTICE

**N**ow that you understand the concepts of community-based nursing, including the importance of a healthy community, understanding cultural surroundings, and care of the family, you are ready to explore how you can develop skills in applying your knowledge. Skills in assessment, teaching, case management, and continuity of care are all important to practice in community-based nursing. Although you probably have studied these concepts previously, they are discussed in this unit in the context of their specific relationship to community-based health care.

Chapter 5 opens with a discussion of the significance of assessment to community-based care. Assessment of the individual client, family, and community is addressed. A section on community assessment includes concepts, methods, and applications. The chapter ends with a discussion of the nurse's role as an advocate in public policy making.

The importance of client teaching along with teaching theory and developmental considerations in Chapter 6 leads to a discussion of the relationship of the nursing process to the teaching process.

Chapter 7 discusses the role of the case manager in community care.

Continuity of care, addressed in Chapter 8, is a concept central to quality of care in the community. It can be easy for the client and family to get lost in the new health care system, but responsible professionals build bridges between settings and people. Entering and exiting the system are covered, along with the skills and competencies involved in continuity of care.

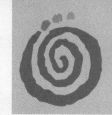

## CHAPTER 5

# Assessment: Individual, Family, and Community

Roberta Hunt

## LEARNING OBJECTIVES

1. Identify components essential to assessment of the individual client in community-based settings.
2. Discuss health needs commonly assessed in community-based settings.
3. Outline the components of a holistic assessment.
4. Identify the components of the 15-minute family interview.
5. Discuss the value of community assessment.
6. Review concepts of people, place, and social systems in a healthy community.
7. Discuss methods for collecting community data.
8. Apply concepts of assessment to a client situation, including the individual client, the family, and the community.

## KEY TERMS

activities of daily living (ADL)
assessment
community assessment
community health need
constructed surveys
demographics
environmental assessment
epidemic
functional assessment

holistic assessment
informant interviews
instrumental activities of daily living (IADL)
participant observations
power systems
secondary data
social system
spiritual assessment
windshield survey

## CHAPTER TOPICS

- **Significance of Assessment**
- **Assessment of the Individual Client**
- **Assessment of the Family**
- **Assessment of the Community**
- **Advocacy in Public Policy Making**
- **Conclusions**

## THE NURSE SPEAKS

I worked as a school nurse in a large high school in a growing school district. The student population came from rural and suburban areas and the small town where the school was located. There were numerous youngsters who had chronic illnesses. Two students had seizure disorders and were having an average of one seizure a week during school hours. These events were traumatic for the student with the seizures, the other students in the class, and the teachers. Several teachers came to my office with questions and obviously had many misconceptions about seizures. Students came into my office after observing one of the seizures with questions and comments. Michelle and Janelle, the students with the seizure disorders, spent a great deal of time in my office and, understandably, were upset about having seizures in front of their friends. Their parents were kept apprised of every event and were diligent about the medical care that their child was receiving, and the children were taking the prescribed medication. I asked Michelle and Janelle if there was anything more that we could do at school that they thought might be helpful. They could not come up with any suggestions.

One day I was talking to one of the counselors about the seizures, and the counselor noted that there were many misconceptions among the teachers and students about this type of condition. I decided to talk to Janelle and Michelle about having a class for interested teachers, counselors, and students on seizure disorders and called the Epilepsy Foundation for some suggestions. They were willing to come to talk to any interested people and had a speaker who liked to visit schools. I then asked Janelle and Michelle how they felt about this idea. One of them really liked the idea, and the other one did not. After talking to several teachers, one of the principals, Michelle and Janelle, and their parents, I decided to go ahead and set up the class. Janelle decided that she did not want to come.

After ambitious publicity for several weeks, only 10 people attended the class. In some ways, I was disappointed with the small turnout, but Michelle was not. She came with several friends and her parents and was enthusiastic about the session. I saw less of Michelle in the next few months as her seizures seemed to be less frequent. In her last 3 years of high school, she was almost seizure free. Janelle transferred to another school soon after the class. I forgot about the simple community assessment I used to develop health promotion classes for students with a seizure disorder.

Eight years later, I ran into Michelle in the grocery store. She hugged me and told me that she had gotten married and had a baby son. "You helped me so much when I was in the ninth grade," she said. I was pleased that such a simple intervention had been so helpful to someone trying to manage a chronic condition.

— **Joan Davis, RN, MPH**

**SIGNIFICANCE OF ASSESSMENT**

Nursing has long understood the significance of the community in the health of the individual and family. Florence Nightingale set the scene early for involvement of health care professionals in assessing and intervening in establishing healthy communities. Her analysis of 1861 census data became the foundation of England's sanitary reform acts (Woodham-Smith, 1950). Much of Nightingale's work focused on assessment of the physical and social environment and its role in causing or contributing to illness. She identified how sanitation, nutrition, and rest contribute to successful recovery from injury and illness. She also determined the relationship among adequate housing, recreation, employment, and health.

**Assessment** is a dynamic, ongoing process that uses observations and interactions to collect information, recognize changes, analyze needs, and plan care. Physicians primarily use assessment to determine pathology. Hospital-based nurses use assessment as the first step in the nursing process, for ongoing monitoring of acute conditions, and as an essential component in ensuring continuity with discharge planning. In community-based settings, assessment provides baseline information to help evaluate physiologic and psychologic normality and functional capacity and to identify environmental factors that may enhance or impair the individual's health status. Because the community-based nurse sees clients only periodically and the status of conditions varies over time, thorough assessment is the cornerstone of quality community care. Assessment of the individual client, family, and community is discussed in this chapter.

 **ASSESSMENT OF THE INDIVIDUAL CLIENT**

To perform an accurate assessment, the nurse must communicate effectively, observe systematically, and interpret the collected data accurately (Carpenito, 2002). Typically, the health assessment consists of the interview and health history. The focus and parameters of the assessment depend on the scope of the service provided by the agency and the role of the nurse in that service. However, the first contact is always extremely important because it acts as the foundation for the nurse–client relationship. Establishing trust beginning with the first contact is imperative.

Community care differs from nursing care provided in tertiary care settings. Because the client and family are in charge of most aspects of care most of the time, the nurse is primarily a facilitator of self-care rather than solely a care provider. Thus, the assessment process is intended to assess the client, whether it be the individual client, family, or community, and to identify needs and strengths and proceed accordingly. It is a continuous process that occurs in the context in which the response occurs. Thus, the response must be considered within the environment, whether it be family, culture, immediate physical environment, or community environment. A holistic assessment often requires collaboration of many professionals. This approach expands the usual definition of holistic assessment—body, mind, and spirit—to an even broader view.

This comprehensive view is used across the life span. The nurse in community-based settings is always diligent to complete a comprehensive assessment but is particularly attentive when caring for vulnerable populations. Thus, when assessing a newborn during a home visit, the nurse will bear in mind that a holistic assessment of the physical and psychologic condition of the newborn, the immediate environment, and the skill of the primary caregivers is essential to the infant's normal growth and development and protection from harm. The newborn is unable to speak on his or her behalf, so a thorough assessment is the primary way the nurse initiates advocacy for the infant. Thus, comprehensive assessment is essential to injury and disease prevention as well as health promotion and maintenance.

## Infants and Children

When assessing the infant and toddler, the nurse should begin by interviewing the primary caregiver. Typically the areas covered include nutrition, growth and development, and vision and hearing. When working with families with infants, it is essential to assess and promote attachment. Box 5–1 presents some helpful suggestions.

Monitoring growth and development is easily done by weighing the infant, measuring length and head circumference, and plotting the results on a growth grid. Psychologic status should also be assessed. Development of the infant, toddler, and preschooler is assessed by using the Denver Developmental Screening Tool (Figure 5-1).

### COMMUNITY-BASED NURSING CARE GUIDELINES

**Box 5–1** ▶ Personalizing Nursing Care
to Promote Attachment

The following are interventions that are directed to parents to assist them to develop an attachment with their newborn.

- Explore the mother and partner's feelings of moving from pregnancy to postpartum.
- Ask the parents what they see in the newborn that were behaviors from the baby in utero.
- Remind the parents that the newborn knows their voices from hearing them when the baby was in utero.
- Tell the parents that newborns like being flexed and close to them as they were positioned before they were born.
- Emphasize the partner's role in nurturing the mother to nurture the newborn.
- Encourage the partner to get support as needed.
- Compliment the mother on her ability to read her newborn's cues, for example, the need for comfort, nourishment, and diaper change. Bring to the mother's attention the infant's response to her care.
- Comment positively regarding the newborn's progress.
- Ask about the mother's well-being.

O'Leary, J. (1998). *After loss: Parenting in the next pregnancy.* Minneapolis: Allina Publishing.

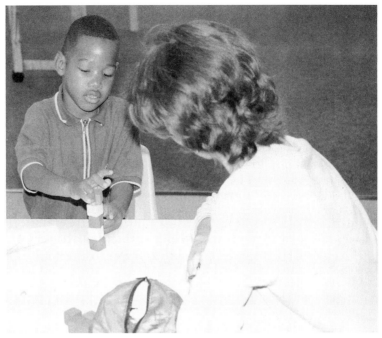

***Figure 5–1.*** ▶ The Denver Developmental Screening Tool uses a series of tasks to screen children for developmental delays.

Infants and toddlers are not routinely screened for vision and hearing until 3 years of age. However, a parent's observations may indicate the possible presence of vision and hearing problems. For assessment of vision with an infant older than 6 weeks of age, ask the parent the following questions:

Does the infant return your smile?

Do the infant's eyes follow you as you walk past or move around the room?

Do you have any concerns that the infant is unable to see?

To assess for evidence of the need to screen the vision of toddlers, ask the parents the following questions:

Does the child cover one eye when looking at objects?

Does the child tilt his or her head to look at things?

Does the child hold toys, books, or other objects very close or very far away to look at them?

Does the child rub his or her eyes, squint, frown, or blink frequently?

Infants at high risk for hearing impairment should be screened at birth. These include infants with the following:

▶ Family history of childhood hearing impairment
▶ Perinatal infection (eg, cytomegalovirus, rubella, herpes, toxoplasmosis)
▶ Anatomic malformations of the head or neck
▶ Low birth weight (<1,500 g)

▶ Hyperbilirubinemia exceeding indications for exchange transfusion
▶ Bacterial meningitis
▶ Birth asphyxia, infants with an Apgar score of 0 to 3, failure to breathe spontaneously in 10 minutes, or hypotonia of 2 hours past birth

To determine if a toddler should be screened for hearing impairment, ask if the child has had frequent ear infections or has the same risk factors listed previously for infant screening. Also assess the child's speech. Hearing impairments often become apparent when the child begins to talk and are evidenced by the child's difficulty with pronunciation, resulting in speech that is hard to comprehend.

Periodic assessment of preschool- and school-age children includes a health history and physical and developmental evaluation. As with the infant and toddler, height, weight, and head circumference are important indicators of growth. Not only do these measurements determine if the child is following a normal growth curve, but they also reflect whether the child's weight is proportional to his or her height. Obesity is on the increase, with more than 15% of children between the ages of 6 and 19 years overweight (Centers for Disease Control and Prevention [CDC], 2002). Because obesity substantially increases the risk of illness from high blood pressure, high cholesterol, type 2 diabetes, heart disease and stroke, arthritis, sleep disturbances, and cancer (breast, prostate, and colon), it is important to identify overweight children early to allow for early intervention. Nutrition assessment is also an important portion of a health assessment.

## Adults and Elderly Adults

Increasingly, the caseload of nurses working in community-based settings will reflect the graying of the population. By 2030, 20% of the population will be older than 65 years, and the number of people older than 85 will triple (AARP, 2001). Because contact with the nurse is intermittent in community-based settings, it is essential that the assessment be comprehensive. A **holistic assessment** includes environmental, cultural, spiritual, and nutritional factors, as well as functional and physical aspects of the client.

### Assessing Function

The **functional assessment** requires the nurse to determine whether there are environmental, cognitive, neurologic, or behavioral barriers to independent function and self-care. Societal and cultural factors may also create barriers. The primary consideration of the functional assessment is whether the client needs the assistance of another person for daily function. The client's ability to conceptualize an activity is just as important as the client's physical ability to perform the activity.

The **environmental assessment**, or evaluation of the client's home and neighborhood environment, is the first component of the functional assessment. The client may be physically, cognitively, or emotionally disabled yet able to function independently except for the limitations created by barriers in the home. The next areas assessed are neurologic status, cognitive and emotional status, integumentary status, and respiratory status. Last, the individual's abilities to complete **activities of daily living (ADL)** and **instrumental activities of daily living (IADL)** should be assessed. Analyzing a client's ADL is a standard method for evaluating ability to perform the activities that are essential for independent living. They include grooming, dressing, bathing, toileting, transferring, walking, and feeding or eating. IADL involve planning and preparing light meals, traveling, doing laundry, housekeeping, shopping, and using the telephone. Box 5–2 presents a complete functional assessment.

### Assessing Nutrition

Nutrition screening is an important part of providing care for clients across the life span in community-based settings. A screening tool that may be used in home settings is found in Box 5–3. This tool screens all types of home care clients for nutritional risk. After assessing the client's nutritional risk, the nurse, client, and family will devise a plan together to address the identified needs. If the client requires a level II assessment, a nurse specially trained in nutrition assesses the client.

### Assessing Medication Knowledge

Assessing medication knowledge and practice is an important aspect of comprehensive assessment. Polypharmacy, the use of multiple medications, is common among older people because of the multiple chronic illnesses they experience. Fifty percent of individuals over the age of 65 have multiple chronic conditions. Studies show that these elderly take an average of two to six prescribed medications routinely and concurrently use one to three (Dunn, 2002). Inappropriate use of medication among the elderly is particularly high, with 30% making medication errors when they have multiple medications prescribed (Meredith, Feldman, & Frey, 2001; Jennings-Sanders, 2001). (See Research Box 5–4.) However, correct use of medication is a concern across the life span. The tool in Box 5–5 can be used in a community-based setting to assess a client's medication use. After assessing the client's knowledge base, the nurse and client then devise a plan to address identified learning needs.

### Assessing Cultural Beliefs

Culture and the impact culture has on health and health beliefs are discussed in Chapter 3. A cultural assessment is always a part of the health history. It is important to start with the client's understanding of health-related issues. One way to begin is to ask the following questions:

> *How is this kind of illness treated in your culture (or home country)?*
> *How would you describe this problem you have?*
> *What does this sickness do to you?*
> *How long have you had this problem?*
> *Why do you think the problem began when it did?*
> *What has been done so far?*
> *What do you think will help your problem clear up?*
> *What does the family think should be done?*
> *What else do you think can be done to help you get better?*
> *How serious do you think this situation/problem is? (Heineken & McCoy, 2000)*

Further, a psychosocial assessment in tandem with the cultural assessment will help the nurse understand the client in the context of family, as defined by the client's culture. This may involve exploring the topics of family decision maker, sick role behavior, language barriers, and community resources as they relate to the client's culture. This assessment may simply address the following issues:

Who is the decision maker in the family?

What are the characteristics of the sick role in the client's culture?

# ASSESSMENT TOOLS

## Box 5–2  Functional Assessment

### Environmental Assessment

**Structural Barriers**

Do stairs in the home limit the client's independent mobility
to reach the bathroom, kitchen, and bedroom?
Check for presence of the following:

Handrails on stairs and in the
bathroom and tub
Narrow doorways
Unsafe flooring or floor covering

Inadequate lighting
Safe gas and electrical appliances
Improperly stored hazardous
materials

### Neurologic Status

**Perceptual Function**

Is the client able to perceive his or her immediate environment?

**Sensory Function**

Does the client have impaired vision?
Does the client have impaired hearing and ability to understand spoken language?
Is the client able to participate in an appropriate conversation 10 to 15 minutes long?
Is the client experiencing chronic pain?

### Cognitive and Emotional Status

Does the client make eye contact with the visitor, greet the visitor, and appear to be well groomed or have made an attempt to be?
Assess if the client is oriented to person, place, and time. Work these questions into the conversation.
Ask the client to perform a simple task such as getting the nurse a glass of water (but without putting the client on the spot or acting as if this is a test).

### Integumentary Status

If the client is unable to perform ADL or IADL because of a wound, dressing, or pain, then the wound impairs the client's functional ability.

### Respiratory Status

Respiratory status is impaired if the client's respiratory status, typically shortness of breath or dyspnea, prevents functioning. Here are some indications:

If the client stops or slows down the activity before it is completed
If the client sits down midway through or after the activity
If the client complains of chest tightness or pain or breathes in quick shallow breaths

Adapted from Neal, L. (1998). Functional assessment of the home health client. *Home Healthcare Nurse, 16*(10), 670–677, and Hunt, R. (Ed.). (2000). *Readings in community based nursing* (pp. 168–177). Philadelphia: Lippincott Williams & Wilkins.

## ASSESSMENT TOOLS

### Box 5–3   Level I Nutrition Screen

| LEVEL I<br>NUTRITION SCREEN | CLIENT | | |
|---|---|---|---|
| | PAYER | TEAM | MR# |
| | DATE | | TIME |

BODY WEIGHT AND HEIGHT (Measure height to the nearest inch and weight to the nearest pound):
PRIMARY DIAGNOSIS: _____ Weight (lbs): _____Height (in): _____
OTHER DIAGNOSIS: _____ Special diet. Type: _____Calorie limitations: _____

Check any boxes that are TRUE for the individual:

■ ☐ Has lost or gained 10 pounds (or more) in the past six (6) months without wanting to.

**EATING HABITS**

| | |
|---|---|
| ■ ☐ Has appetite changed? | ● ☐ Has difficulty chewing or swallowing. |
| ■ ☐ Consumes dairy or dairy products once or not at all daily (and does not take calcium supplement). | ◆ ☐ Has pain in mouth, teeth, or gums. |
| | ☐ Anorexia. |
| ■ ☐ Consumes fruits or drinks fruit juice once or not at all daily. | ☐ Has more than one alcoholic drink per day (woman); more than two drinks per day (man). |
| ■ ☐ Does not have adequate fluid intake (less than 4 glasses [8 oz] per day). | ☐ Usually eats alone. |
| ◆ ☐ Eats vegetables two or fewer times daily. | ● ☐ Does not have enough food to eat each day. |
| ◆ ☐ Eats breads, cereals, pasta, rice, or other grains five or fewer times daily. | ◆ ☐ Does not eat anything on one or more days each month. |

**LIVING ENVIRONMENT**

| | |
|---|---|
| ◆ ☐ Lives alone. | ☐ Does not have a stove and/or refrigerator. |
| ■ ☐ Are there more than six people living in household? | ☐ Lives in a home with inadequate heating or cooling. |
| ■ ☐ Is housebound. | ● ☐ Is unable or prefers not to spend money on food (< $25–$30 per person spent on food each week). |
| ■ ☐ Does not have significant caregiver. | |

**FUNCTIONAL STATUS**

| Usually or always needs assistance with these activities: (check each that apply) | Other Problems: |
|---|---|
| ◆ ☐ Walking or moving about. | ● ☐ Nausea.   ☐   Vomiting. |
| ■ ☐ Eating. | ● ☐ Diarrhea (> 3–5 per/day for > 2 days). |
| ■ ☐ Preparing food. | ◆ ☐ Constipation (> 2 weeks). |
| ● Shopping for food or other necessities. | ◆ ☐ Over 80 years of age. |

INSTRUCTIONS: To be completed within 5 days from start of care date.                    TOTALS:
Repeat Level I screen at least every 120 days (every other recertification).
HIGH RISK:
● Proceed to Level II Nutritional Screen.                                              ● _____
◆ 5 or more "◆," proceed to Level II Nutritional Screen.                                ◆ _____
■ 8 or more "■," go to Level II Nutritional Screen.                                     ■ _____
Categories left blank should be addressed by the signature nutrition screener or go to Level II.

Signature of Screener:                                                  Date:

**RESEARCH IN COMMUNITY-BASED NURSING CARE**

**Box 5–4** ▶ Examining Medication Knowledge and Behavior of Older African-American Adult Day Care Clients

The purpose of this study was to examine medication knowledge and behavior of older African-American adult day care clients and describe how community health nurses working in adult day care centers can improve medication regimen compliance. Forty older African-Americans from an adult day care in two urban geriatric centers were surveyed using the Debrew, Barba, and Tesh medication assessment tool. The author found that the older African Americans sampled needed assistance from adult children or other caregivers to follow their medication regimen evidenced by an inability to open medication bottles, lack of a system for taking the medication, having trouble swallowing pills and difficulty obtaining prescribed medications from the pharmacy. In addition, there was a significant knowledge deficit regarding the side effects and usefulness of medication. To enhance medication knowledge and safe use, the author suggests that community health nurses identify motivational factors of the client and caregiver regarding medication regimen compliance by providing client education, advocacy, and case management.

Source: Jennings-Sanders, A. (2001). Examining medication knowledge and behavior of older African-American adult day care clients. *Journal of National Black Nurses Association, 12*(2),23–29.

Do any language barriers exist?

What resources are available in the community that are sensitive to the client's culture?

A simple cultural assessment guide is seen in Box 5–6. After the assessment is complete, the nurse, client, and family devise a plan of care, which is built around the identified cultural considerations.

### Assessing Environment

An environmental assessment is an essential aspect of any assessment across the life span and across settings. Figure 5–2 and Box 5–7 are useful when completing an environmental assessment.

The primary consideration of any environmental assessment is to identify safety concerns. Again, vulnerable populations, the very young and very old, and those with serious chronic conditions are most at risk for safety issues. Many communities have home safety check kits available through the Red Cross or local fire department to assess for unsafe conditions in the home.

### Assessing Spirituality

Numerous studies show that religious practice is correlated with greater health and longer life. Assessing spiritual health and intervening according to the client's

*(text continues on page 128)*

## ASSESSMENT TOOLS

### Box 5–5   Medication Assessment

Note to administrator: The sequence of the interview, along with the instructional statements, are merely suggestions, and should be considered guidelines when using the interview. It is acceptable to reword statements or change the format to better meet the needs of the individual, yet all topics must be included in the assessment.

Start Time: _____

Who is the respondent?   ☐ Client   ☐ Spouse   ☐ Other (list) _____

**Please Check the Appropriate Response.**

Administrator: "*I need to see all of your medications. Please show me those you take every day and those you take occasionally. Don't forget to show me eyedrops, insulin, laxatives, vitamins, antacids, ointments, or any over-the-counter drugs you sometimes use. Are there any other medications that you regularly take that are not here today?*" (Attach copies of medication profiles to document drugs.)

### I. Medication Administration and Storage

☐ Yes   ☐ No   Can client open a pill bottle? (Have client demonstrate.)
☐ Yes   ☐ No   Can client break a pill in half? (Have client demonstrate. Omit if not applicable.)
☐ Yes   ☐ No   Does someone help you take your medicine?
☐ Yes   ☐ No   Do you use any type of system to help you take your pills, such as a pillbox or a calendar?
List: _____
☐ Yes   ☐ No   Do you have problems swallowing your pills?
Where do you store your medicines? _____

### II. Medication Purchasing Habits

What drugstore do you use? _____
☐ Yes   ☐ No   Does the drugstore you use deliver the medications to your home?
If no, then how do you get your medications? _____
☐ Yes   ☐ No   Do you always use the same drugstore? If no, explain: _____
☐ Yes   ☐ No   Do financial difficulties ever prevent you from buying your medications?

### III. Attitudes

☐ Excellent     How would you describe your health? _____
☐ Good          What do you see as your health needs? _____
☐ Fair
☐ Poor
☐ Yes   ☐ No   Does taking your medications upset your daily routine? If yes, explain:
_____
☐ Yes   ☐ No   Do side effects from your medications upset your daily routine?
☐ Yes   ☐ No   Do your medications help you?
☐ Don't know
☐ Yes   ☐ No   Do you ever share your medications with anyone else? _____

*(continued)*

## IV. Lifestyle Habits

TIMES PER WEEK

_____ How often do you drink coffee, tea, or colas or eat chocolate?
_____ How often do you use cigarettes, snuff, or tobacco products?
_____ How often do you consume beer, wine, or liquor?
_____ How often do you use recreational drugs such as marijuana?

## V. Home/Environment

Who else stays at your residence? (List relationship and age) _____

_____

If someone else lives in your home, does that person participate in your health care?

_____

## VI. Medication Profile

Record each medication separately on the following form: (Attach additional sheets as necessary.) _____

_____

_____

*(Medicine Name, Dosage, Route, Expiration Date Exactly as Printed on Label)*

☐ Yes  ☐ No  Can you read the name, dosage, and expiration date of this medicine? Why

do you take the medication? _____

_____

How long have you taken this dosage? _____

When do you take the medicine and how many do you take? _____

Do you know what the side effects are? List: _____

_____

☐ Yes  ☐ No  Does the medicine cause you any problems or side effects?_____

_____

What do you do if you experience side effects? (Stop the pills, call the doctor, etc.) _____

_____

Adapted with permission from DeBrew, J., Barba, B., & Tesh, A. (1998). Assessing medication knowledge and practice in older adults. *Home Healthcare Nurse, 16*(10), 686–692.

## ASSESSMENT TOOLS

### Box 5–6   Cultural Assessment Guide

Client _____ Client Number _____ Team_____
Cultural/Ethnic Identity_____ Religion _____
Etiquette and Social Customs _____
_____

Nonverbal Communication Patterns _____
_____

Client's Explanation of Health Problem _____
_____
_____

Traditional Treatments/Healers _____
_____

Expectations of Nurse/Care Providers _____
_____

### Pain Assessment
Cultural Patterns/Client's Perception of Pain Response _____
_____

### Nutrition Assessment
Meal Patterns_____
_____

Sick Foods _____
_____

Food Intolerances/Taboos _____

### Medication Assessment
Client's Perceptions of Medications _____
_____

Possible Pharmacogenetic Variations_____
_____

### Psychosocial Assessment
Family Structure and Decision-making Patterns _____
_____

Sick Role Behavior_____
_____

Language Barriers and Resources _____
_____

Cultural/Ethnic/Religious Resources/Supportive Systems _____
_____

Adapted with permission from Curry, M. (1996). Cultural assessment in home healthcare. *Home Healthcare Nurse, 15*(10), 664–671.

## Environmental Assessment Checklist

Patient _____ Patient Number _____ Team/Person Completing Form _____

Date and initial as each assessment area is addressed. Describe unsafe/unmet needs. Suggest modifications.

| Assessment Areas | Safe/Meets Client's Needs | Unsafe/Needs Adaptation | Recommended Modifications and Possible Referral |
|---|---|---|---|
| **Physiologic and Survival Needs** Food/Fluids/Eating | | | |
| Elimination/Toileting | | | |
| Hygiene/Bathing/Grooming | | | |
| Clothing/Dressing | | | |
| Rest/Sleeping | | | |
| Medication | | | |
| Shelter | | | |
| **Safety and Security** Mobility and Fall Prevention | | | |
| Fire/Burn Prevention | | | |
| Crime/Injury Prevention | | | |
| **Love and Belonging** Caregiver | | | |
| Communication | | | |
| Family/Friends/Pets | | | |
| **Self-Esteem, Self-Actualization** Enjoyable/Meaningful Activities | | | |

***Figure 5–2.*** ▶ Environmental assessment checklist (see Box 5–7 for questions for each category). Adapted with permission from Narayan, M., & Tennant, J. (1997). Environmental assessment. *Home Healthcare Nurse, 15*(11), 799–805.

### Physiologic and Survival Needs

#### Food and Fluids/Eating

What does the client plan to eat? Drink? Who will prepare the food?
Is there food in the home? Who will do the grocery shopping?
Is the food properly stored? Does the refrigerator work?
Is there drinkable water?
Does the kitchen have barriers to the client actually preparing the food?
Are the pathways clear? Can the items be reached? Are there clean dishes?

#### Elimination/Toileting

Can the client get to the bathroom? Is the pathway clear? Is a bedside com-
  mode indicated?
Do assistive devices (wheelchairs, walkers) fit through the doorways and can
  the client turn?
Will the client have a hard time getting up and down from the commode?
  Would a raised toilet seat help? Grab bars? (Towel racks, if used for steady-
  ing, can pull away from the wall.)
Will the client be able to wash hands? Able to turn water off and on?

#### Hygiene/Bathing/Grooming

What is the plan for bathing? Bathtub? Shower? Shower chair? At the sink?
  Requires help?
Is there hot and cold running water? Is the water temperature 120° or less?
Are there grab bars next to the tub and shower?
Are there nonskid tiles/strips/appliques/rubber mats on tub bottom and
  shower floor?
Are the bathroom and fixtures clean?
What provisions are there for mouth care? Hair care?

#### Clothing/Dressing

Does the client have shoes or slippers that are easy to put on, fit properly
  with nonskid soles?
Will the client be able to change clothes?
Are the clothes so baggy that they could trip the client?
Are there clean clothes? How will the laundry be washed?

#### Rest/Sleeping

Where will the client sleep? Would the client benefit from a hospital bed? A
  trapeze?
How far is the bed from the floor? Can the client get in and out of
  the bed?
How much time will the client spend in bed? Does the client need a special
  mattress?
How far is the bed from the bathroom? From other family members?

*(continued)*

### *Medications*

Does the client have a plan for taking the right medications at the right time?
Is there a secure place to store the medications? Are they safe from children
  and the cognitively impaired?
Can the client reach the medications needed? Open the container? Read the
  label?
Is there adequate lighting where the client will be preparing medications?
Is there a safe way to dispose of syringes? Medical supplies?

### *Shelter*

Is the house clean and comfortable for the client? Who will do the housework?
Are the plumbing and sewage systems working?
Is there a safe heat source? Are space heaters safe? Are the electrical cords in
  good condition?
Is there adequate ventilation?
Is the house infested with roaches, other insects, or rodents?

## Safety and Security

### *Mobility/Fall Prevention*

Is the client able to get around the home? Does the client have good
  balance? Steady gait?
Is the caregiver thinking of using restraints? What sort of restraints? Are they
  necessary?
Does the client use assistive devices (walkers, canes) correctly? Are they the
  right height?
Do the devices fit through the pathways without catching on furnishings?
Are the pathways, hallways, and stairways clear? Are there throw rugs?
Are there sturdy handrails on the stairs? Are the first and last steps clearly
  marked?
Is there adequate lighting in hallways and stairways? Is the path to the
  bathroom well lighted at night?
Are the floors slippery? (Floors should not have a high gloss or be highly
  waxed.)
Are there uneven floor surfaces?
Are the carpets in good repair without buckles or tears that could cause
  tripping?
Can the client walk steadily on the carpets? (Thick pile carpets can cause trip-
  ping if the client has a shuffling gait.)
Are the chairs the client uses sturdy? Are they stable if the client uses them to
  prevent a fall?
Does the client use furniture or counters for balance when walking? Are
  these sturdy enough to withstand the pressure?
Are there cords or wires that could cause the client to trip?

*(continued)*

### *Fire/Burn Prevention*

Is there a smoke detector on each level of the home? Is there a fire extinguisher?

Is there an escape plan for the client to get out of the house in case of fire?

Is the client using heating pads and space heaters safely?

Are wires and plugs in good repair?

If the client smokes, are there plans to make sure the client smokes safely?

Are there signs of cigarette burns? Burns in the kitchen?

Are oxygen tanks stored away from flames and heat sources?

### *Crime/Injury Prevention*

Are there locks on the doors and the windows?

Can the client make an emergency call? Is the telephone handy? Are emergency numbers clearly marked?

Are firearms securely stored in a locked box? Is the ammunition stored and locked away separately?

Is there evidence of criminal activity?

## Love and Belonging

### *Caregiver*

Is there a caregiver? Is the caregiver competent? Willing? Supportive?

Does the caregiver need support?

Can the caregiver hear the client? Should there be an intercom? "Baby monitor?" Handbell?

### *Communication*

Is the telephone within easy reach of the client?

Should the telephone have an illuminated dial? Oversized numbers? Memory feature? Audio enhancer?

Are needed numbers clearly marked? Police? Fire? Ambulance? Nurse? Doctor? Relatives? Neighbors?

Is there a daily safety check system? Should there be an alert system like Life-line?

How will the client obtain mail?

### *Family/Friends/Pets*

Are the neighbors supportive?

Does the client have family, friends, church/synagogue/mosque members to help and visit?

Is the client able to take proper care of any pets? Are pets well behaved?

*(continued)*

**ASSESSMENT TOOLS**

Box 5–7    Questions to Complete: Environmental Assessment
Checklist *(Continued)*

**Self-Esteem and Self-Actualization**

Are there meaningful activities the client can do? Listening to music/book
tapes? Interactive activities?

What kind of activities does the client enjoy? Are there creative ways that
these activities can be brought to the client?

Adapted with permission from Narayan, M., & Tennant, J. (1997). Environmental assessment.
*Home Healthcare Nurse, 15*(11), 799–805.

values may be one of the most important areas to address in community-based
care. A **spiritual assessment** allows the nurse to determine the presence of spiritual distress or identify other spiritual needs. A spiritual needs protocol is shown
in Box 5–8. The nurse, client, and family can mutually use the results of this assessment to identify spiritual issues and incorporate them in the plan of care. Another
reason for completing a spiritual assessment on all clients stems from the require-
ment by the Joint Commission on Accreditation of Healthcare Organizations
(JCAHO) that all clients cared for by accredited health care organizations must
have a spiritual assessment (JCAHO, 2001).

## ASSESSMENT OF THE FAMILY

Changes in health care delivery, budget constraints, and staff cutbacks have all
contributed to enormous pressure on nurses to do more in less time. A simple
family assessment, completed in 15 minutes or less, may actually save the nurse
time, allowing the nurse to identify issues early and prevent problems later. The
key ingredients to a simple family interview are speaking politely and respectfully,
using therapeutic communication, constructing a family genogram, asking therapeutic questions, and commending the family and individual on their strengths
(Wright & Leahey, 1999).

In many ways, modern culture has experienced a decline in civility and good
manners. Nursing has not been immune to this phenomenon. The professional relationship requires that the nurse introduce himself or herself to the client and
family and set a contract with the client and family. Following basic elements of establishing a therapeutic relationship, such as calling the client and family by name
and involving the client and family in the care, are essential to establishing a trusting relationship with the client (Wright & Leahey, 1999).

Therapeutic communication is the second element of a simple family assessment. From the start of a brief family assessment, conversation is purposeful and
time limited. Often, listening, showing compassion, and emphasizing strengths are
the most powerful therapeutic interventions that a nurse can use. Some of the

## ASSESSMENT TOOLS

### Box 5–8  Spiritual Needs Protocol

Illness often triggers spiritual wrestling in addition to emotional, mental, and physical pain. Spiritual care is an integral part of holistic care. The health care team must be comfortable with and receptive to these needs for them to emerge and be addressed. The concept of presence implies self-giving by the health care provider to the client. It means being available and listening in a meaningful way. It also means having an awareness that it is a privilege to be invited into a person's life in this way, as well as an ethical responsibility.

### Assessment

*Assess* spiritual or religious preference and note any request to see the chaplain. Use admission database.
*Listen* for verbal cues regarding spiritual or religious orientation:

* Client refers to God or higher power
* Client talks about prayer, church, synagogue, mosque, spiritual or religious leader

*Look* for visual cues on the client and in his or her room regarding spiritual or religious orientation:

* Bible, Torah, Koran, or other spiritual books
* Symbols such as the cross, Star of David or prayer rug
* Articles such as prayer beads, medals, or pins

*Listen* for significant comments, such as, "It's all in God's hands now" or "Why is this happening to me?"
*Assess* for signs of spiritual concerns:

* Discouragement
* Mild anxiety
* Expressions of anticipatory grief
* Inability to participate in usual spiritual practice
* Expressions of concern about relationship with God or higher power
* Inability to obtain foods required by beliefs

*Assess* for signs of spiritual distress:

* Crying
* Expressions of guilt
* Disturbances in sleep patterns
* Disrupted spiritual trust
* Feeling remote from God or higher power
* Moderate to severe anxiety
* Anger toward staff, family, God, or higher power
* Challenged belief or value system
* Loss of meaning and purpose in life

*(continued)*

## ASSESSMENT TOOLS

### Box 5–8   Spiritual Needs Protocol *(Continued)*

*Assess* for signs of spiritual despair:
- Loss of hope
- Refusal to communicate with loved ones
- Loss of spiritual belief
- Death wish
- Severe depression
- Flat affect
- Refusal to participate in treatment regimen

*Assess* for special religious concerns such as diet, refusal of blood.

### Interventions

*Convey* a caring and accepting attitude.
*Provide* support, encouragement, and respect.
*Provide* presence.
*Listen* actively.
*Use* therapeutic communication techniques such as restatement, clarification, or silence.
*Join* in prayer or reading scripture if comfortable.
*Use* therapeutic touch with the client's permission.
*Include* family or significant other in spiritual care.
*Consult* physician for medications as needed for anxiety or depression.

### Reportable Conditions

*Notify* physician of severe anxiety or depression that may require pharmacologic or psychiatric intervention.
*Notify* chaplain, priest, rabbi, pastor, or spiritual leader of spiritual concerns, distress, or despair with client's permission.

### Documentation

*Document* assessment on database and flow sheet.
*Document* in nurse's notes significant comments, behaviors of client, family, or significant other; interventions; physician notification; and referrals to chaplain or other religious leader.
*Document* initiation of protocol on plan of care.

Adapted with permission from Sumner, C. (1998). Recognizing and responding. *American Journal of Nursing, 48*(1), 26–31.

most basic suggestions include the following (adapted from Wright & Leahey, 1999, p. 264):

▶ Invite families to accompany the client to the unit/clinic/hospital.
▶ Involve families in the admission procedure or interview.
▶ Encourage families to ask questions during the client orientation or first visit.
▶ Acknowledge the client and family's expertise in self-care or assisting in self-care.
▶ Ask about routines at home and incorporate them in the plan of care.
▶ Encourage the clients to practice interactions that may come up in the future related to health regimens (eg, have a parent practice telling a diabetic child that she may not eat ice cream at a birthday party).
▶ Consult with clients and family about their ideas for treatment and discharge.

A genogram is an essential element of the quick family interview. See Chapter 4 for detailed information on completing genograms.

Asking therapeutic questions is the next element of the brief family interview. Numerous examples are found in Chapter 4. Additional questions are listed below (Wright & Leahey, 1999):

> Of your family or friends, who would you like us to share information with, and who should we not?
▶ How can we be most helpful to you and your family or friends as we provide care for you?
> What has been most or least helpful to you in past hospitalizations, home visits, or clinic visits?

The last aspect of the simple family interview is to focus on strengths rather than on needs and problems. Strength-based nursing validates the client and family's assets. In every encounter with a family, the acknowledgment of the resources, competencies, and efforts observed allows the family and client to realize their strengths and develop new perspectives of themselves and their abilities.

In summary, this framework recommends the following steps:

1. Use good manners to engage or reengage the client's family; introduce yourself by offering your name and role and orienting family members to the purpose of a brief family interview.
2. Assess key areas of internal and external structure and function; obtain
▶ genogram information and key external support data.
3. Ask three key questions to family members.
4. Commend the family on two strengths.
5. Evaluate the usefulness of the interview and conclude (Wright & Leahey, 1999, p. 272).

## ASSESSMENT OF THE COMMUNITY

All nurses have a role in community assessment, ranging from identifying appropriate resources for referral to determining the need for a new hospital. Because community assessment varies in levels of complexity, the role of the nurse depends on the nurse's educational preparation and expertise. The person with an associate's degree in nursing (ADN) uses community assessment primarily as it relates to the care of the individual client in the context of the community. For example, a nurse working in the acute care setting may want to find placement for a client with mental illness, but the agencies generally used by the referring facility are not appropriate. Thus, the nurse may conduct a simple community assessment to determine available, accessible, and appropriate community resources for referral.

Public health nurses typically use community assessment to determine needs for particular services or programs in a given geographic area or neighborhood. An example is the community health nurse who uses community assessment to determine the need for flu shot clinics in a neighborhood.

A more complex example is the use of community assessment in influencing public policy. The nurse with a graduate degree, or a nurse statistician or epidemiologist, may be contracted by a state or local government to do a community assessment to determine the number and percentage of citizens in a particular geographic area who are uninsured or underinsured.

Through community assessment, the nurse determines how a community influences the health of its residents. Community assessment is a technique that may be used to determine the health status, resources, or needs of a group of individuals. Similar to basic nursing process, **community assessment** consists of information about the physiologic, psychologic, sociocultural, and spiritual health of the community. Community assessment allows the nurse to explore the relationship between a variety of community variables and the health of its occupants. Professionals from a number of disciplines participate in community assessment activities. These professionals include nurses, social workers, therapists, community health workers, public health nurses, physicians, epidemiologists, statisticians, and public policy makers.

## Components of Community Assessment

Chapter 1 describes the community as an entity made up of people, a place, and social systems, and it discusses the characteristics of a healthy community. Just as the characteristics of healthy families can be used in assessment, the characteristics of a healthy community can be used as a simple tool to assess a community's level of health.

Community assessment reflects a problem-solving process similar to the nursing process and uses steps similar to those used to assess the individual client or family. All three dimensions of the community are assessed: the people, the place, and the social systems.

### People

A community can be assessed by analyzing the characteristics of the people in that community. These characteristics are defined through the **demographics** of the community, which include the number, composition by age, rate of growth and decline, social class, and mobility of the people in the community. Other vital statistics include the birth rate, overall death rate, death rate by cause and by age, and infant mortality rate. Of these, the infant mortality rate is considered to be the most important statistical indicator regarding the level of maternal–infant health in a community. These vital statistics are the "vital signs" of the community.

### Place

Place or location is where the community is located and its boundaries. It may include the type of community, such as rural or urban; location of health services; and climate, flora, fauna, and topography. Assessment of location is important because it determines what services are accessible and available to the people living within that area.

### Social Systems

**Social systems** are assessed as economic, educational, religious, political, and legal systems. Further, human services, opportunities for recreation, and communication systems are components of a community's social systems. **Power systems** within a community must also be assessed as part of the overall social system—how power is distributed throughout a particular social system. Determining how decisions are made and how change occurs is essential in planning.

## Methods in Community Assessment

Many methods can be used to collect data in a community. Five methods are discussed here: windshield survey, informant interviews, participant observations, secondary analysis of existing data, and constructed surveys. These assessments are typically in the domain of the public health nurse; however, it is helpful for community-based nurses to understand these methods because they may be asked to participate in community assessment.

### Windshield Survey

A common method of community assessment is a windshield survey. The **windshield survey** is the motorized equivalent of a simple head-to-toe assessment. The observer drives through a chosen neighborhood and uses the five senses and powers of observation to conduct a general assessment of that neighborhood. Conclusions from a windshield survey show common characteristics about the way people live, where they live, and the type of housing that exists in a given neighborhood. An example of a windshield survey is seen in Box 5–9.

### Informant Interviews

**Informant interviews** involve community residents who are either key informants or members of the general public. Key informants are individuals in positions of power or influence in the community, such as leaders in local government, schools, and the religious or business community. General public interviews may include random telephone or person-on-the-street interviews. Interviews are typically unstructured and are conducted to collect general information.

Nurses working in acute care settings use the equivalent of informant interviews to elicit information from the client, family members, social workers, and spiritual leaders. Nurses may also use this technique as they talk to other nurses about potential community resources that may be appropriate for referral purposes. If the hospital or agency uses follow-up telephone calls after discharge, informant information about referral sources is elicited.

### Participant Observations

The third method of data collection is **participant observations**. The nurse observes formal and informal community activities to determine significant events and occurrences, leading to conclusions about what is happening in selected set-

This assessment has been designed to assist the nurse traveling around the neighborhood to identify objective data related to people, places, and social systems that help define the community. This information may help identify trends, stability, and changes that may affect the health of the individual living in the community.

## People

Who is on the street (eg, women, children, men)?
How are they dressed?
What are they doing?
Are the people African American, White, Asian?
How are the different racial groups residentially located?
How would you categorize the residents: upper, upper middle, middle, lower class? How did you come to this conclusion?
Is there any evidence of communicable diseases, alcoholism, drug abuse, mental illness? How did you come to this conclusion?
Are there animals on the street? What kind?

## Place

### Boundaries

Where is the community located?
What are its boundaries?
Natural boundaries?
Human-made boundaries?

### Location of Health Services

Where are the major health institutions located?
What health institutions may be necessary for a community of this size but are not located in the community (eg, a large community with few or no acute care or ambulatory care facilities)?
Are there geographic features that may pose a threat?
What plants or animals could pose a threat to health?

### Human-Made Environment

Do you see major industrial areas with heavy industrial plants?
Do the roads allow easy access to health institutions? Are those roads marked by easily seen and understandable signs?

### Housing

What is the quality of the housing?
How old are the houses?
Are there single or multifamily dwellings?
Are there signs of disrepair and decay? If so, explain.
Are there vacant dwellings? If so, explain.

*(continued)*

**ASSESSMENT TOOLS**

Box 5–9   **Windshield Survey** *(Continued)*

**Social Systems**

Are there schools in the area? Are they in good repair?

Are there parks and outdoor recreation opportunities?

What churches are located in the community?

What schools, community centers, clinics, or other services for the community
   are provided by the churches?

Does the community have public transportation that provides accessible service?

What supermarkets and stores are available in the neighborhoods?

Is there evidence of police and fire protection in the area?

Are there social agencies, clinics, hospitals, dentists, or other health care
   providers?

tings. Formal gatherings would include government, city council, county board, and school board meetings. Informal gatherings occur at the local coffee shop or cafe, barbershop, or school. This type of assessment can be effective in determining the values, norms, and concerns of a community. It may also offer an opportunity to identify the power systems within the community. Recognizing how power is distributed throughout the community social system and how decisions are made provides important insight into how change occurs in a community.

Nurses in inpatient settings use this technique when they observe a client in physical therapy, occupational therapy, or any activity off the unit. These observations may tell the staff nurse something about the client's values and behavior. Home visits, conducted with clients after discharge from the acute care setting to assess their ongoing needs or before admission to an acute care setting, are examples of participant observation. During the home visit, the nurse collects information about the client in the context of the family and the community.

### Secondary Data

Sources of **secondary data** for analysis include records, documents, and other previously collected information. Depending on the community, an abundance of demographic data may be available to describe the health status of its members. These may include databases from schools, departments of health at the city and state levels, county data, private foundations, and state universities. Health data kept by the state may be thought of as the health record of the citizens of that state. Secondary data provides the statistics that are the vital signs of the community.

An example of secondary data may be seen in a clinic setting. Last week you noticed that many of the adults seen in the clinic where you work were admitted with the diagnosis of bronchitis. You calculate that last week 30 of 100 clients who came to the clinic had bronchitis. You wonder if this is an **epidemic** (the occurrence of a disease that exceeds normal or expected frequency in a community or region). To determine if it is, you look at the clinic statistics for the year before and find that during the same week last year, 20 of 60 adults were admitted for bronchitis.

Are you seeing an epidemic this year? Nurses in acute care and clinics use secondary data when they consult old charts and past notes, vital signs, orders, and other indicators of client progress documented in the client's chart.

### Constructed Surveys

**Constructed surveys** may be used to collect information about communities. This model is typically time consuming and expensive. A random sample of a targeted population asks a list of specific questions. Data collected are analyzed for patterns and trends.

## Application

Community assessment may be accomplished by using any one, or a combination, of the methods discussed. These methods are applied to the three dimensions of community: people, place, and social systems. One simple method of assessment is to use the characteristics of a healthy community. Another way to assess a community is to use an assessment guide with specific assessment questions. Once information is collected, the nurse reviews it for repeating patterns that may appear in all three areas of assessment. At this point, a community health need may be identified. A third way to assess people, place, and social systems is to use the components of community-based care, as outlined in Table 5–1.

**TABLE 5–1** • Examples of Community Assessment in Community-Based Care

| People | Place | Social Systems |
|---|---|---|
| **Self-Care** | | |
| Assess the client related to people in immediate environment and surrounding community to determine ability to enhance or detract from the client's ability to maintain self-care. | Determine where the client lives and how the home, neighborhood, and community may contribute to the client's ability to maintain self-care. | Assess available, appropriate, and accessible community resources to support self-care. |
| Context of Client, Family, and Community | | |
| Assess the values, attitudes, and norms of people in the client's immediate environment and surrounding community. | Determine where the client lives, both the immediate environment and surrounding community. | Identify if social systems provide support or detract from the individual's potential for recovery. |
| **Prevention** | | |
| Consider the people in the immediate environment and surrounding community to determine support or disregard for a preventive focus. | Assess the location and whether it supports or disregards a preventive focus. | Assess the social systems for evidence of a preventive focus. |
| **Continuity** | | |
| Determine if the people in the immediate and surrounding community support continuity. | Identify if the location enhances or detracts from continuity. | Describe the available, accessible, and appropriate community resources that support continuity. |

## CLIENT SITUATIONS IN PRACTICE

### ▶ Addressing Community Needs in the School

Maria is the school nurse for Harmony High School, which has an enrollment of 2,300 students. To determine the health needs of the students attending Harmony, she is conducting an assessment of the school community. She has collected the following information about the school district and the students at Harmony High.

*Windshield Survey*

First, Maria spent time traveling around the school district completing a windshield survey. This is what she discovered.

Most of the people on the street during the day are women and small children. Based on the way they are dressed and the cars they are driving, they appear to be middle class. Most of the people are Mexican American or White. There is no evidence of drug abuse or blatant sale of drugs on the street observed and no problems with communicable diseases, as may be evidenced by people with hacking coughs or a wasted appearance.

Harmony is a community of 20,000 people located at the outer suburban ring of Metropolitan City, which has a population of 3,000,000; it is a predominantly suburban community with 10% of the citizens in rural areas. There is little pollution of any type in the area. There are no hospitals or clinics in the community. The houses are primarily well-kept, single-family dwellings between 5 and 20 years old.

In evaluating the social systems, Maria found that there are primary, secondary, and tertiary health care services nearby. However, because there is no public transportation, it is difficult for students to gain access to these services. In addition, none of the health services is targeted at adolescents. For instance, 100% of the prenatal classes are attended by suburban, middle-class couples. The closest facility in which adolescents can receive confidential pregnancy testing, prenatal care, or prenatal classes is 45 minutes away by car.

*Informant Interviews*

Maria then interviews some of the key informants in the community. She asks them what they think are the primary health issues among high school students in their community. The county public health nurses, counselor, principal of the high school, and parish nurse all agree that many pregnant adolescents do not receive prenatal care. The fire chief and mayor believe there is a need for more emergency medical services.

*Participant Observations*

Based on the students who come to her office for care, Maria has identified two categories of students who frequently need health care. One group consists of students with somatic complaints related to personal or family stress. The second group consists of students who have questions about sexuality or who are pregnant and need referral. The girls who are pregnant have a great deal of difficulty getting early prenatal care.

Maria attends the school board meetings where issues of health are occasionally discussed. All of the school board members are concerned about cost containment, and two members are particularly sensitive about including sexuality in the school's curriculum. The superintendent is committed to curricula sensitive to community values. She is reluctant to consider curricula that may include sexuality if the board members' concerns are representative of the community.

### Secondary Data

Maria collects secondary data on the community from the state health department. She discovers demographic facts about Harmony and compares them with data on all the high school students in the state. Harmony has a lower rate of prenatal care among adolescents and a higher percentage of infant mortality and low-birth-weight newborns.

### Community Health Need or Problem Statement

Maria decides that the community health need in Harmony High School is early identification of pregnancy and provision of prenatal care for pregnant adolescent girls.

### Outcome and Interventions

Maria defines the outcomes she hopes to establish and the interventions as follows:

### Outcome after 6 months

Establish a task force made up of a teacher, a counselor, a public health nurse, and a member of the school board to determine how the school and community can address this need.

### Interventions after 6 months

1. Establish and convene a task force every 2 weeks.
2. Present a summary of the results of the community assessment to the school board, public health nurses, teachers, and counselors.
3. Keep the key players apprised of the progress of the task force.

### Outcome after 1 year

1. Develop a method for referring all pregnant adolescents seen by school and community personnel to the school's prenatal program.
2. Develop a prenatal course to be offered in the school.
3. Develop a list of community referral sources for prenatal adolescents.
4. Develop a mechanism for follow-up after birth.

### Interventions during year 1

1. Present the results of the task force to the school board, public health nurses, teachers, and counselors.
2. Ask for input and involvement of all key players.

### Interventions after year 2

1. Streamline a method for referral.
2. Evaluate the prenatal program including the number and percentage of pregnant students attending the classes, satisfaction with the program, and total percent now receiving prenatal care, infant mortality rate, and rate of low-birth-weight infants.
3. Increase community awareness about the prenatal program.

### Evaluation

Are the outcomes met?

1. Yes: Continue with the interventions.
2. No: Revise the interventions: Reconvene the task force; reassess the community.

*Reassessment*

To reassess the community, Maria answers the following questions:

1. What additional data do we need to collect to evaluate the program?
2. Did the problem statement focus on the most important problems for the individuals living in the community?
3. What other problems are important to this community?
4. Were the problem statement, expected outcome, and interventions realistic and appropriate for this community?
5. Are the individual members of the community satisfied with the outcome?

## CLIENT SITUATIONS IN PRACTICE

### ▶ Concluding the Assessment

Formatting statements of the community's health concerns or problems, as well as its strengths, concludes the assessment phase. It is important to document the data that support the problem and the overall processes used for the identification of the problem.

*Statement of a Concern or Problem and Expected Outcomes*

From the problem statement, the nurse defines expected outcomes. These outcome statements are specific and based on measurable criteria. Examples with possible outcomes are given here.

*Example 1:* When the Individual is the Client

Nursing diagnosis: Ineffective Airway Clearance related to asthma as manifested by a respiratory rate of 28 breaths/min and wheezes in all lung fields.

Expected outcome: The client will demonstrate a respiratory rate of 16 breaths/min and cessation of wheezes in all lung fields.

*Example 2:* When the Community of the School District is the Client

Problem statement: The number of children between the ages of 5 and 18 years with asthma in the school district of Rosie Mountain increased from 3/1,000 in March 1995 to 6/1,000 in March 2005.

Expected outcome: Reduce the number of children between the ages of 5 and 18 years in Rosie Mountain with the diagnosis of asthma from 6/1,000 in 2005 to 3/1,000 by the year 2010.

*Example 3:* When the Community of the County is the Client

Community problem: The infant mortality rate for Normaldale County was 11/1,000 births in 2005, compared with the state infant mortality rate of 8/1,000 and the national rate of 7/1,000.

Expected outcome: Reduce the infant mortality rate for Normaldale County to 9/1,000 births by 2010.

*Example 4:* When the Community of the Hospital is the Client

Community problem: In March 2007, at Normaldale County Hospital, 65% of the nursing staff washed their hands between clients. The recommended percentage is 90%.

Expected outcome: By March 2003, 85% of the nursing staff will wash their hands between clients.

### Interventions

Interventions at the community level are directed primarily toward health protection, health promotion, and disease prevention. These interventions fall under the categories of education, enforcement, or engineering (Salmon-White, 1982). Educational interventions are programs aimed at achieving the expected outcome, including programs that give information or seek to change attitudes about health issues. Enforcement interventions include legislated mandates such as seat-belt laws or restricted smoking in public places. Engineering interventions protect by design. Toys are engineered to be safe for specific age categories. Air bags are designed for the safety of the automobile driver; the intervention has been engineered into the product.

### Evaluation

Community interventions are evaluated, just as nursing interventions for individual clients and families are evaluated. The expected outcome is compared with the outcome achieved at the end of the established time frame. Similar to the nursing process, community assessment is cyclical and continuous. Evaluation is not an end point. It usually begins the assessment step of the next phase of community assessment.

##  ADVOCACY IN PUBLIC POLICY MAKING

Public policy may appear, at first glance, to evolve primarily from the government. However, policy makers consider many sources when developing public policy. Nurses are valued professionals whose opinions and input are often sought by those who participate in the policy-making process. The nurse may participate in policy making in a variety of ways. These activities may range from calling or sending a letter to a city, state, or federal lawmaker, to testifying at a public hearing, to informing a client about proposed changes in the law related to health care. Often, through public education, the nurse may influence public opinion and, in turn, public policy. It is a professional responsibility of the graduate nurse to stay current on health care issues and to share that expertise with other members of the community.

Evidence of public opinion affecting public policy is seen in maternal care (Fig. 5–3). Until the late 1970s, third-party payers allowed a postpartum woman to stay in the hospital from 3 to 5 days. Gradually, reimbursement reduced the length of stay to 2 to 4 days and, eventually, to 24 hours to 3 days. As the negative consequences of early discharge on the mother and newborn became common knowledge through the medical and nursing community's disapproval and advocacy for longer stays, this policy was changed. By the late 1990s, many states extended the 24-hour stay to 48 hours.

Numerous issues offer nurses the opportunity to act as advocates for individuals, families, and communities. Through advocacy and education, the nurse may influence public opinion and health care public policy.

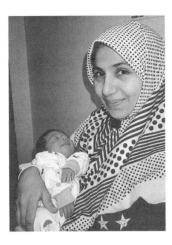

***Figure 5–3.*** ▶ Public opinion and advocacy led to increased postpartal care.

 **CONCLUSIONS**

Assessment in community settings has long been a part of nursing practice. Assessment is directed toward individual clients across the life span, families, and communities. Holistic assessment considers not only physical and psychosocial factors, but also cultural, functional, nutritional, environmental, and spiritual aspects of the client. Family assessment may be abbreviated but is always essential to quality community care. Community assessment helps the nurse become aware of problems in the community that directly or indirectly affect the lives of clients and their families. Although the community-based nurse is infrequently asked to do a formal community assessment, the nurse may, along with other health care professionals, participate in some aspect of community assessment. Communities are assessed by using the nursing process to determine how people, place, and social systems influence health. As health care and nursing shift from the acute care setting to the community setting, the role of the nurse in community assessment will continue to expand.

### References and Bibliography

AARP. (2001). *A profile of older Americans–2001*. Retrieved January 15, 2003, from http://research.aarp.org/general/profile_2001.html

Carpenito, L. (2002). *Nursing diagnosis: Application to clinical practice* (9th ed.). Philadelphia: Lippincott Williams & Wilkins.

Centers for Disease Control and Prevention, National Center for Health Statistics. (2002). *Prevalence of overweight among children and adolescents: United States, 1999–2000*. Retrieved March 2, 2003, from http://www.cdc.gov/nchs/

products/pubs/pubd/hestats.overwght99.htm

Curry, M. (1996). Cultural assessment in home healthcare. *Home Healthcare Nurse, 15*(10), 664–671.

Debrew, J., Barba, B., & Tesh, A. (1998). Assessing medication knowledge and practices of older adults. *Home Healthcare Nurse, 16*(10), 686–692.

Dunn, C. (2002). Assessing and preventing medication interactions. *Home Healthcare Nurse, 20*(2), 104–111.

Heineken, J., & McCoy, N. (2000). Establishing a bond with clients of different cultures. *Home Healthcare Nurse, 18*(1), 45–51.

Jennings-Sanders, A. (2001). Examining medication knowledge and behavior of older African-American adult day care clients. *Journal of National Black Nurses Association, 12*(2),23–29.

Joint Commission on Accreditation of Healthcare Organizations (2001). Spiritual assessment. Retrieved January 19, 2003, from http://www.jcaho.org/

Lindell, D. (1997). Community assessment for the home healthcare nurse. *Home Healthcare Nurse, 15*(9), 618–627.

Meredith, S., Feldman, P. H., Frey, D., Hall, K., Arnold, K., Brown, N.J., Ray, W. A. (2001). Possible medication errors in home health care patients. *Journal of American Geriatric Society, 49*(6), 719–724.

Narayan, M., & Tennant, J. (1997). Environ-

mental assessment. *Home Healthcare Nurse, 15*(11), 799–805.

Neal, L. (1998). Functional assessment of the home health client. *Home Healthcare Nurse, 16*(10), 670–677.

O'Leary, J. (1998). *After loss: Parenting in the next pregnancy.* Minneapolis: Allina Publishing.

Salmon-White, M. S. (1982). Construct for public health nursing. *Nursing Outlook, 30,* 527–530.

Sumner, C. (1998). Recognizing and responding. *American Journal of Nursing, 98*(1), 26–30.

Woodham-Smith, C. (1950). *Florence Nightingale.* London: Constable.

Wright, L., & Leahey, M. (1999). Maximizing time, minimizing suffering; the 15 minute (or less) family interview. *Journal of Family Nursing, 5*(3), 259–274.

# LEARNING ACTIVITIES

## LEARNING ACTIVITY 5-1

Nhu is a home care nurse who is making a home visit to Marion, an 85-year-old woman who has just been discharged from a transitional hospital after a hip replacement. After completing the agency admission intake interview, Nhu takes a few minutes to assess Marion's functional capacity.

*What areas will Nhu assess?*

Nhu learns that Marion is able to perform all ADL, her home environment is basically safe, her sensory and perceptual function is intact, and her cognitive, emotional, integumentary, and respiratory status are all within normal limits and sufficient to allow her to live independently. However, as Nhu is assessing function, Marion tells her, "I was doing fine until the physician changed my medication for high blood pressure. Now I am dizzy all the time."

*What does Nhu assess next?*

## LEARNING ACTIVITY 5-2

Conduct a windshield survey of your community. Consider people, place, and social system using Box 5–9.

**LEARNING ACTIVITY 5-3**

Complete a functional assessment (See Box 5–2) for a vulnerable client in his or her home or apartment. Determine one or more appropriate nursing diagnoses, short- and long- term outcomes, and nursing interventions. Summarize the safety concerns you identified for this client as well as the client's strengths. Identify resources in the community that provide safety devices, such as the safety council. Share all of the information with the client and his or her family and suggest that he or she share it with the appropriate community providers, such as the client's physician, nurse practitioner, or public health nurse.

**LEARNING ACTIVITY 5-4**

Make a home visit to a family with a newborn baby. Use the Community-Based Nursing Care Guidelines in Box 5–1 to assess and intervene with issues related to attachment. Identify family strengths and needs and formulate one or more short- and long-term nursing diagnoses. Use at least one of the nursing interventions listed in the guidelines and evaluate how well it worked, why it did or didn't work, and what other things you would do on the next visit. Document your care plan.

**LEARNING ACTIVITY 5-5**

*Individual Client Assessment*

In your clinical journal, describe a situation in which you used an assessment guide from this chapter to assess a client in a community-based setting.

> What did you learn from this activity?
> What benefit do you think you created for your client?
> What did you do that didn't work?
> What will you do differently next time?

*Family Assessment*

In your clinical journal, describe a situation in which you used an assessment guide from this chapter to assess a family in a community-based setting.

> What did you learn from this activity?
> What benefit do you think you created for the family?
> What did you do that didn't work?
> What will you do differently next time?

*Community Assessment*

In your clinical journal, describe a situation in which you used an assessment guide from this chapter to assess a community.

> What did you learn from this activity?
> What benefit do you think you created for the community or could create for the community?
> What did you do that didn't work?
> What will you do differently next time?

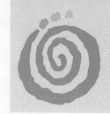

# Client Teaching

Roberta Hunt

At no other time in nursing history has client teaching been so important. Owing to the decreased length of stay in all acute care settings and increased amount of care provided in community settings, teaching is a central role for nurses in all settings. One example is seen in teaching of clients who will soon be discharged from acute care settings. As many as 20% of clients discharged from hospitals do not even fill their prescriptions after discharge. Of those who do, between 40% and 60% do not follow the prescribed regimen, either increasing or decreasing the dose, not taking the correct dose at the prescribed time, or not taking the entire dose. For example, of people that are prescribed high blood pressure medication, only 50% continue to take it after 1 year, and of those, only 75% take enough to fully control their blood pressure (Consumer Health Information Corporation [CHIP], 2003). These errors may result in serious health complications as well as unnecessary hospitalization, treatment, and lost work time. In the United States, as much money is spent treating the complications of home medication errors as is spent to purchase all the medications in the United States. In 2000, $76 billion was spent to purchase medication and another $76 billion to treat the complications that people have when they do not understand how to take their medications (CHIP, 2001). As care is more community based, our clients provide most of their own health care, with up to 80% of all illnesses managed by clients or family members (London, 1999). Studies repeatedly show that client education prevents up to 50% of medication errors for clients in community settings where they self-administer their medications. Further, clients have fewer side effects, doctor visits, and hospital admissions when they are given enough education to take medication correctly (CHIP, 2001). It is the nurse's responsibility to promote quality self-care through teaching. Quality teaching is essential in community-based nursing care.

With this in mind, this chapter addresses quality teaching. The benefits of teaching are presented in light of the current health care system. Teaching and learning theory are discussed along with learning domains. A large section of the chapter is devoted to helping the nursing student develop skills and competencies in teaching, discussing teaching as it follows the nursing process, and sharing useful teaching techniques. The chapter ends with activities to be used in further developing understanding and skills in teaching. Because of its importance, teaching is also addressed in other chapters.

## SIGNIFICANCE OF TEACHING

In the 21st century, more care will be provided outside the acute care setting. Clients are discharged from the hospital "quicker and sicker," or they are not being admitted to an acute care facility at all. The days of progressive teaching in the acute care setting are past. Teaching now begins at whatever point the client enters the system. In fact, many clients and families receive their initial teaching from the home care nurse. Table 6–1 gives examples of important teaching opportunities. Benefits of quality teaching include better outcomes, improved satisfaction, continuity of care between settings, and cost containment while maintaining quality care.

The first and most important goal of teaching in community-based care is to assist the client and family in achieving independence. Quality teaching enhances the ability of the client and family to be successful in providing for their own needs. When client learning needs are considered within the context of the client, family, and community, better outcomes will result. These outcomes include improved care, facilitated recovery, reduction of postoperative complications, and resumption of activities of daily living.

Good teaching improves client and family satisfaction. Clients and families are more likely to feel confident about discharge and follow-up care if they believe they have some knowledge about their condition and their questions have been answered satisfactorily. Teaching often increases a client's sense of control through mutual participation in care planning. Staff satisfaction improves when teaching results are positive. It is professionally satisfying to prepare a client for

| TABLE 6–1 • Important Teaching Opportunities in Community-Based Nursing Care | |
|---|---|
| **Opportunity** | **Possible Learning Need** |
| Admission | Facility policies, how to work call light and bed, specific treatments that have been ordered and why |
| New medication | Action of drug, possible side effects, frequency, and any special considerations |
| Diagnostic procedure | Preparation that is necessary *before* procedure, what will be experienced during procedure, any restrictions or special considerations after procedure |
| Surgery | Preoperative preparation, postoperative protocols (eg, deep breathing, leg exercises), pain control, how to get out of bed and turn easily |
| Discharge | Limitations on activity or diet, procedures such as wound care, when to call the physician |

discharge and receive subsequent feedback that the discharge was satisfactory. Likewise, it is professionally satisfying for the home care nurse to prepare a client to successfully manage self-care at home. On the other hand, it is stressful when a nurse sees a client with inadequate preparation trying to manage home care unsuccessfully.

Quality health education provides continuity between settings of care. When they give clear instructions, health care professionals in one setting can confidently discharge a client into another setting.

A final benefit to quality instruction is more efficient use of resources. One national report indicates that 2% of all hospital readmissions are a result of a need to reeducate caregivers (Leske & Pelczynski, 1999). Rehospitalization of clients is costly to the client, family, and third-party payers. It is frustrating to the client, family, and care providers when teaching has to be repeated several times because it was not done well the first time. Furthermore, concern for cost containment while maintaining quality care requires that all teaching incorporate prevention strategies, which further allow resources to be used efficiently.

 **TEACHING AND LEARNING THEORY**

To be a successful teacher in any setting, the nurse must understand and apply basic teaching and learning principles. Learning depends on both the **need to learn** and the **readiness to learn** and is influenced by the individual's life experiences (Knox, 1985).

### Need to Learn

Learning is facilitated when the client perceives information as needed or relevant for immediate application. For example, a postoperative client is scheduled to go home in 2 hours with a client-controlled analgesia pump. The client learns quickly how to use the pump and administer medication to control postoperative pain. This learning is facilitated by the need for pain relief and the immediate application of learning.

### Readiness to Learn

Learning depends on readiness. Readiness involves such factors as emotional state, abilities, and potential. Examples of these are listed in Box 6–1.

An example of lack of learning readiness follows. You are doing preadmission teaching with a 30-year-old woman, an attorney with a busy law practice who has outpatient surgery scheduled for the next day. She is thinking about the important trial she has beginning the afternoon following surgery. She may not hear you when you tell her she should not drive or make important decisions for a full day after surgery with general anesthesia. Because of her distracted mental state, she is not ready to learn.

Motivation is a strong determinant of learning readiness. Motivation starts with the client's need to know and then provides the drive or incentive to learn. Because so many things can affect motivation, it can change from day to day. For instance a young woman who drinks alcohol becomes pregnant, and her health care provider tells her alcohol is harmful for the fetus. Because she is concerned for her baby's welfare, she discontinues drinking. The motivation is strong enough to

## COMMUNITY-BASED TEACHING

### Box 6-1 ▶ Factors That Affect Readiness to Learn

- Physiologic factors: Age, gender, disease process currently being treated, intactness of senses (hearing, vision, touch, taste), preexisting condition
- Psychosocial factors: Sociocultural circumstances, occupation, economic stability, past experiences with learning, attitude toward learning, spirituality, emotional health, self-concept and body image, sense of responsibility for self
- Cognitive factors: Developmental level, level of education, communication skills, primary language, motivation, reading ability, learning style, problem-solving ability
- Environmental factors: Home environment, safety features, family relationships/problems, caregiver (availability, motivation, abilities), other support systems

make her stop. However, at a party her friends insist that she join them in a drink. "One drink won't hurt you," they say. Now the woman is motivated to drink. Her decision depends on which motivation is stronger.

### Life Experiences

Both differences and similarities between past and present life experiences influence learning. For example, you are doing discharge planning from a maternity center for a multipara who delivered her second child yesterday evening. Her delivery was complicated by a 1,000-mL blood loss and a fourth-degree laceration. She has an 18-month-old toddler at home. Her husband is an accountant. It is tax season, and he presently works 12 or 13 hours a day. Neither set of grandparents nor any other family nor friends live nearby. Your client is going home this afternoon and insists that she does not need help at home because she did not need help after her first child. The client does not understand the difference between her first delivery and the circumstances complicating the second one.

## LEARNING DOMAINS

Teaching and learning occur in three **learning domains:** cognitive, affective, and psychomotor. Teaching strategies are listed in Box 6–2. All three domains must be considered in all aspects of the teaching and learning process. Thus, the nurse must assess the client's need, readiness, and past experience in the cognitive, affective, and psychomotor domains.

Cognitive learning involves mental storage and recall of new knowledge and information for problem solving. Sometimes this domain is referred to as the critical thinking or knowledge domain. An example is the client who has recently been diagnosed with insulin-dependent diabetes. Not only will this client need informa-

## COMMUNITY-BASED TEACHING

**Box 6–2** ▶ Suggested Teaching Strategies
for the Three Learning Domains

| **Cognitive Domain** | **Affective Domain** | **Psychomotor Domain** |
|---|---|---|
| Lecture or discussion | Role modeling | Demonstration |
| Panel discussion | Discussion | Discovery |
| Discovery | Panel discussion | Audiovisual materials |
| Audiovisual materials | Audiovisual materials | Printed materials |
| Printed materials | Role playing | |
| Programmed instruction | Printed materials | |
| Computer-assisted instruction programs | | |

Adapted from Taylor, C., Lillis, C., & LeMone, P. (2001). *Fundamentals of nursing: The art and science of nursing care* (p. 395). Philadelphia: Lippincott-Raven.

tion about diet, insulin, and exercise, but he will also need to use the information to formulate menus and an exercise plan. In addition, as blood sugar levels fluctuate, a client with diabetes must alter food intake and exercise. All this requires cognitive learning.

**Affective learning** involves feelings, attitudes, values, and emotions that influence learning. This is also referred to as the attitude domain. For example, the client who has just been identified as having diabetes may have to talk about his feelings about having diabetes before he is ready to learn about insulin.

**Psychomotor learning** consists of acquired physical skills that can be demonstrated. This may be referred to as the skill domain. For example, the newly diagnosed insulin-dependent client must learn to give self-injections, which will require learning the skill of using syringes.

## DEVELOPMENTAL CONSIDERATIONS

It is helpful for the nurse to understand various theories of development. Appendix 6-1 (p. 473), Implications for teaching at Various Developmental Stages, outlines intellectual development as well as other developmental stages and nursing implications related to them. Just as the need to learn will be different at various age levels, the cognitive domain will differ and life experiences will differ. For example, teaching a 6-year-old girl about insulin administration will be different from teaching a 24-year-old woman, which would in turn be different from teaching a 69-year-old woman. The nurse must consider these factors.

Affective learning and psychomotor learning will also differ. The 6-year-old girl will approach insulin administration differently emotionally than will the 24-year-old woman. The 6-year-old girl may not have the fine motor skills needed to administer insulin. On the other hand, the older woman may have arthritis and not have the dexterity needed to fill the syringe or insert the needle in the site. Figure

**TABLE 6–2** • Relationship Between Nursing Process and Teaching and Learning

| Steps | Nursing Process | Teaching and Learning |
|---|---|---|
| Assessment | Assessment of client/family/caregiver determines need for nursing care. | Assessment of client/family/caregiver determines need for nursing care. |
| Diagnosis | Statement of nursing problem | Statement of learning need |
| Expected outcome | Expected outcome for client or family | Learning objectives/goals for the learner |
| Planning | Nurse and client work together to develop plan of nursing care. | Nurse and client work together to develop learning plan. |
| Interventions | A variety of actions can be used to implement the plan. | A variety of actions in cognitive, affective, and psychomotor learning are used to augment plan. |
| Evaluation | Nurse and client evaluate success of outcomes; nurse determines why plan was not successful (if so); nurse and client revise and set new objectives and plan. | Nurse and client evaluate success of outcomes; nurse and client determine weakness of plan; new objectives and plan are written. |

ferent from the nurse's own culture. A nonjudgmental attitude is enhanced when the nurse does the following:

▶ Recognizes and accepts differences between the nurse and client
▶ Tries to understand the cultural or value basis for the client's behavior
▶ Listens and learns before advising or teaching
▶ Empathizes with the client regardless of differences in attitudes and values

A cultural assessment tool will help the nurse determine how learning need is influenced by culture. Various types of cultural assessment tools are discussed in Chapter 3.

A learning assessment guide can be used to assess the learning need of the client. Such a guide is printed in Box 6–3. Documentation is integral to the teaching process. All assessment is documented. After assessments on the client, family, and caregiver needs; readiness to learn; and past life experiences have been assessed and documented, the learning need can be determined.

## Identification of the Learning Need

The nurse draws some inferences and conclusions based on the assessment. Table 6–3 shows this process. A list of **learning needs** and problems emerges, which leads to identification of priority needs. When lack of knowledge, attitude, or skill hinders a client's self-care, a nursing diagnosis can be used to name the problem or strength. The list of the North American Nursing Diagnosis Association (NANDA) diagnoses can help identify the learning needs of the individual, family member, or caregiver.

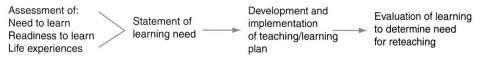

*Figure 6–2.* ▶ Diagram of the teaching process. The nursing process and the teaching process have some similarities.

## ASSESSMENT TOOLS

### Box 6–3    Learning Assessment Guide

Client name _____

Health condition requiring health education_____

Primary caregiver _____

Learner_____ Relationship to client _____

Age _____ Gender _____ Occupation _____

Developmental Stages and Implications for Learner _____

Psychosocial stage _____

_____

Cognitive stage_____

Language _____

_____

How does the caregiver or client feel about the responsibilities of self-care?

_____

_____

Describe any disabilities or limitations of the learner (including sensory

disabilities) _____

_____

Describe any preexisting health conditions of the learner _____

_____

List sociocultural factors that may impede learning_____

_____

State learner behaviors that indicate motivation to learn _____

_____

_____

Can the learner read and comprehend at the reading level required by the

task? _____

_____

Does the learner show an ability to problem solve at a level that provides

safe care in the home? _____

_____

*(continued)*

**ASSESSMENT TOOLS**

Box 6–3  **Learning Assessment Guide** (*Continued*)

Is the home environment conducive to the learning required by the care?

_____

_____

If not, what modifications are necessary?_____

_____

If the learner is not able to carry out the care, are other caregivers available for backup support? _____

_____

If so, please name._____

Phone number _____

Address_____

What other support is available for the client and caregiver? _____

_____

_____

According to Carpenito (2002), knowledge deficit does not represent a human response, alteration, or pattern of dysfunction, but rather a related factor. All nursing diagnoses incorporate teaching as a part of the diagnosis, as follows:

- ▶ Risk for Ineffective Management of Therapeutic Regimens related to lack of knowledge of management, signs, and symptoms of complications of diabetes mellitus
- ▶ Decisional Conflict related to lack of knowledge about advantages and disadvantages of infant circumcision
- ▶ Risk for Impaired Home Maintenance Management related to lack of knowledge of home care and community resources
- ▶ Risk for Injury related to lack of knowledge of bicycle safety

It is also useful to consider learning domains. Learning needs can be determined in one, two, or all of the learning domains. Consider the learning domains in the following example.

## CLIENT SITUATIONS IN PRACTICE

### ▶ Newborn Circumcision

Pat, a primipara, delivered a boy yesterday afternoon. The newborn is to be circumcised this afternoon before Pat and her newborn are discharged. Despite the fact that you have gone over the teaching outline about circumcision twice with

TABLE 6–3 • Examples of Inferences Made From Assessment Data

| Factors to Consider When Assessing Readiness to Learn | Data | Inference |
|---|---|---|
| **Physiologic Factors** | | |
| Age | 85 | Elderly client may have special needs |
| Gender | Male | Men and women each have special needs |
| Disease process currently under treatment | Newly diagnosed diabetic | New diabetics have many teaching needs |
| Intactness of senses—hearing, vision, touch, taste | Hearing and vision are impaired | Teaching must be modified considering sensory deficit |
| Preexisting conditions | Cataract surgery 2 y ago | Vision may still be partially impaired or may be corrected |
| **Psychosocial Factors** | | |
| Sociocultural | Hmong refugee | Teaching must consider diet common to this culture |
| Occupation | Retired | |
| **Cognitive Factors** | | |
| Motivation | Learner states, "I am interested in learning about _____" | Learner is motivated |
| Reading ability | Observed reading the newspaper | Shows ability to read |
| Learning style | Observer, doer, or listener | Tailor teaching to style |
| Problem-solving ability | Learner can come up with concepts and alternatives | Learner can problem solve |
| **Environmental Factors** | | |
| Home environment | Home cluttered with no place to sit or set up teaching | Environment must be modified before teaching |
| Caregiver | | |
|   Availability | Client is a widow or spouse works full time | No caregiver available |
|   Motivation | Caregiver states, "I can't handle hearing about that device" | Caregiver not motivated |
|   Abilities | Caregiver is unable to follow simple instructions or directions | Caregiver has limited ability to provide care |
| Other support | Client is active in his or her church | Church may be another source of care and support |

Subject: client
Action verb: state
Performance criteria: signs and symptoms of infection
Target time: (date)
Special conditions: when to contact the nurse on call

Pat, she states, "How will the penis look in 3 days?" She is also unable to demonstrate the application of the dressing to the site and states, "Maybe we shouldn't have the baby circumcised if it will hurt the baby."

For this scenario, the following is an example of a learning need in the affective domain:

---

## ▶ Box 6–4   Medicare Guidelines ◀

". . . activities which require skilled nursing personnel to teach a benefici- ary, the beneficiary's family or care givers how to manage his treatment regimen constitutes skilled nursing services. Where the teaching or train- ing is reasonable and necessary to the treatment of the illness or injury, skilled nursing visits for teaching would be covered. The test of whether a nursing service is skilled relates to the skill required to teach and not to the nature of what is being taught. . . . Skilled nursing visits for teaching and training activities are reasonable and necessary where the teaching or training is appropriate to the beneficiary's functional loss, or his illness or injury." From *Medicare Guidelines Coverage of Services* Revision 222, Sec- tion 205.13.

### Summary of Medicare Reimbursement Requirements for Teaching

Teaching is reimbursed when it is considered in these ways:
* Teaching how to manage treatment
* Reasonable and necessary to the treatment of the illness or injury

"Reasonable and necessary" means teaching to the client's functional loss or his or her illness or injury.

To determine the number of necessary and reasonable visits, use the following criteria:
* Initial teaching = number of visits depends on the *complexity* of the tasks and the *ability* of the learner
* Reinforcement teaching = number of visits depends on *retained knowl- edge* and *anticipated learning* progress

Teaching is not generally reimbursed under these conditions:
* It becomes apparent after a reasonable period of time the client, fam- ily, or caregiver is *not* able to learn.
* The reason that learning did not occur is *not* documented.

---

Adapted from *Medicare Guidelines Coverage of Services*, Revision 222, Section 205.13.

---

*Anxiety related to lack of knowledge as manifested by the mother's state- ment, "Maybe we shouldn't have the baby circumcised if it will hurt the baby."*

Here is an example of a learning need in the psychomotor domain:

*Risk for Impaired Home Maintenance Management related to lack of knowl- edge and ability to demonstrate dressing change.*

The following is an example of a nursing diagnosis in the cognitive domain:

*Altered Parenting related to lack of knowledge and inexperience as manifested by the mother's statement, "How will the penis look in 3 days?"*

After the learning need is identified, the nurse determines if the teaching needed by the client is reimbursable. Referral may depend on reimbursement. In most situations, nurses providing teaching to clients in the home are restricted by **reimbursement requirements.** Medicare, Medicaid, and most other third-party payers reimburse skilled nursing care. The specific requirements are defined in the Medicare Guidelines, Revision 222, Section 205.13. Box 6–4 summarizes the guidelines.

It is imperative that the nurse knows the reimbursement requirements of the various third-party payers for teaching at the agency where he or she works. Agencies will not receive payment for teaching if the nurse does not follow the requirements specified by the particular payer.

## Planning

Planning for learning involves developing a teaching plan. Teaching plans are similar to nursing care plans—both follow the steps of the nursing process. Some agencies use standardized teaching plans and may include a computerized teaching plan. If standardized teaching plans are used, the plan must be individualized to the client and his or her needs. Teaching plans are also incorporated into critical pathway documentation.

Planning skills are essential in the development of individualized teaching plans. The teaching plan identifies learning objectives that reflect the specifics of the ongoing care at home. Often, the goal of teaching is to ensure the client's safety and total reliance on self-care. The planning of the care is a mutual process among the nurse, client, and family caregivers. Planning is based on the three learning domains.

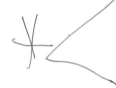

▶ *Cognitive objectives:* Relate to learning activities that strengthen comprehension regarding the illness and its treatment
▶ *Affective objectives:* Relate to learning activities that enhance the acceptance of the illness and subsequent treatment
▶ *Psychomotor objectives:* Relate to learning activities that demonstrate management of the treatment procedures

A **learning objective** is the same as a client goal or expected outcome used in the nursing process. Each objective includes a subject, action verb, performance criteria, target time, and special conditions.

The following learning objective contains these components:

Client will state three signs and symptoms of infection by (date)_____ and know which complications require contacting the nurse on call.

Subject: client

Action verb: state

Performance criteria: signs and symptoms of infection

Target time: (date)

Special conditions: when to contact the nurse on call

Examples of learning objectives in the three learning domains are as follows:

▶ *Cognitive objectives:* Family or caregiver will state three signs and symptoms of infection by (date)_____.
▶ *Affective objectives:* Family or caregiver will express feelings about having to be in charge of client's Port-a-Cath care by (date)_____.
▶ *Psychomotor objectives:* Family or caregiver will demonstrate aseptic technique when cleaning and flushing sites on Port-a-Cath by (date)_____.

> ▶ **Box 6–5**   Active Verbs for Learning Objectives ◀

| Cognitive Domain | Affective Domain | Psychomotor Domain |
|---|---|---|
| categorize | answer | adapt |
| compare | choose | arrange |
| compose | defend | assemble |
| define | discuss | begin |
| describe | display | change |
| design | form | construct |
| differentiate | give | create |
| explain | help | manipulate |
| give example | initiate | move |
| identify | join | organize |
| label | justify | rearrange |
| list | relate | show |
| name | revise | start |
| prepare | select | work |
| plan | share | |
| solve | use | |
| state | | |
| summarize | | |
| write | | |

Action verbs that can be used when writing learning objectives are listed in Box 6–5.

In most situations, the nurse and the client plan a series of small, incremental learning objectives through a series of lessons based on the specific needs of the client. The overall goal of planning is to assist the client to have enough understanding to be safe with self-care. For many clients, the ultimate goal of independence is achieved through reliance on family or other caregivers. The goal of teaching is to maximize individual potential or quality of life.

## Intervention

The nurse carries out the teaching plan according to the client or family caregiver's learning needs. This is accomplished in one or more teaching sessions. Interventions may vary according to learner readiness, perceived need, and past life experience, all of which fluctuate throughout an individual's life span. Specific interventions for children are shown in Box 6–6, and nursing implications for various developmental stages are given in Appendix 6-1 (p. 473). It is essential to incorporate nursing interventions that are designed to deal with existing barriers to successful teaching. Some of these barriers are discussed in the next section.

The basic principles of teaching and learning discussed so far apply in both community-based and acute care settings. However, there are some differences between the two settings. These differences are discussed in relation to discharge

## COMMUNITY-BASED TEACHING

**Box 6–6** ▶ Cognitive Stages and Approaches to
Patient Education With Children

| Cognitive Stage | Approach to Teaching |
|---|---|
| ***Ages Birth to 2 y—Sensorimotor Development*** | |
| Begins as completely undifferentiated from environment | Orient all teaching to parents. |
| Eventually learns to repeat actions that have effect on objects | Make infants feel as secure as possible with familiar objects in home environment. |
| Has rudimentary ability to make associations | Give older infants an opportunity to manipulate objects in their environments, especially if long hospitalization is expected. |
| ***Ages 2–7 y—Preoperational Developments*** | |
| Has cognitive processes that are literal and concrete | Be aware of explanations that the child may interpret literally (eg, "The doctor is going to make your heart like new" may be interpreted as, "He is going to give me a new heart"); allow child to manipulate safe equipment, such as stethoscopes, tongue blades, reflex hammers; use simple drawings of the external anatomy because children have limited knowledge of organs' functions. |
| Lacks ability to generalize | Do not compare child to other children; this is not helpful, nor is it meaningful to compare one diagnostic test or procedure to another. |
| Has egocentrism predominating | Reassure child that no one is to blame for his pain or other problems; belief that he causes events to happen may result in guilty thoughts that he caused his own pain, hospitalization, and so forth; |
| Has animistic thinking (thinks that all objects possess life or human characteristics of their own) | Anthropomorphize and name equipment that is especially frightening. |

*(continued)*

## COMMUNITY-BASED TEACHING

**Box 6–6** ▶ Cognitive Stages and Approaches to
Patient Education With Children *(Continued)*

| Cognitive Stage | Approach to Teaching |
|---|---|
| *Ages 7–12 y—Concrete Operational Thought Developments* | |
| Has concrete, but more realistic and objective, cognitive processes | Use drawings and models; children at this age have vague understandings of internal body processes; use needle play with dolls to explain surgical techniques and facilitate learning. |
| Is able to compare objects and experiences because of increased ability to classify along many different dimensions | Relate his or her care to other children's experiences so he or she can learn from them; compare procedures to one another to diminish anxiety. |
| Views world more objectively and is able to understand another's position | Use films and group activities to add to repertoire of useful behaviors and establish role models. |
| Has knowledge of cause and effect that has progressed to deductive logical reasoning | Use child's interest in science to explain logically what has happened and what will happen; explain medications simply and straightforwardly (eg, "This medicine [insulin] unlocks the door to your body's cells just as a key unlocks the door to your house. By unlocking the door to the cell, the insulin can deliver the food and energy in your blood to the cell."). |

Sources: London, F. (1999). *No time to teach: A nurse's guide to patient and family education.* Philadelphia: Lippincott Williams & Wilkins. Adapted from Petrillo, M., & Sanger, S. (1998). *Emotional care of hospitalized children* (pp. 38–50). Philadelphia: Lippincott-Raven, and Kolb, L. C. (1977). *Modern clinical psychiatry* (9th ed., pp. 90–91). Philadelphia: Saunders.

planning and teaching. Barriers to successful teaching are presented first and followed by characteristics of successful teaching.

### Discharge Teaching in the Acute Care Setting
Because clients are discharged from the hospital "quicker and sicker" or have complicated procedures done on an outpatient basis and are sent home, the need for comprehensive discharge teaching is accentuated.

#### BARRIERS TO SUCCESSFUL TEACHING
Discharge teaching does not always result in learning. In a questionnaire designed to evaluate the quality of discharge teaching, only one of five family caregivers re-

### TABLE 6–4 • Combating Barriers to Successful Discharge Teaching

| Barriers | Sample Nursing Interventions |
|---|---|
| Timing is not conducive to learning (client's physical or psychological conditions do not allow learning to occur) | Document client's lack of mastery of the material. Update physician or nurse practitioner on an ongoing basis to plan discharge. Refer for follow-up if learning is not adequate for safe self-care. |
| Past experiences impede perceived learning readiness or need. | Identify past experiences. Determine and clarify misconceptions. Determine if past experience will interrupt or enhance new learning. |
| Retention of information impeded by anxiety of going home or leaving security of health care environment. | See interventions for timing. Break learning into small, easily mastered segments. Use positive reinforcement and praise. |
| Cultural differences between nurse and client or family impede learning or understanding. | Work to build a trusting relationship with client and family. Show respect for the client's culture and incorporate it in discharge planning. Use resources to overcome a language barrier. |
| Lack of adherence | Establish trust. Identify reasons for lack of adherence. Clarity misinformation. Use formal and informal contracting. |

ported feeling adequately prepared to care for the client at home (Leske & Pelczynski, 1999). Their retention of information may diminish owing to the anxiety experienced with the client's homecoming. Barriers to successful discharge teaching are shown in Table 6–4.

The average length of stay for all clients in acute care settings has decreased significantly in the past 10 years. A postpartum client's stay has decreased from 5 days to 24 hours. Many procedures that used to be performed in the acute care setting are now performed on an outpatient basis. Consequently, time for teaching is now grossly limited in the acute care setting.

Women in the immediate postpartum period are not receptive to learning (Rubin, 1984). The typical postpartum client who has just delivered is not ready to learn because of normal physical and psychologic conditions of the postpartum status. Seventy-two hours after delivery, mothers are in a stage where they need reinforcement from professionals. Now, because of early discharge, 72 hours falls after they have left the hospital and are at home. As a result of the unreadiness to learn and the shortened stay, almost no teaching or learning occurs. In addition, limiting postpartum stay to 24 hours has resulted in an increased incidence of serious complications for newborns. These complications include an increase in hyperbilirubinemia and dehydration, which frequently require hospitalization or clinic follow-up. Inadequate breast-feeding and weight loss have also resulted from early postpartum discharge.

Clients may speak a language different from the nurse's or have sight, comprehension, or retention problems (see Boxes 6–7 and 6–8). There are several community-based guidelines that should be followed when providing health informa-

## COMMUNITY-BASED NURSING CARE GUIDELINES

**Box 6–7** ▶ Working With Interpreters

- Determine the language the client speaks at home.
- Use qualified, professional interpreters.
- Avoid using interpreters from rival tribes, states, regions, or nations.
- Use an interpreter of the same gender as the client, if possible. In general, an older interpreter is preferred to a younger interpreter.
- Allow enough time for the interpreted session.
- Look directly at the client, addressing your questions to him or her.
- Speak in a normal tone of voice, clearly and slowly, using words and not just gestures.
- Keep your sentences simple and short; pause often to permit interpretation.
- Ask only one question at a time.
- Give the interpreter freedom to interrupt for clarification.
- Ask the interpreter to take notes if needed when the interview gets too complex.
- Be prepared to repeat yourself, use different words and rephrase as necessary for understanding. Be patient.
- Use the simplest vocabulary; avoid slang, jargon, and unfamiliar medical terminology.
- Check to see if the information has been understood. Have the interpreter tell you what the client has said he or she understands. Be direct and expect directness.

Adapted from Andrews, M., & Boyle, J. (2003). *Transcultural concepts in nursing care* (4th ed., p. 32). Philadelphia: Lippincott Williams & Wilkins.

tion to a client or family member who uses English as a second language (Wilson, & Robledo, 1999).

- ▶ Listen carefully to what the client and family are telling you. Present one idea at a time, use simple, uncomplicated sentences, and use concrete examples to enhance learning.
- ▶ Assess the client and family members' understanding of the illness being treated.
- ▶ Include the client and family in the plan of care.
- ▶ Assess the client and family members' understanding of the agreed-on treatment plan.
- ▶ Use materials printed in the client or family members' first language, when possible.
- ▶ Validate the correct use of folk medicines and home remedies.
- ▶ Be aware of and discuss the contraindications for concurrent use of medications with the client and family.

# COMMUNITY-BASED NURSING CARE GUIDELINES

**Box 6–8** ▶ Communicating With Clients With Special Needs

## Strategies for Visually Impaired Clients
- Speak to the client when approaching.
- Avoid speaking from behind the client.
- Identify yourself by saying your name or gently touching the client to alert him or her to your presence.
- Ask other people in the room to introduce themselves—this allows the client to hear each person's voice.
- Describe the room and the position of furniture to familiarize the client with the surroundings.
- Explain procedures precisely.
- Inform the client when you are leaving the room; let the client know what you are doing and where you are located at all times.
- Use adaptive devices for the partially impaired client such as large-print materials (telephone dials, thermostat dials) and a magnifying glass.

## Strategies for Hearing Impaired Clients
- Provide a well-lit environment.
- Face the client; speak slowly and deliberately.
- When entering a room, place yourself in front of the client so he or she can see you, or lightly touch the client.
- Always ask if the client uses a hearing aid and if it is working properly; ask if the client needs assistance with inserting the hearing aid and if he or she wears the aid.
- Ask the client if he or she desires an auditory amplifier in the telephone, a TDD telecommunications device for the hearing impaired, or a light on the telephone to alert client of a caller.
- Write down points you make and give the list to the client.

## Strategies for Clients With Speech and Language Deficits (Aphasia)
- Provide services for communication such as a letter board so the client can spell words, word boards (nurse or client points to word), picture charts (nurse or client points to object), or a computer.
- Be patient; supply needed support when the client falters in communication attempts.
- Provide regular mental stimulation.
- Praise all efforts and encourage practicing what is learned in treatment.

Adapted from Anderson, C. (1990). *Patient teaching and communication in an information age.* Albany, NY: Delmar, Arnold & Boggs. (1995). *Interpersonal relationships; Professional communication skills for nurses* (2nd ed.). Philadelphia, Saunders.

A major area of discharge teaching that has been identified as problematic is compliance with medications after discharge. Fifty percent of individuals over the age of 65 have multiple chronic conditions. Studies show that these elderly routinely take an average of two to six prescribed medications and concurrently use one to three medications. Therefore, there is great need for teaching in this age group (Dunn, 2002). Numerous studies have shown a high rate of nonadherence with the medication regimen after discharge from an inpatient setting. This may result in rehospitalization, clinic follow-up, or admission to home care. Comprehensive discharge teaching regarding medication management at home prevents or reduces this problem. Box 6–9 lists strategies to help clients get the full benefit from drug therapy. As the primary client educator, the nurse is in a vital position to promote adherence to prescribed treatment regimens.

### SUCCESSFUL TEACHING

The first and most essential component of successful teaching is building a trusting relationship with the client and family. As trust is built, barriers to accurate communication between the nurse and the client and family are removed. This results in increased client adherence to the prescribed regimen and enhanced learning. It is important that the nurse and client jointly determine the learning plan. Joint planning leads to better adherence to treatment regimens. This process requires forming a partnership, building an alliance, and working together toward a shared goal. It takes time to build trust and know the client, but this is the only way to individualize care (London, 2001). Strategies for better adherence to treatment regimens are shown in Box 6–10

Meticulous documentation is an essential component of a successful discharge teaching program. Methods of documentation vary, but the trend is toward the use of clinical pathways that outline teaching needs by diagnosis or procedure and include learning outcomes, content, methods, and strategies for teaching.

Successful discharge teaching also involves care of the client in the context of the community (see Box 6–11). Careful assessment of the family, its culture, and the community environment can result in a comprehensive teaching plan. Discharge teaching objectives must focus on all levels of prevention. Continuity of teaching strengthens discharge teaching and improves outcomes.

### Teaching in the Community-Based Setting

The primary difference between teaching in the acute care setting and the community-based setting is the need for independent decision making in the unstructured community-based setting. The nurse's role changes from client care manager to health care facilitator. Because of this difference, nurses may feel as if they have lost control of outcomes. The nurse has to focus on enhancing self-care for the client rather than giving care to the client, which is the norm within the structured context of the acute care setting.

### BARRIERS TO SUCCESSFUL TEACHING

A number of barriers to successful teaching in community-based care exist (Table 6–5). These barriers interrupt the coordination of and consistency in teaching and communication with the caregiving team.

Client resistance to following the treatment regimen is a barrier to successful teaching in the home. Nursing students often express dismay over their diminished control of client behavior when providing care in settings other than the

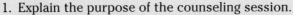

> ▶ **Box 6–9** Effective Medication Counseling: 26 Steps ◀

1. Explain the purpose of the counseling session.
2. Obtain pertinent initial drug-related information (eg, allergies, other medications, age).
3. Warn client about taking other medications, including over-the-counter medications, herbals or botanicals, and alcohol, that could inhibit or interact with the prescribed medication.
4. Assess the client's understanding of the reason(s) for therapy.
5. Assess any actual or potential concerns or problems of importance to the client.
6. Discuss the name (generic and trade) and indication of the medication.
7. Explain the dosage regimen, including scheduling and duration of therapy, when appropriate.
8. Assist the client in developing a plan to incorporate the medication regimen into his or her daily routine.
9. Explain how long it will take for the drug to show an effect.
10. Discuss storage recommendations and ancillary instructions (shake well, refrigerate, etc).
11. Inform the client if and when the medication is to be refilled.
12. Emphasize the benefits of completing the medication as prescribed.
13. Discuss potential (significant) side effects.
14. Discuss how to prevent or manage the side effects of the drug should they occur.
15. Discuss precautions (activities to avoid, etc).
16. Discuss significant drug–drug, drug–food and drug–disease interactions.
17. Explain in precise terms what the client should do if a dose is missed.
18. Explore with the client potential problems in taking the medication as prescribed.
19. Use language that the client is likely to understand.
20. Use appropriate aids to enhance teaching.
21. Respond with understanding or empathy.
22. Use open-ended questions.
23. Display effective nonverbal behaviors.
24. Verify that the client understands via feedback.
25. Summarize by acknowledging and/or emphasizing key points of information.
26. Provide an opportunity for final concerns or questions.

———
Effective medication counseling: 26 Steps. (2000). *Home Healthcare Nurse, 18*(3), 157–160.

acute care setting. For instance, teaching in the home often requires adaptation to the particular home environment, with the client in control.

The need to bring all necessary supplies to the home interferes with successful teaching. Unlike the acute care or inpatient settings where all teaching supplies

---

▶ **Box 6–10**   Steps to Improve Treatment Adherence ◀

Assess for potential problems
- Past adherence issues
- Presence of psychologic stress
- Present knowledge base

Start teaching during hospitalization
- Review medications during each administration
- Begin discharge planning at admission
- Introduce self to family members at admission

Discuss typical schedule at home and requirements of treatment
- Determine how regimen can fit into typical schedule

Promote self-monitoring
- Include family in teaching
- Use techniques to enhance compliance (eg, calendar, pamphlets, teaching sheets, phone numbers)

Follow up after discharge
- Follow-up phone call
- Referral to home care follow-up

---

Adapted from Dunbar-Jacob, J. (1999). Five steps to better treatment adherence. *Nursing 99, 29*(11), 32hm14.

---

are on the unit, teaching in the home requires the nurse to carry a supply of teaching materials.

Another barrier relates to difficulty in coordinating client teaching among multiple providers. Often, many care providers are involved with the client's care. Other professionals may include other nurses, physical therapists, social workers, home health aides, nurse practitioners, and physicians. It is difficult to maintain ongoing communication among multiple caregivers in several diverse settings.

Wide age variations among clients and family members create differences in cognitive and developmental levels. This makes teaching difficult in community-

**COMMUNITY-BASED NURSING CARE GUIDELINES**

**Box 6–11** ▶ Characteristics of Successful Discharge Teaching

- Use varied teaching techniques.
- Provide a follow-up visit.
- Plan telephone calls after discharge to review learning objectives.
- Provide hands-on practice before discharge.
- Structure home visit to reduce anxiety and enhance learning.
- Promote self-care.
- Provide link between acute care facility and community-based care.

---

**TABLE 6–5** • Combating Barriers to Successful Home Teaching

| Barriers | Sample Nursing Interventions |
|---|---|
| **Home Environment** | |
| *Examples:* | |
| Home setting is nonstructured. | Involve client and family in all stages of planning. |
| Environment is the client and family's home turf. | Build trusting relationship with client and family, maintaining respect for family's culture and values. |
| Equipment and setting are inadequate for teaching. | Adapt the home environment to facilitate learning and compliance. |
| **Nurse Caregiver** | |
| *Examples:* | |
| Nurse has less control over the outcomes of the teaching. | Approach the client with a nonjudgmental attitude. |
| Nurse may have inadequate preparation for providing teaching in the home. | Acquire specific knowledge and skill in community-based care. |
| Nurse must bring all the teaching supplies to the home. | Plan and organize ahead and bring all supplies. |
| Nurse must coordinate client teaching among many providers. | Facilitate communication and documentation among caregivers. |
| Nurse role shifts from client care manager to health care facilitator. | Focus on enhancing client's self-care instead of providing care to the client. |
| **Client/Family/Recipient of Teaching** | |
| *Examples:* | |
| Wide variation in family members' ages and cognitive and developmental stages | Carefully assess learning need, learning readiness, and past learning experiences of all recipients of teaching. Involve family and client in all stages of planning and teaching. |
| Lack of adherence unless client/family are involved in the teaching plan | |

---

based nursing. Further, most home care clients are older; consequently, their particular learning needs are different. Cultural barriers also impede successful teaching in the community-based setting.

Lack of time is a barrier to home care teaching. The time factor in acute care settings may prohibit teaching, and many home care referrals come from clinics or physicians' offices. As a result, the first teaching, in many cases, may be done in the home. Home care nurses are often pressed for time. It may be difficult for the home care nurse to feel teaching is ever complete or even adequate.

**SUCCESSFUL TEACHING**

The first and most essential component of successful teaching, as in the acute care setting, is building a trusting relationship with the client and family. Successful teaching also requires the nurse to function as the interdisciplinary team member who furnishes a link between the referral source and community-based setting. The nurse has the responsibility of being the client's advocate, providing a critical communication channel between community organizations and providers who are members of the team. Coordinating communication among many care providers ensures consistency in teaching and reinforcement of learning and enhances continuity of care. Ongoing communication is the foundation of good teaching and the key to maintaining safe, effective care. Following the suggestions in Box 6–12 can foster communication and enhance continuity and learning (Long, Ismeurt, & White, 1999).

Frequently, clients and family caregivers may only need reinforcement that the client is progressing normally in the recovery process. In these situations, the focus should include care for the caregiver as well as care for the client. Affirming the quality of care provided by the family caregiver by listening to the concerns and frustrations of the caregiver should be a priority of the nurse. Table 6–5 presents other interventions to combat barriers to successful home teaching.

An advantage to teaching in the home is the reduction of anxiety in the learner. One of the basic principles of teaching is that when anxiety is reduced, learning is enhanced. The client is on "home turf" and has more control of the environment and the situation, thus helping to lessen anxiety (Fig. 6–3). As part of the original and ongoing assessment process, the nurse assesses the learner's anxiety level. If the learner exhibits anxiety that is interrupting learning, the learning plan must be modified. It is also important to plan lessons that include "digestible" segments that build on information shared in previous teaching sessions.

Research Box 6–13 describes a study that examined the effect of preprocedure teaching prior to outpatient gastrointestinal endoscopy (Salmore & Nelson, 2000). This is an example of how successful teaching promotes self-care. Home nursing visits increase client and family compliance with both appointments and medication management. In the home, the nurse can vary the environment and timing of instruction. The caregiver also has an opportunity to discuss fears and stresses, and the nurse has an opportunity to assess the caregiver for cultural tendencies, past experiences, and coping ability.

Behaviorally oriented client education, which emphasizes a change of environment to facilitate client self-care, is the most successful method for improving the

---

▶ **Box 6–12    Characteristics of Successful Discharge Teaching ◀
Through Ongoing Communication**

Encourage the client to schedule the follow-up telephone call or office visit. Have the client write down the name of the contact person at the clinic or pharmacy, or other appropriate caregiver.

Keep the health care provider informed regarding any progress, or lack of it, when a new medication or treatment is started.

Be sure to identify any unexpected effects of treatment or drug interactions, even if they appear to be minor.

Encourage clients to ask questions until they understand what they need to know. Emphasize that there are no "stupid questions" regarding a client's health.

In asking the questions, have the client insist on answers in "layman's terms" in the most basic form of language used to communicate with any health care provider.

Adapted from Long, C., Ismeurt, R., & White, P. (1999). Preventing drug interactions in the home: A five-step approach for client teaching. *Home Healthcare Nurse, 17*(2), 106–112.

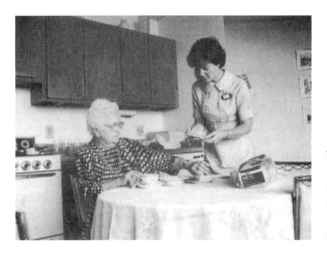

*Figure 6–3.* ▶ A teaching/
learning experience in the
home often is more successful
because the client is in his or
her own territory. The nurse is
responsible for teaching and
coordinating care.

clinical course of chronic disease. In addition, behavioral education contributes to
care that is more easily managed in the home. An example is rearranging furniture
so that it is in the field of vision for a client with hemianopsia.

Although changing the environment can enhance self-care, this must be accomplished within the context of the client and family's value system. When the nurse
provides teaching in the context of these values and norms, learning is enhanced.
Because care in the home is provided on the client and family's "turf," it is particularly important to consider what the family values are when formulating a teaching plan.

### Successful Teaching Techniques

Because of the increased workload of the nurse, decreasing length of stay in the
acute care setting, and limited visits in home care, teaching time is limited. The
nurse needs to be familiar with a variety of teaching techniques and feel competent to choose which technique is most suitable for the circumstance.

For example, demonstration of a new skill is used to change behavior, whereas
videotapes are used to increase knowledge. Video use supplements one-on-one
and group teaching. Videos can be viewed several times by anyone with access to
a videotape player.

Many acute care settings use closed-circuit television to display successful
teaching programs and to reinforce learning. Before discharge, the client as well
as the family or caregiver may watch programs several times if reinforcement is
necessary. The videotape can be used the same way in the home.

Learning is always enhanced by use of a variety of methods. Successful teaching strategies include showing as well as telling. Much teaching occurs while the
nurse is providing client care—taking blood pressure or a temperature, giving a
bath, examining a newborn or infant, weighing the client, and changing wound
dressings. Client education seldom is the formal process one experiences in a
classroom.

A variety of teaching methods and materials are available. Box 6–14 lists some
of them. Choices depend on the developmental level of the client, the availability
of materials, the setting for the educational opportunity, the time available for
teaching, and the nurse's abilities to use various methods. In addition, teaching

### RESEARCH IN COMMUNITY-BASED NURSING CARE

**Box 6–13** ▶ The Effect of Preprocedure Teaching, Relaxation Instruction, and Music on Anxiety as Measured by Blood Pressures in an Outpatient Gastrointestinal Endoscopy Laboratory

Abnormally elevated blood pressure and pulse caused by anxiety often are present on admission to the hospital. These elevated vital signs are then used as baseline vital signs for the client's hospital stay. This study sought to determine whether vital signs are elevated because of anxiety on admission to the hospital and how much they decrease after sedation. A second purpose of this study was to explore the effect of instruction about relaxation and the use of music relaxation audiotapes in decreasing client anxiety.

Clients undergoing gastrointestinal endoscopy for the first time were randomly assigned into two groups. Those in the treatment group received a home visit by an RN, where they were given brief instruction in relaxation and provided with an audiotape player and relaxation music. Statistical analysis comparing differences between control and treatment groups over time reflected a difference in diastolic blood pressure. Those in the treatment group had significantly lower blood pressure throughout the entire procedure. This study revealed no significant difference between the groups related to the amount of medication used.

There were several unintended benefits from the home visits. The home visits contributed to feelings of increased satisfaction for the nurses who reported they offered an opportunity to provide teaching about the upcoming exam in a more relaxed atmosphere. Further, the nurses provided other health-related information about blood pressure and heart disease. Nurse–patient interaction enhances job satisfaction and is important for nurse retention.

Salmore, R., & Nelson, J. (2000). The effect of preprocedure teaching, relaxation instruction, and music on anxiety as measured by blood pressures in an outpatient gastrointestinal endoscopy laboratory. *Gastroenterology Nursing, 23*(3), 102–110. Retrieved January 18, 2003 from the CINAHL database.

methods have to be acceptable and nonthreatening to the client and family or caregiver.

Actual equipment and objects can be used for effective teaching, including the catheter, tubing, port, monitor, or other devices. Picture cards can be made to illustrate each item in a procedure. Photos can be made of each key step or diagrams can be drawn for the cards. Quizzes can be developed with short statements related to the procedure in true or false categories. The nurse can design

## COMMUNITY-BASED TEACHING

### Box 6–14 ▶ Sampling of Teaching Techniques

One-on-one teaching
Group teaching
Self-evaluation/worksheet
Discussions/questions
Explanations/examples
Demonstrations/return demonstrations
Charts/graphs/diagrams
Pictures/photos/picture cards
Reading materials (pamphlets/books)
Role modeling/role playing
Audiovisuals (computer programs/movies/slides/TV/videotapes)
Equipment (such as catheters/tubing/port/monitors)
Models (such as fetus and uterine models/breast models)
Web page and Internet
Games
Health fairs

posters with information the client needs to learn. Work sheets can be developed to use with a videotape or audiotape.

A new teaching method for health education is the use of Web sites on the Internet. For example, one innovative program provides presurgical preparation for adolescent clients prior to tonsillectomy and adenoidectomy. Interactive content provides preparation without the client having to leave the home (O'Conner-Von, 2001). This method could be used for any type of teaching for clients who are computer literate and have access to a computer at home, school, or the public library.

### Teaching the Challenging Client

When the teaching plan is unsuccessful, special teaching strategies are used. Strategies include the use of good interpersonal communication, problem-solving, and contracting skills. Common reasons why clients do not follow treatment regimens stem from lack of information, lack of skill, and lack of client value for the treatment. It is not uncommon for individuals to not follow a treatment plan because of anxiety or fear. It is important to ascertain why the client is not following the prescribed treatment. The first problem-solving technique that can be used is to ask the client about his or her perception of progress made with the teaching plan. Once the cause of nonlearning is identified, the nurse can tailor interventions accordingly. Barriers to compliance include client factors, home environment, and the teaching plan itself.

#### THE CLIENT

In some cases, client anxiety or fear may impede learning. Before any teaching occurs, the nurse must address the anxiety or fear of the learner.

Learning needs may come from lack of information or skills. These needs are easily met by identifying and providing information and by providing opportunities to practice skills.

The nurse, however, may interpret a learning need as an impediment, when the client's behavior simply reflects the values and attitudes of the client and the client's community. If lack of adherence stems from the client's attitudes and values, the appropriate intervention is different from interventions used when adherence problems arise from lack of information.

Lack of adherence will result if the client does not value the treatment. Consequently, the nurse must address this lack of valuing by attempting to modify the teaching regimen to better fit the client's value system. The revised learning plan that reflects the client's value system will differ based on whether the problem stems from lack of knowledge, skill, confidence, fear, or values. On the other hand, no individual is totally compliant. The nurse must use professional judgment to gauge what level of adherence to treatment is acceptable.

### THE HOME ENVIRONMENT

Behaviorally oriented client education, which emphasizes the change of the environment in which the client does self-care, is often the most successful strategy. Changing the home environment is credited with improving the clinical course of clients instructed in the home. Careful assessment of the home environment allows the nurse to identify and modify problematic issues and enhance learning outcomes. These interventions may be as simple as providing better light for a teaching session by opening the drapes, moving a lamp, or replacing a burned-out lightbulb.

### THE TEACHING PLAN

As previously mentioned, effective teaching requires sound interpersonal skills. When care is provided in the client's home, the nurse's nonjudgmental attitude is essential.

Contracting is important to effective teaching. The most logical resolution for clients who are not following treatment is to set up a mutual plan of action for adherence to the treatment plan. This can be accomplished through use of a learning contract, such as the one shown in Box 6–15. A learning contract may include a date, names of those involved, specific expected behaviors, date of achievement,

---

▶ **Box 6–15** Sample Learning Contract ◀

Steve Hunt agrees to monitor his blood sugar by using the One Touch monitor at 8:00 am and 6:00 pm for 1 week from June 1 through June 8. If this contract is not abided by, Best Home Healthcare will discharge Steve Hunt back to Dr. Berger of Neighborhood Clinics. This discharge relieves Best Home Healthcare from any further responsibility for the care of Steve Hunt.

Signed _____

Date _____

Signed by Case Manager _____

Date _____

action that will be taken if the contract is not followed, and the date and signatures of those involved.

The nurse and the client can set a contract at the first visit and each subsequent visit. Contracting can be done at the beginning of a therapeutic relationship through use of both formal and informal techniques. This may prevent some lack of adherence to the treatment plan from the outset. Most agencies have formal contracts such as a "Bill of Rights" or "Client Responsibilities." Review and implementation of the content of these standards on the first visit is one way to encourage compliance with all clients and their families.

### Teaching Related to Levels of Prevention

Teaching, whether it is in the acute care or community-based setting, occurs at all levels of prevention.

#### PRIMARY PREVENTION

An important goal of teaching is to prevent the initial occurrence of disease or injury through health promotion and prevention activities. A nurse teaching a nutrition class to parents and day care providers is an example of health promotion. A school nurse teaching parents about preventing childhood injuries is focusing on health protection. Teaching parents and day care providers about the importance of immunization is primary prevention, as is teaching about community resources that provide free or inexpensive immunization.

#### SECONDARY PREVENTION

Secondary prevention is teaching targeted toward early identification and intervention of a condition. A home care nurse teaching the parents of a ventilator-dependent child about early signs of upper respiratory infection and when to contact the nurse on call is focusing on secondary prevention.

#### TERTIARY PREVENTION

Most teaching in the home setting addresses tertiary prevention because most home care clients have chronic conditions. Tertiary prevention arises from teaching that attempts to restore health and facilitate coping skills (Fig. 6–4). The home care nurse provides clients with a new diagnosis of diabetes instruction in chang-

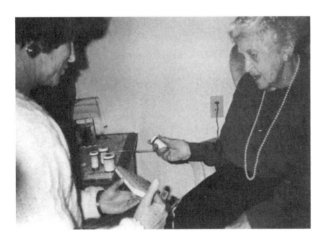

***Figure 6–4.*** ▶ Tertiary prevention involves helping restore the client to health. On this visit, the nurse uses a weekly medication container to help an older woman with limited vision devise a plan for compliance in taking her medications.

ing the diet, handling syringes, giving themselves injections, and measuring their blood sugar. Teaching family or caregivers about community resources that are available for respite care facilitates coping skills and falls in the category of tertiary prevention.

## Evaluation

The last phase of the teaching and learning process is evaluation. Both learning and teaching are evaluated to determine if the learning outcomes were met and if the teaching methods were effective. The plan is then modified as necessary.

Learning is evaluated by deciding if the learning outcomes were met. The following questions may be asked to assess the level of learning:

> What additional data do I need to collect to evaluate the progress made toward the learning objectives?
>
> What other learning needs apply to this client and family?
>
> Were the objectives met? If not, why not?
>
> How do I know that my client learned what I planned to teach?
>
> Did the timing of the teaching impede or enhance learning?
>
> Is the nurse, client, and family satisfied with the outcome? If not, what would provide satisfaction?

Second, evaluation of teaching appraises the efficacy of the teaching plan and methods. Evaluation of teaching considers the barriers to, and characteristics of, successful teaching. The nurse may ask these questions:

> Did the teaching focus on the most important problem for this family in relation to the potential of the client for self-care?
>
> Was the plan collaborative?
>
> Was there reinforcement?
>
> Was the home environment appropriate? If not, how was it modified?
>
> Was the equipment adequate?
>
> Was the nurse prepared?
>
> Did the nurse use a variety of teaching methods?
>
> Did the learner have the opportunity for hands-on practice?
>
> Was the visit structured to reduce anxiety and enhance learning?
>
> Was the teaching plan realistic?
>
> Were the learning objectives, teaching plan, and methods realistic and appropriate for this client and family?
>
> Were the family strengths considered when determining the learning objectives and teaching methods?
>
> If this session were to be repeated, which strategies or tools could be used?

Evaluation must always consider what the client and family believe they need to know, as well as what the nurse considers essential. It is also important for the nurse to recognize when the learning needs of the client, family, or caregiver are beyond the educational preparation of the nurse so that a referral to appropriate resources can be made.

## Documentation

Documentation of teaching is essential (1) as a legal record, (2) as communication of teaching and learning to other health care professionals, and (3) for determination of eligibility for care needed and for reimbursement of care provided. The following parts of the teaching process should be documented:

- ▶ Assessment of the learner's readiness, need, and life experiences
- ▶ Identification of learning needs
- ▶ Identification of barriers to successful learning
- ▶ Plan for teaching and learning outcomes
- ▶ Content taught
- ▶ Teaching techniques used
- ▶ Evaluation of teaching and learning, including learner response and recommendations for the next step

An additional component of documentation is confidentiality. Box 6–16 displays guidelines for maintaining client confidentiality.

## CLIENT SITUATIONS IN PRACTICE

### ▶ Teaching in the Home Setting

*Assessment*

Kathy is the home care nurse assigned to care for Ina, a 76-year-old widow recently diagnosed with insulin-dependent diabetes. On Friday, November 1, Ina visited the clinic with complaints of polyuria, polydipsia, and polyphagia. Her blood sugar was 456 mg/dL. The clinic educator saw her on November 1 and charted the following on the referral form:

Client stated, "I have not slept well for 2 weeks because I have to get up so often to go to the bathroom." After the initial teaching session, which covered the basics of the diabetic diet and the action of insulin, the client was unable to demonstrate retention of knowledge or skills from any of the topics covered."

## COMMUNITY-BASED NURSING CARE GUIDELINES

### Box 6–16 ▶ Confidentiality

- Maintain confidentiality in consultation, teaching, and writing.
- Ensure privacy before engaging in a discussion of content to be entered into the record.
- Release information only with written consent.
- Use professional judgment regarding confidentiality when the information may be harmful to the client's health or well-being.
- Use professional judgment when deciding how to maintain the privacy of a minor. Be aware of your state's legal ramifications of the parent or guardian's right to know.

Recommendation to home care: Client requires diabetic teaching in the areas of following a diabetic diet, drawing up insulin, giving injections, and monitoring blood sugar. Client will receive insulin in the clinic until the home visit on Tuesday to teach about injections.

Reimbursement: This client requires teaching to manage home treatment of insulin-dependent diabetes diagnosed on 11/1. This teaching meets the criteria of Section 205.13 of Medicare Guidelines for Coverage of Services Revision 222.

On Tuesday, November 5, Kathy visits Ina at home. Ina greets Kathy at the door with the statement, "When I was at the clinic on Friday, I was so nervous about all of the things they were telling me, but I am more relaxed today. I talked to my friend Richard who is a diabetic and manages really well. When my granddaughter Karen was a little girl, I gave her shots and got along just fine."

Ina's home is dark so Kathy asks if she can open the drapes and move two chairs closer to the window before they start to talk. Kathy begins visiting with Ina and attempts to begin developing a trusting relationship. Kathy learns that Ina has some knowledge about diabetes from talking to her friend Richard, and she has also asked her son Mark, who is a nurse, to pick up some pamphlets about diabetes at the hospital.

Ina states that she learns best by doing. She does not drive but states that her son will be able to pick up her medication and syringes, or she can take the bus to the pharmacy. Kathy notices a magnifying glass on the table and a large-print book on a bookshelf. Kathy asks Ina about her vision. She responds that she has had three cataract surgeries and has difficulty reading, so she frequently uses the magnifying glass.

Kathy concludes that Ina sees a need to learn and is ready to learn. Kathy also believes that Ina's past experiences will enhance her learning, not impede it. Concerned about Ina's restricted vision, Kathy makes a note to continue to assess this aspect. At this point, Kathy completes the learning assessment guide, as shown in Box 6–17.

### Identification of Learning Need

Kathy and Ina conclude that Ina's overall learning need is as follows:
*Risk for Injury related to lack of knowledge regarding diabetic self-care*
For this visit, Kathy identifies the following priority need:
*Risk for Injury related to client's lack of knowledge and inability to manage diabetes for the next 24 hours until the home visit the next day, as manifested by visual impairment*

### Planning

Kathy and Ina decide upon the following learning objectives for today:
1. Cognitive objective: Client will state when insulin is given and how much to draw up by the end of the visit on 11/5.
2. Psychomotor objective: Client will identify three sites for subcutaneous injection of insulin and demonstrate proper technique for injection by the end of the visit on 11/5.
3. Affective objective: Client will state that she is comfortable injecting insulin by the end of the visit on 11/5.

### Implementation

1. Cognitive objective: Client will state when insulin is given and how much to draw up by the end of the visit on 11/5.

## ASSESSMENT TOOLS

**Box 6–17   Sample Learning Assessment Guide**

Client name *Ina*

Health condition requiring health education *Insulin-dependent diabetes diagnosed on November 1, 2002.*

Primary caregiver *Home care nurse, client, and Mark*

Learner *Ina*                          Relationship to client _____

Age *76*                     Gender *Female*          Occupation *Retired legal secretary*

**Developmental Stages and Implications for Learner**

Psychosocial stage— *The client is in the integrity versus ego despair stage. She describes her life as follows:*

*"I have been blessed. I have 10 wonderful children, 25 grand, and 10 great-grandchildren. I loved my work after my kids grew up. My husband and I had a good relationship."*

Cognitive stage— *no evidence of cognitive impairment*

Language— *speaks English, visual impairment, stated "I was writing a novel about Ireland until I started to have problems with my eyes."*

How does the caregiver or client feel about the responsibilities of self-care?
*States she is more relaxed than 11/1 when diagnosed.*

Describe any disabilities or limitations of the learner (including sensory disabilities)
*Visual impairment and statement "I am afraid that I will not be able to see the numbers on the syringes."*

Disabilities— *arthritis in left knee and left hip*

Describe any preexisting health conditions of the learner
*Client has had multiple cataract surgeries and has visual impairment.*

List sociocultural factors that may impede learning *None*

State learner behaviors that indicate motivation to learn
*Client stated she was more relaxed about her diagnosis, asked her son to get her information about diabetes, contacted a friend with diabetes.*

Can the learner read and comprehend at the reading level required by the task? *Yes, but may not have visual acuity to see the calibrations on the syringe.*

Does the learner show an ability to problem solve at a level that provides safe care in the home?
*Client has managed health problems in her home with her granddaughter's illness 10 years ago.*

*(continued)*

**ASSESSMENT TOOLS**

Box 6–17   **Sample Learning Assessment Guide** *(Continued)*

Is the home environment conducive to the learning required by the care?
*Home is very dark with poor lighting.*

If not, what modifications are necessary?   *Need better lighting in the kitchen.*

If the learner is not able to carry out the care, are other caregivers available
for backup support?   *yes*

If so, please name.   *Mark (son), Karen (granddaughter), Richard (friend)*

Phone number   *555-5555*

Address   *3400 Belmont, White Kitty Lake, PA*

What other support is available for the client and caregiver?   *Client has ten*
*children, three of whom live in the area. Client is active in her church, which has a parish*
*nurse and a befriender program.*
*There is a support group for newly diagnosed diabetics, which meets at a hospital near*
*client's home. Client lives on the bus line with service to the clinic, hospital, and church.*

Together Kathy and Ina review the written material on insulin, when it is given,
and how much to draw up. Kathy proceeds at a slow pace as she teaches, repeats
the information frequently, and does not rush Ina. The teaching sheet is on white,
nonglossy paper with bold, black print. After the teaching session, Ina states, "Insulin should be given before meals and as the schedule states. I am to give myself
insulin according to the schedule." Kathy leaves a videotape that covers the information in the teaching session.

2. Psychomotor objective: Client will identify three sites for subcutaneous injection of insulin and demonstrate proper technique for injection by the end of
   the visit on 11/5.

Kathy demonstrates injecting the insulin into a model and identifies three sites
for subcutaneous injection. Then Ina injects into the model. Kathy draws up the insulin as ordered before dinner and Ina injects herself at 5:00. Ina is unable to see
the numbers on the syringe.

*Evaluation*

Learning objectives 1 and 2 met: Ina identifies three sites for injection and injects
herself correctly. Teaching focused on the most important problem for this client,
the plan was collaborative, and reinforcement was provided with a videotape. The
learner had the opportunity for hands-on practice, and a variety of teaching methods were used.

*Implementation*

3. Affective objective: Client will state that she is comfortable injecting insulin by
   the end of the visit on 11/5.

Ina discusses her feelings with Kathy regarding the teaching session. Kathy asks her if she feels comfortable giving herself an injection, and she says, "No, but I think it will come." Kathy leaves a short videotape on injecting insulin for Ina to review before the next visit.

### Evaluation

Learning objectives met at this time.

Teaching: Kathy encourages Ina by stating how well she has done the first time handling the syringe. Kathy tells Ina specifically what she did well: she did not hesitate before putting in the needle, she found a correct site, and she charted it accurately on the flow sheet. However, she is unable to identify the correct number of units on the syringe. She adds this objective to the list of the next lesson's objectives.

### Assessment and Planning for the Next Teaching Session

Kathy noted Ina's problems with her eyesight in the initial assessment, suggesting that Ina might have difficulty drawing up insulin with a syringe. Kathy discussed her concern with Ina and asked to come back the next day. She also asked Ina if there was a friend or family member who might be available to assist with her care. Ina responded that her son Mark had indicated that he was willing to help with the injections. Kathy requested that Ina contact Mark and ask that he be present at the next home visit.

### Identification of Learning Need

Together, Kathy and Ina decided on the following learning need for the home visit the next day:

> ▶ Risk for Injury related to client's lack of knowledge and inability to read the calibrations on the syringe, as manifested by client's statement, "I have to use the magnifying glass to see print. I can't see the numbers on the syringes. Is it okay if I just estimate?"

### Planning

Kathy and Ina decided that the learning objectives for tomorrow would be as follows:

1. Cognitive objective: Client will state when insulin is given, how much to draw up, and how to use the Magni-Guide syringe.
2. Psychomotor objective: Client will demonstrate how to draw up an accurate amount of insulin with the Magni-Guide syringe.
3. Affective objective: Client will state that she feels confident in her ability to draw up an accurate amount of insulin.

As Kathy leaves Ina's home, Ina hugs her and says, "Thanks for all your help today. You have helped me so much!"

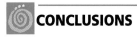

## CONCLUSIONS

Because of circumstances in the current health care system, quality teaching has become essential. There are benefits to quality teaching in all settings. Good teaching improves client self-care and independence. Client, family, and staff satisfaction is improved if teaching results are positive. Another benefit to quality instruction is the more efficient use of resources.

Avoiding barriers and incorporating characteristics of successful teaching can enhance teaching in community-based nursing. Including learning theory in community-based teaching ensures quality instruction. Comprehensive assessment of the client and family safeguards accurate identification of learning needs. Collaborative planning preserves successful learning outcomes because clients and families are more likely to learn when they have participated in the planning. Following these principles protects the teaching process in community settings.

The first and most important goal of teaching in community-based care is to assist the client and family to achieve independence in self-care. Self-care is provided in the context of the values and resources of the client and family with a prevention focus. Continuity requires documentation and interdisciplinary communication, which augment teaching efficacy. Successful teaching in community-based care meets all of these goals.

# What's on the Web

Centers for Disease Control and Prevention (CDC)
**Internet address:** *www.cdc.gov*
This site offers abundant resources about topics related to disease prevention and health promotion. You can find information on any health topic on the Health

Topics A–Z site.
**Internet address:** *www.cdc.gov/ publications.htm*
This CDC site offers an unlimited number of publications, software, and other products for teaching or research.
**Internet address:**
*www.cdc.gov/aboutcdc.htm*
This site outlines all of the components of the CDC and the centers to assist you to find teaching materials for various topics.

Healthfinders
**Internet Address**:
*http://www.healthfinder.gov/*

This is your guide to reliable health information with three versions of the site, one for consumers and professional health providers, one for children, and one in Spanish. Each site includes a health library, health topics, information about health care providers, and a directory of healthfinder organizations.

Mayo Clinic
**Internet Address:** *http://www.mayo.edu*
This site has reliable information for a healthier life. You can find information quickly on the A–Z index of various conditions. You can also ask a specialist any questions that you may have about your client's conditions. There are timely topics, as well as slides on various subjects— lots of materials to use as you teach in community-based settings.

## References and Bibliography

Barry, C. (2000). Teaching the older client in the home: Assessment and adaptation. *Home Healthcare Nurse, 18*(6), 374–385.

Carpenito, L. J. (2002). *Nursing diagnosis: Application to clinical practice* (9th ed.). Philadelphia: Lippincott Williams & Wilkins.

Consumer Health Information Corporation (CHIP). (2001). Preventing home medication errors. Retrieved January 17, 2003, from http://www.consumer-health. com/services/cons-preventerrors. htm

Dunn, C. (2002). Assessing and preventing medication interactions. *Home Healthcare Nurse, 20*(2), 104–111.

Effective medication counseling: 26 steps. (2000). *Home Healthcare Nurse, 18*(3), 157–160.

Haynes, R., Montague, P., Oliver, T., Mckibbon, K., Brouwers, M., & Kanani, R. (2000). Interventions for helping patients to follow prescriptions for medications. *The Cochrane Library, 2,* 2000. Oxford: Update Software.

Jarvis, C. (1996). *Physical examination and health assessment* (2nd ed.). Philadelphia: Saunders.

Knox, A. B. (1986). *Helping adults learn.* San Francisco: Jossey-Bass.

Leske, J., & Pelczynski, S. (1999). Caregiver satisfaction with preparation for discharge in a decreased-length-of-stay cardiac surgery program. *Journal of Cardiovascular Nursing, 14*(1), 35.

London, F. (1999). *A nurse's guide to patient and family education.* Philadelphia: Lippincott Williams & Wilkins.

London, F. (2001). Take the frustration out of patient education. *Home Healthcare Nurse, (19)*3, 158–163.

Long, C., Ismeurt, R., & White, P. (1999). Preventing drug interactions in the home: A five-step approach for client teaching. *Home Healthcare Nurse, 17*(2), 106–112.

Magoon, L. (2002). Parents and medication errors. *American Journal of Nursing, 102*(9), 24A–24C.

O'Conner-Von, S. (2001). *Preparation of adolescents for outpatient surgery: A comparison of methods.* Unpublished doctoral dissertation. Rush University of Chicago, Illinois.

Rubin, R. (1961). Basic maternal behavior. *Nursing Outlook, 9,* 683–684.

Salmore, R., & Nelson, J. (2000). The effect of preprocedure teaching, relaxation instruction, and music on anxiety as measured by blood pressures in an outpatient gastrointestinal endoscopy laboratory. *Gastroenterology Nursing, 23*(3), 102–110. Retrieved January 18, 2003, from the CINAHL database.

Sitzman, K. (2001). Tips for teaching older adults. *Home Healthcare Nurse, 19*(3), 141.

Stanley, M., & Beare, P. (1999). *Gerontological nursing: A health promotion/protection approach* (2nd ed.). Philadelphia: Davis.

Steps for effective medication counseling. (2000). *Home Healthcare Nurse, 18*(3), 157–160.

Stone, J., Wyman, J., & Salisbury, S. (1999). *Clinical gerontological nursing* (2nd ed.). Philadelphia: Saunders.

Taylor, C., Lillis, C., & LeMone, P. (2001). *Fundamentals of nursing: The art and science of nursing care* (4th ed.). Philadelphia: Lippincott Williams & Wilkins.

Weber, J. (2001). *Nurses' handbook of health assessment* (4th ed.). Philadelphia: Lippincott Williams & Wilkins.

Wilson, A. H. & Robledo, L. (1999). Role play. Listening to Hispanic mothers: Guidelines for teaching. *Journal of Society of Pediatric Nurses, 4*(3), 125–127.

# L E A R N I N G   A C T I V I T I E S

## JOURNALING: ACTIVITY 6–1

1. In your clinical journal, discuss a situation in your clinical experience in which you observed or were the caretaker for someone who had several teaching needs. Outline the process used to assess, plan, and teach the client and family members.
2. Using theory from this chapter, identify what was successful and what was not successful related to teaching and learning for this client and family.
3. What would you do differently next time? From this experience, what did you learn about yourself and teaching clients and families?

## CLIENT CARE: ACTIVITY 6–2

Jennifer is a nurse working on a postpartum unit. She is caring for Joan, a 35-year-old primipara (normal spontaneous vaginal delivery [NSVD]), who delivered a boy yesterday and is going home at noon today. Joan states she has been working full time since she graduated from law school. She is the youngest of three siblings. She and her husband Tim took prenatal classes, and she describes him as being very excited about the baby.

Jennifer interviewed Joan and Tim to determine their learning needs. They both tell Jennifer that they are wondering about having their baby circumcised. They also wonder how they are going to take care of the surgery site after the procedure on their newborn. Joan had a sitz bath and pain medication 45 minutes ago. Both parents have good eye contact and relaxed postures as Jennifer interviewed them.

1. Determine the behaviors that show that Joan and Tim are ready to learn.
2. List the factors Jennifer should assess regarding Joan and Tim's readiness to learn.
3. Recognize what indicates to Jennifer that Joan and Tim show a need to learn.
4. Examine Joan and Tim's prior experience and knowledge base related to the topic.
5. Identify Joan and Tim's learning need in each domain: cognitive, affective, and psychomotor.
6. State one learning outcome for Joan and Tim for each learning need.
7. Discuss how the principles of community-based care apply to the learning needs of Joan and Tim.

## CLIENT CARE: ACTIVITY 6–3

Hazel is a 65-year-old woman whose husband is blind and was recently diagnosed with early signs of dementia. Shannon is doing preadmission teaching with Hazel, who is scheduled for outpatient surgery tomorrow morning. Shannon knows it is important to assess Hazel's readiness to learn. If Hazel is thinking about her husband's care during the time she is preparing for surgery, she may not hear Shannon tell her that she should not drive or make important decisions for at least 24 hours after receiving general anesthesia.

Explain how Shannon will assess Hazel's readiness to learn.

## PRACTICAL APPLICATION: ACTIVITY 6–4

Volunteer to teach a health-related class at a local elementary, middle, or high school. Ask the school nurse or the class teacher to recommend a topic, or go to the class and survey the students to find out what topics they would like to cover. Use the content in this chapter to plan and develop the class. After you teach the students, use some of the following questions to evaluate your class.

- Were the objectives met? If not, why not?
- How do you know that students learned what you planned to teach?
- Did the timing of the teaching impede or enhance learning?
- Were the students satisfied with the outcome? If not, what would provide satisfaction?
- Did the teaching focus on the most important problem for the students?
- Was the plan collaborative?
- Was there reinforcement?
- Was the environment appropriate? If not, how was it modified?
- Was the equipment adequate?
- Were you prepared?
- Did you use a variety of teaching methods?
- Did learners have the opportunity for hands-on practice?
- Was the session structured to reduce anxiety and enhance learning?
- Was the teaching plan realistic?
- Were the learning objectives, teaching plan, and methods realistic and appropriate for students?
- If this session were to be repeated, what other strategies or tools could be used?

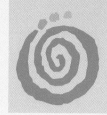

# CHAPTER **7**

# Case Management

Roberta Hunt

**THE NURSING STUDENT SPEAKS**

While working in the community setting, I learned a lot about nursing presence. I had read about it but had never seen the power of it until I was working at the shelter. I realize that listening to someone is important, but what caring does is amazing. Some of the people I worked with never had anyone willing to listen to them. There was always some reason they couldn't talk to people in their lives. Their relationships were just a mess. They were always hiding something from somebody or they were in an abusive relationship. They didn't have anyone that would sit down and listen to them without getting into an argument. Nursing presence is so powerful.

During postclinical discussion one day, a resident came in to talk to us. She was one of my classmate's clients. She praised the nursing student she was meeting with. She talked about how her life had turned around when she started seeing this student. Somebody cared and was helping her, probably for the first time. All this nursing student had done was listen and point the client in a few directions. The student had really done very little time-wise, and yet it was so powerful.

— **Brende Radford, RN**
  Student completing a BSN
  The College of St. Catherine

 **SIGNIFICANCE OF CASE MANAGEMENT**

In this era of short length of stay in acute settings, where clients are discharged sooner than ever before, case management has become an even more important aspect of community-based nursing care. However, it is not a new concept to nursing in community settings. The origins of this intervention date back to the turn of the century, when nurses staffed settlement houses. An article by Tahan (1998, p. 56) describes a system of cards used by nurses at the settlement houses, which stated that the duties of the staff were to " . . . list family needs, establish a mechanism for follow-up, facilitate the delivery of services and ensure that families were connected with appropriate resources."

This same focus on a continuum of care was used to facilitate the return of discharged World War II soldiers to civilian life (Lyon, 1993). Other examples of this framework are seen in the management of clients with long-term rehabilitation needs. The concept of case management as it is commonly thought of today springs from the insurance industry's interest in cost containment. Case management is now common in a variety of settings and situations as more health care is provided in the community.

 **DEFINITIONS AND MODELS**

**Case management,** also known as care management or **care coordination,** is a complex concept with many definitions. This often leads to confusion about what is the correct or best definition. Case management is defined by the American

Nurses Association (ANA) as "an organized system or process for delivering health care to a client or group of clients, including assessment, development of a plan of care, initiation and coordination of referrals and services, and evaluation of care" (ANA, 1999, p. 19). According to Mitchell and Reaghard (1996), the purpose of case management is to serve as a client advocate by enhanced coordination of services.

Although numerous definitions of case management exist, the goals typically aim to achieve a balance between quality and cost. These goals include the following:

- Improve the quality of client care by emphasizing the importance of health restoration and maintenance and increased continuity of care
- Decrease the cost of care by empowering clients and their families to maximize self-care capabilities and prevent unnecessary or lengthy admissions
- Improve client, nurse, and physician satisfaction and professional development by promoting multidisciplinary collaborative practice and coordinated care (Lee, Mackenzie, Dudley-Brown, & Chin, 1998)

Note how closely these goals parallel those of community-based nursing, which are to facilitate continuity and self-care in the context of the clients, family, culture, and community by considering the principles of disease prevention, health promotion, and collaboration.

Case management results in direct outcomes for the client and family. First of all, case management facilitates the provision of information about health benefits, service parameters, the disease process, and plan of treatment for clients and families. Successful case management involves the client in the decisions and actions of self-care. Case management allows for realistic evaluation in cases where there is low adherence to treatment plans. Finally, case managers provide consistency of care across the continuum of care (Zink, 2001).

There are several case management models. Understanding these may help clarify why the case manager has one set of responsibilities in one situation and a different set in another. The **brokerage model** defines the role of the case manager as a coordinator of care, mediating among all parties. The **interdisciplinary team model,** built on the concept of collaboration, allows each professional on the team to offer his or her particular specialty. One member of the team is often the primary or lead manager, usually depending on the needs of the client (Chan, Mackenzie, Tin-Fu, Leung, & Ka-yi, 2000).

In some models, unlicensed assistive personnel provide care, with the nurse acting as case manager. In these models, appropriate delegation is the key element. This text will primarily focus on the foundational models—the interdisciplinary team model and the models that use the nurse as care manager of nonprofessional caregivers.

In some settings, a case manager's only role is to manage a number of cases, whereas in other settings the nurse has many roles, with case manager being one. For example, a nurse working in an emergency department (ED) may function as a staff nurse and also call clients for follow-up the day after their ED visit. A home care nurse may be the client's case manager, as well as the direct care provider and health educator. The ways this role is operationalized differ by geographic area, provider, payment restriction, and setting.

Thus, case management is a term with many definitions and implementation models. In community-based care, case management is the vehicle to care coordi-

---

### ► Box 7–1   Steps of Case Management ◄

1. Involve clients and families in assessing their level of functioning.
2. Determine the resources and services necessary to maximize quality of life.
3. Involve clients and families in identifying, exploring, and accessing available resources.
4. Have clients and families identify the most appropriate referral for their needs.
5. Make referrals and supply services with needed information.
6. Act as an advocate or troubleshooter as necessary.
7. Evaluate progress toward the health outcomes and revise plan accordingly.

---

nation and continuity of care. Some argue that the nurse is the best professional to act as a case manager for clients in all health care settings (Kesby, 2002).

To accomplish this end, the nurse uses collaboration, consultation, delegation, advocacy, referral, and follow-up. Case management in community-based settings reflects a commitment to facilitate self-care in the context of the client's family, culture, and community.

## NURSING SKILLS AND COMPETENCIES IN CASE MANAGEMENT

Case management follows several prescribed steps similar to the nursing process (Box 7–1). It is essential to assess the client's level of functioning to determine the resources and services necessary to maximize quality of life. The nurse involves the client and family in the design and implementation of the plan of care. Collaboration plays a central role in coordinating the services as the nurse serves as client advocate, troubleshooting to resolve barriers. Last of all, progress toward achievement of outcomes is evaluated, revising the plan accordingly.

Case management has long been an important role for the nurse providing care in community settings. Betsy Rodgers explored what nurses who work in the community say about care coordination, from old letters by Lillian Wald and Mary Brewster, nurses who worked in the settlement houses in New York City at the turn of the century, to nurses currently practicing. She studied stories of these case managers through old records and interviews with practicing nurses. The nurse–client relationship and outside connections were the central elements to successful care coordination (Rodgers, 2000). Box 7–2 summarizes Rodgers's research.

### Forming the Nurse–Client Relationship

According to Rodgers's research, several components work together to build the nurse–client relationship. The first is establishing a pact in which the relationship becomes the foundation of coordination (Fig. 7–1).

> ► **Box 7–2**   Essentials of Care Coordination ◄

**Nurse–Client Relationship**

Establishing a pact
Talking and listening
Building trust
Giving back control
Holding it together
Dealing with absent families

**Outside Connections**

Nurse's knowledge of the community
Effort beyond the job description
Optimization of the client's environment

—————

Adapted from Rodgers, B. (2000). Coordination of care: The lived experience of the visiting nurse. *Home Healthcare Nurse, 18*(3), 301–307.

> ► I don't care what color you are, or where you come from or who you are or where you have been in your life, if you are my patient, I am going to do the very best that I can. I have a commitment. It's like when you walk into somebody's home and you form a bond with that person. It's like a pact that I'm going to be there for you until you die, and I'm going to take you through it, we're going to go through it together. (Rodgers, 2000, p. 303)

The second theme within the nurse–client relationship is talking and listening. Most basic to good therapeutic communication, listening allows the nurse to assess the client's most immediate needs and is often a powerful nursing intervention.

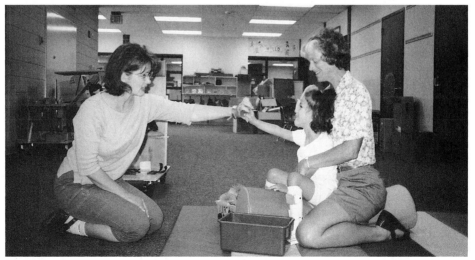

*Figure 7–1.* ►  A strong and trusting nurse–client relationship is the foundation of coordinated care.

> ▶ **Box 7–3** Trust-Building Strategies ◀
>
> - Begin cultivating the client's trust with the first contact.
> - Establish credibility with the client.
> - Use an empathic, nonjudgmental approach.
> - Guard the client's privacy.
> - Expect testing behavior from clients.
> - Learn to trust the client.
> - Persevere with the nurse–client relationship.
>
> ———
> Wendt, D. (1996). Building trust during the initial home visit. In R. Hunt (Ed.), *Readings in community-based nursing* (pp. 154–160). Philadelphia: Lippincott Williams & Wilkins.

> ▶ Five years ago, my baby daughter died of SIDS. The nurse in the clinic just sat with me and let me cry. That was so helpful. I will always be thankful that she took the time to sit with me. (Julie, a nursing student)

Building trust is the third element found in Rodgers's research. Box 7–3 presents strategies to build trust.

Giving back control is the next step in forging the nurse–client relationship. From the first chapter, this text has emphasized mutual care planning and self-care. The ultimate in successful nursing care is the plan that leads the client to independent self-care.

The fifth component of the nurse–client relationship found in Rodgers's research is holding it all together. This may seem like an almost impossible task for some of the complex individuals and families we care for in community settings.

> ▶ Jack is one of the more difficult clients I have ever cared for. He is 80 years old with very brittle diabetes. His wife died last year. She was the one who could drive, cook, and check his blood sugar. His daughter said she would help by dropping by with a meal every day. He has refused Meals On Wheels, says that welfare is for old people, and will only eat what his daughter brings for him. Now his daughter is in the hospital having a spinal fusion, so I don't think he is eating. I am trying to problem solve with him about alternatives, hoping we will be able to uncover an option he is comfortable with before he ends up back in the hospital. (Kathy, a home health care nurse)

The last theme in care coordination considers the nurse–client relationship when the family is absent. It is not uncommon for family members to become estranged from one another or unable or unwilling to assist one another during illness. In some situations, when an individual has a chronic illness over a long period of time, everyone is exhausted from managing the work of the illness. In other cases, estrangement may have continued for many years.

> ▶ Ernest has no family or social support. He has three children, but they all live on the West Coast. Ernest and his wife separated 15 years ago because of his substance abuse. When we called to see if she would be able to assist with his care, she gave the nurse an earful! His family has been totally unwilling to assist with his care. (Phyllis, a home care nurse)

## Outside Connections: Working With Community Resources

The second pattern that emerged from Rodgers's research involves community connections essential to providing effective care management. The nurse must know the community and the resources available within it. Often nurses in community settings act as client advocates or participate in activities that may not be in their job descriptions. Several factors are essential for outside connections to result in care coordination.

The first factor is the nurse's knowledge about the community. To provide comprehensive, coordinated care, the nurse must know the client, the client's family and culture, and the broader community in which they live. To make appropriate referrals to ensure continuity, the nurse must know what services are available. For these outside connections to be accessed, the client and family first must know about the service and then must be willing to accept help.

> I had been making home visits to a client after the birth of her twins. She was about to be evicted from her home. Her relationship with the father of her babies was volatile. He was not living with her and not supportive. Every visit, she talked about the lack of progress she had made in finding a place to live. "Nobody will take someone with five kids," she would say over and over again. "I am going to be homeless with my kids," she exclaimed. In our community, there is virtually no low-cost housing. We had explored every option available to her, with no success. One day, when I went to make my weekly home visit and weigh the twins, she didn't answer the door. I could hear the kids inside and knew she must be home. I knocked and waited. She finally opened the door. Both of her eyes were black, and her face was bruised and swollen. She shamefully said, "He beat me up in front of the kids. I am never going to see him again, but I have no place to go." I knew about special housing available in our county for those experiencing domestic violence. I explained to her that she would have to go to a shelter for domestic abuse, but from there she could get into the housing program. Her mother helped her pack up her kids, and she moved to the shelter the next day. (Mary, a senior nursing student)

Another element of community connections is client advocacy. **Client advocacy** is defined as intervening for or acting on behalf of the client to provide the highest quality health care obtainable. Sometimes our health care system is characterized as uncaring, impersonal, and fragmented. Clients become frustrated, often feeling devalued and unable to cope with the system. A community-based nurse acts as an advocate for the client and family, providing information to the client to help ensure uninterrupted care. In many situations, the client is vulnerable, which often results in the nurse contacting a community service, other caregivers, or a physician on the client's behalf.

For example, a school nurse notices that a 13-year-old child often comes to the nurse's office on Monday mornings complaining of a stomachache. When the girl comes in for the third week in a row, the nurse asks her, "Tell me about your weekend." The child starts crying and says, "My dad doesn't live with us anymore. My mom drinks beer and yells at me." The nurse and the child discuss the child's feelings and fears about her family situation. Then the nurse explains to the child that with her permission, she would like to talk to the school counselor about their conversation, to learn about some groups that may help her. Second, the nurse tells the child that she would like to call her mom and talk to the two of them about her stomachaches. In this situation, the nurse is acting as an advocate for the child, with the goal of facilitating self-care in the context of the student's family. The nurse is collaborating with other professionals to enhance care.

The client advocate role involves informing clients about the nature of their health problems and the choices they have in seeking to resolve or alter their health care needs. This role is activated whenever clients are unable to take responsibility for their own health care, lack knowledge or skill, or do not have the financial or emotional basis from which to act. The advocacy role is also one of support after clients have been informed, made choices, and need to implement these choices. Clients have an inherent right to make their own decisions and to take responsibility for those decisions. The nurse lends support and respect for clients, whether or not the nurse agrees with their decisions.

To advocate for clients, the nurse must consider all aspects of the clients' lives. Advocacy is often used with vulnerable populations who have a weak voice within a system. Some people, because of age, cognitive abilities, lack of sophistication, or other factors need assistance in speaking for themselves. Clarification of a do-not-resuscitate order on behalf of an elderly client who is unaware of the need to explicitly state his or her preference is one example of a nurse acting as a client advocate.

Sometimes visiting nurses do things that are an extension of their usual role responsibilities, as Rodgers's research revealed. For example, Celia is 62 years old, living at home alone in her apartment. She has diabetes and had surgery last month for breast cancer. She just started chemotherapy this week. She takes the bus to an outpatient clinic for her treatment, but she must pick up her insulin at a drugstore that is six blocks away and not on a bus line. She would like to get her medication at the pharmacy at the outpatient clinic, but her insurance company will pay only if she fills it at the drugstore. Her home health care nurse knows that the insurance company makes exceptions in some situations. She calls the customer relations representative at the insurance company and arranges for Celia to pick up her medication at the outpatient clinic.

Health is related to the environment, and sometimes our environment is detrimental to our health. Chapter 6 discussed the benefits of altering the environment to enhance learning. The same is true with case management because the nurse may use interventions that indirectly affect the client or family's health. For example, with the client's consent, the nurse arranges for the home health aide to dispose of piles of old magazines and papers. This eliminates a fire hazard, prevents a potential fall, and may improve the client's psychologic status by making the environment more pleasant.

## Intervention Strategies

Several intervention strategies that have not been discussed may enhance case management. They include case finding, referral and follow-up, collaboration, consultation, and delegation.

### Case Finding

**Case finding** is a set of activities used by the nurse working in community settings that identifies clients who are not currently receiving health care but could benefit from such care. The nurse, of all members of the interdisciplinary team, usually has the most contact with the client and family. This contact allows the nurse to assess and identify client service needs that, if addressed, would enhance care coordination or case management. In some cases, this may be a simple process, with the nurse making one contact or giving the client one suggested referral. Case finding happens in every setting where care is provided, and it requires an open attitude and skillful assessment by the nurse.

### Referral and Follow-up

**Referral and follow-up** is the process by which nurses in all settings assist individuals and families in identifying and accessing community resources to prevent, promote, or maintain health. To be skilled in this competency, the nurse must know the community and the resources available in it. Obviously, just knowing what resources are present in the community is only the first step. For example, when caring for a client who has just had a knee replacement, the nurse learns that the client lives alone and does not have friends or family living nearby. It will be difficult for the client to cook for several weeks. Giving the client the telephone number for Meals On Wheels is one nursing intervention. In addition, the client is concerned about getting to the grocery store. There is a grocery delivery service that has a reduced rate for senior citizens. A second intervention is giving the client the name and telephone number of the service. Box 7–4 lists the steps in the referral process. Chapter 8, Continuity of Care, provides a more in-depth discussion of the referral process.

### Collaboration

Frequently a client requires services from many different disciplines. The case manager often initiates referrals and requests these services. Some of the various professionals the nurse will work with are physicians, social workers, nutritionists, physical and occupational therapists, and pharmacists. One of the many roles the case manager must assume is that of collaborator. **Collaboration** means working jointly with others in a common endeavor—to cooperate as partners (Allender & Spradley, 2001). It takes a team effort to care for a client well, and the team leader is often the nurse. The nurse must take the following steps of coordinating multiple disciplines to facilitate continuity of care:

- ▶ Notify all disciplines involved when there is a change in the client's health.
- ▶ Coordinate visits with the client to avoid two professionals visiting at the same time and tiring the client.
- ▶ Integrate services to provide maximum benefit to the client; for example, have the physical therapist measure blood pressure when he or she visits the home to ambulate the client.
- ▶ Problem solve jointly with other team members and include the client when appropriate.

## COMMUNITY-BASED NURSING CARE GUIDELINES

**Box 7–4** ▶ Steps in the Referral Process

1. Establish the need for referral.
2. Set objectives for the referral.
3. Explore the resources that are available.
4. Have the client make decisions concerning the referral.
5. Make the referral to the selected service.
6. Supply the agency with needed information.
7. Support the client and family in pursuing the referral.

The role of the case manager is often viewed as that of a gatekeeper. Often the manager is a broker for services. For example, Margaret, an occupational health nurse who served worker's compensation clients, described her role as "interpreting the insurance company's medical information and working with health care providers to find the most efficient means of helping people return to the workplace." Other nurse case managers describe their roles as "assessing and evaluating delivery systems and benefit criteria . . . making sure that resources are available . . . stretching the dollar . . . client advocacy . . . and making sure the client and family are fully involved in the decision and care."

### Consultation

**Consultation** is an interactive problem-solving process between the nurse and the client. From a list of alternative options generated by the nurse and client, the client selects those most appropriate for the situation. The case manager uses basic steps in the consultation intervention (Box 7–5).

### Delegation

Delegation is a key intervention in successful case management. **Delegation** is a management principle used to obtain desired results through the work of others and is a legal concept used to empower one person to act for another (National

---

▶ **Box 7–5** **Steps in Consultation for the Case Manager** ◀

1. Establish a trusting relationship with the client and family.
2. Clarify the client's perception of the problem, causes, and anticipated results.
3. Assess all issues in a mutual process with the client.
   - Determine the impact the issue has on the client's experience.
   - Identify everyone involved in the issue and how they are affected.
   - Determine how the client and family's attitudes, beliefs, and behaviors may be contributing to the issues.
   - Explore environmental aspects.
   - Identify strengths and barriers for the client and family.
   - Anticipate what may be gained or lost by solving or addressing the issue.
   - Consider how a solution might affect the client and family.
4. Through mutual planning, the nurse and client perform the following functions:
   - Identify the desired outcome.
   - Consider the advantages and disadvantages of each.
   - Support the client as they choose the preferred option.
5. Determine support essential to facilitate implementing the plan.
6. Evaluate the process and outcome.

Adapted from Minnesota Department of Health, Section of Public Health Nursing. (2000). *Public health nursing interventions II. Basic steps to the consultation intervention.* Minneapolis: Author.

Council of State Boards of Nursing [NCSBN], 1997). **Unlicensed assistive personnel** (UAP) are any unlicensed workers, regardless of title, to whom nursing tasks are delegated (NCSBN, 1997). As more UAP are providing care to individuals in community settings, the case manager becomes central to the issues related to delegation.

According to the NCSBN (1997), all decisions related to delegation of nursing activities must be based on the fundamental principle of public protection. Licensed nurses have the ultimate accountability for the management and provision of nursing care, including all delegated decisions and tasks. This accountability is outlined in the Five Rights of Delegation, shown in Box 7–6.

### Managed Care Skills

Managed care is an organized system of health care that carefully plans and monitors the use of health care services so that standards are met while costs are minimized (Ludwig-Beymer, 1999). Many health maintenance organizations (HMOs) and insurance companies use managed care. Preferred provider organizations (PPOs) are another form of a managed care organization. An increasing segment of the population receives health care through managed care. Box 7–7 lists skills needed for nurses to work effectively in a managed care environment.

Often a nurse is the person responsible for evaluating what care is necessary. Sometimes this puts the nurse in the difficult position of seeing firsthand the needs of the client but discovering that coverage limitations of the managed care contract prohibit the provision of the needed care. Sometimes, this is the point where the nurse acts as an advocate for the client to secure the service.

### Documentation

Documentation of care management is essential as a legal document, as means of communication to other health care professions and UAP, and for determination of eligibility of care.

## BARRIERS TO SUCCESSFUL CASE MANAGEMENT

There are countless barriers to successful case management, all contributing to lack of continuity for the client and family. One barrier is the lack of a consistent definition of case management. With so many definitions, case management is not a concept that is easily understood or operationalized. Because it is not easily understood, nurses may not know where their job responsibilities begin and end related to case management. There are numerous models of case management, adding to the confusion about who does what for the client and when is it done.

A second barrier to case management is lack of time. Each year, with cost-containment concerns dictating who gets what care, nurses in all settings are pressed to care for more clients with more complex needs. "The problem is that it's hard for case managers to focus on the tasks of the day and get patients through episodes of care if they're also trying to run teams and coordinate data" (Moore, 1999, p. 28). In these situations, only the most essential and immediate aspects of care are addressed.

Lack of preparation for the case manager role is another barrier. There is little literature on how to best prepare nurses for this role. Often, case management is a minor aspect of theory content and absent altogether from clinical experiences in nursing programs.

> ▶ **Box 7–6**   The Five Rights of Delegation ◀

1. **Right task**

   Is this a task that may be delegated?
   - Depending on the state, assessment may or may not be delegated to others.
   - Does the task require extensive training to reliably, consistently, and safely perform it? If so, it should not be delegated.
   - Does the task require alteration based on the client response during the task? If so, this need for professional judgment deems that the task should not be delegated.

2. **Right circumstances**

   Are the care settings, available resources, and other relevant factors conducive to ensuring client safety?
   - Is there potential for harm to the client?
   - Is the complexity of the nursing activity low?
   - Are problem-solving and innovation requirements minimal?
   - Is the outcome of the task predictable?
   - Is there ample opportunity for client interaction?
   - Is an RN available to adequately supervise?

3. **Right person**

   Is the right person delegating the right task to the right person to be performed with the right client?
   - An RN may delegate all functions to another RN as long as that individual agrees.
   - Others to whom an RN delegates should have reasonable knowledge, training, and experience to ensure consistent and safe performance of the task.
   - Likewise, an RN should not accept the responsibility for carrying out tasks for which he or she has not had the proper training or experience to ensure safe and effective care.
   - The client's stability and response to the task must be predictable and not require professional judgment for the administrator to respond effectively.

4. **Right direction/communication**

   Are expectations clearly and concisely stated, including objectives, limits, and expectations?
   - If the task is new to the RN or developmental in nature or if the description requires complex or multiple steps, the task is probably not delegable.

5. **Right supervision**
   - Is the supervising RN accessible for answering questions and directly supervising?
   - Are appropriate monitoring, evaluation, and feedback activities ensured? As a rule, the more complex the task, the less experienced the delegate should be, and the more unstable or unresponsive the client, the closer the supervising RN should be.

---

Adapted from Minnesota Department of Health, Section of Public Health Nursing. (2000). *Public health nursing interventions II. The five rights of delegation*[AQ] . Minneapolis: Author.

Adapted from National Council of State Boards of Nursing. (1997). *The Delegation Resource Folder* [Data file]. Available from http://www.ncsbn.org/regulation/vap_delegation_documents_delegation.asp.

---

▶ **Box 7–7   Skills Needed by Nurses ◀
in a Managed Care Environment**

- Negotiation skills
- Delegation skills
- Ability to analyze care in terms of cost and benefit
- Ability to understand the process of care provision across the continuum
- Ability to look at and predict outcomes
- Ability to collect and evaluate outcome data
- Business understanding, or ability to understand and use financial data
- Advocacy skills
- Assessment skills
- Ethical decision-making skills
- Collaboration skills

Kersbergen, A. (2000). Managed care shifts health care from an altruistic model to a business framework. *Nursing and Health Care Perspectives, 21*(2), 81–83.

---

 **ELEMENTS OF SUCCESSFUL CASE MANAGEMENT**

Successful case management requires the nurse to function as an interdisciplinary team member who furnishes the link between the referral source and the client. An ED in Alabama is using case managers in a multidisciplinary team with clients with asthma. A standardized care plan and follow-up telephone calls have resulted in a decreased length of stay and fewer repeat visits by clients receiving the case management care (Zimmerman & Pierce, 1998). In addition, staff members consult the ED case manager when patterns of frequent visits result from nonadherence with treatment or drug-seeking behavior.

Another ED works to manage care at both admission and discharge. At admission, for clients who are denied care at that facility but must go to another for the presenting condition, the nurse provides the client with information that lists treatment sites, reinforces the information, and verifies that the client knows the location. At discharge, the case manager provides for client needs, whether a home health referral or follow-up physician referral is given. This model has improved customer relations as well as appropriate utilization of community services (Zimmerman & Pierce, 1998).

Successful case management programs demonstrate that with nursing leadership, client outcomes and quality of care can be enhanced by following the basic interventions of case management. Box 7–8 presents an example of nursing research related to interdisciplinary case management.

### Case Management and Self-Care

The community-based nurse must be able to understand what promotes and what inhibits the abilities of others. This is evident when the nurse recognizes the ability of a client to irrigate and dress his or her own wound. Using this as a starting

## RESEARCH IN COMMUNITY-BASED NURSING CARE

**Box 7–8** ▶ Effect of a Standardized Case Management Telephone Intervention by Nurses on Resource Use in Clients with Chronic Heart Failure

Although it is believed that case management promotes continuity of care and decreased hospitalization rates, few case control studies have tested this approach. This study assessed the effectiveness of a standardized case management intervention, using telephone calls to decrease resource use in clients with chronic heart failure. Clients were identified while hospitalized and assigned to either the treatment group or the control group. For 6 months the treatment group received telephone case management by a nurse using a support software program. The nurse called them 5 days after discharge and more or less frequently depending on the symptoms they reported. Case managers also spoke to family members, other professionals (eg, physicians, dietitians, social workers, and physical therapists), and individuals from community agencies in the course of case management. Printed educational materials were mailed to those in the treatment group on a monthly basis. Those in the treatment group, who received standardized telephone calls from an RN case manager, required significantly fewer resources over the 6 months of the study. Significant cost savings were demonstrated with this intervention. The cost of acute care for each client in the usual care group was $2,186, while the average cost per client in the intervention group was only $1,192. This difference computes to about $1,000 less per client over the 6 months of the study. This savings is more than twice the cost of the intervention, which was $443 per patient for the 6-month case management intervention. It is important to note that few other investigators have scientifically tested an intervention of this type with chronically ill populations despite the fact that telephone case management is used widely in disease management programs across the country.

Source: Riegel, B., Carlson, B., Kopp, Z., LePetri, Glaser, D., & Unger, A. (2002). Effect of a standardized nurse case-management telephone intervention on resource use in patients with chronic heart failure. *Archives of Internal Medicine, 162*(6), 705–712.

point, the nurse coaches and encourages the client to take charge of his or her own care. The nurse also uses the techniques of establishing trust, making appropriate referrals, advocating, consulting, and collaborating to facilitate self-care.

## Case Management and Prevention

Significant economic changes in health care have dramatically altered the role of the nurse. Large areas of responsibility are delegated to nurses' aides, who, on the average, have 6 weeks or less of training. Nursing care in the acute and long-term care settings and in home health care is being assigned to less-prepared providers, families, and UAP.

The case management model of care delivery places a large burden on the RN who works in community-based care. People living with a chronic condition often require a great deal of assistance with health promotion to help maximize the quality of their lives. Because chronic diseases are the major cause of morbidity and mortality in developed countries, nurses are increasingly involved with illness prevention and health promotion.

## Case Management in the Context of Community

Community-based nursing occurs within the context of the client's community. The nurse is responsible for identifying resources and constraints or limitations for care that exists in the community. This can occur when the nurse states clearly and coherently to the client the purpose of the nursing care and how all the care needs will be met with organizational and community resources. For example, a 76-year-old client living in a rural community was originally treated for metastatic cancer of the prostate in a large, urban medical center 175 miles away from his home. Now he needs 6 weeks of daily radiation treatments for his metastasis. The nurse recognizes a problem with the client being so far away from his original primary care institution and arranges treatment at a hospital 40 miles from the client's home. When arranging care, the nurse coordinates care between the two facilities so continuity is not lost and the client is ensured the best care possible within the constraints of his community.

## Case Management and Continuity of Care

Collaboration and acting as an advocate on behalf of the client are important aspects of ensuring continuity of care. Using an analytical approach to make referrals and follow up on client progress is another strategy to promote continuity.

## CLIENT SITUATIONS IN PRACTICE

### ▶ Case Management

Steve, age 40, and Barb, age 37, are a young couple with three children: Brook, 15, Jane, 13, and Jack, 11. Both parents are professionals. Steve works at the Veterans Administration, where he is in charge of the information systems, and Barb is a professor at a small liberal arts college. Because Steve has a family history of colon cancer (his paternal grandfather died of colon cancer at age 41 and his father and uncle had surgery for colon cancer at ages 65 and 60, respectively), he was advised to have a colonoscopy at age 40. One month after his 40th birthday, Steve scheduled a test. He was diagnosed with colon cancer 3 days after the test, on Christmas Eve day. He has no symptoms. Because of the size of the tumor, Steve's physician recommends he have the surgery at a large medical center 200 miles from Steve's home. Two days after Christmas, he has a colon resection without a colostomy at Methodist Hospital. At that time, it is determined that the cancer is class C2 according to Dukes classification system (or stage 4 with the other commonly used classification). Although he was a candidate for a colostomy, he and Barb decided they wanted to try the more conservative approach, with the option of a colostomy later, if necessary.

Barb has been with Steve throughout his hospital stay while their three children have been home, 200 miles away, staying with Barb's elderly mother. It is 14 days after the operation, and he is to return home the day after tomorrow. He will begin chemotherapy at the rural hospital close to his home next week.

- *You are a staff nurse caring for Steve in the hospital. What strategies to manage care would you use, starting from the first day?*
  The first step in care management is establishing a relationship with the client and family by listening and talking. By doing this, you hope to build trust.

By now you would have established a very open relationship with Barb and Steve. You ask Barb and Steve how they anticipate the homecoming will go when they arrive home. Barb says, "We have both really missed the kids. I really want to have a normal life again—sleep in my own bed and make breakfast for everyone. Just normal stuff."

Steve says, "I can't wait to get out of here. But I am worried about the chemo. We had one conversation with the nurse at the clinic, and she said that we have to have the chemo in the morning. I have most of my meetings at work in the morning and would rather do the chemo in the afternoon."

- *How could you, as a staff nurse, respond to this comment?*
  To help give some control back to the client, you might encourage him to call the clinic that day and explore whether chemotherapy could be scheduled at a time more convenient for his work schedule.

You are working in a clinic as an oncology nurse, providing chemotherapy for Steve. This is the third week of his treatment, and you have established a relationship with both Barb and Steve. During Steve's visit, you ask them how things are going. Barb tells you, "Awful. Brook was picked up for shoplifting, and her grades are dropping in school." You note that Steve is unusually quiet and does not make eye contact with you. You ask, "Steve, you look down today. Are you doing okay?"

"It feels like it is all coming apart. I can't keep up at work, the kids are having trouble . . .," Steve shares.

"He won't listen to me about resting. And he's throwing up all the time. That medication you gave him doesn't work," Barb reports.

- *What are some interventions you could use at this point in your care of Steve and his family?*
  *Possible interventions include the following:*
  Using the steps of the referral process to find some community resources to support the family with the issues the family is facing, including the daughter's shoplifting and falling grades
  Advocating for the client by calling the physician to identify additional antiemetics that may be helpful in controlling the nausea and vomiting
  Contacting a social worker (with the family's knowledge) to begin to collaborate and problem solve regarding the family's issues and stress

Ten months later, Steve has completed chemotherapy and radiation therapy. Because of the intensity of the radiology treatment, he has developed interrupted bowel function. He has been to the clinic and the ED several times in the past weeks with severe cramps. You receive a call late in the afternoon from Barb. She states that the medication given at the last clinic visit is not helping; Steve has been throwing up all day, has severe abdominal cramps, and has a temperature of 103°. You tell them to go to the local ED.

At the ED, Steve is diagnosed with a bladder and kidney infection and bowel obstruction, and he is admitted to the hospital. A complete workup is performed while he is in the hospital, and liver cancer is discovered throughout his liver, with lesions in the brain as well. He is discharged home unable to eat, with a central line and hyperal for total parenteral nutrition.

You are Steve's home care nurse. On the first home visit, his functional capacity for activities of daily living is clearly impaired. He is homebound and needs a home health care aide to help him bathe and shave. Barb is working two jobs to try to make ends meet. The plan is for the home health aide to come every other day, with you coming once a day to start the hyperal. Two months later, at one of your visits, Steve says, "The home aide says he can do the hyperal and clean the site on the days when he is here. Then you don't have to come every day."

- *Can you delegate the administration of hyperal to the home health aide?*
  According to the Five Rights of Delegation from the NCSBN (Box 7–6), this task may not be delegated for the following reasons:

  Assessment may be needed.
  The task requires extensive training.
  The task requires professional judgment regarding client response.
  There is potential for harm.

  The RN would not be immediately available for assistance or direct supervision.
  Steve's condition continues to deteriorate over the next month. As you are getting ready to leave after a visit, Barb asks you, "Do you think we should be making plans for Steve's death?"

- *You conclude that Barb and Steve may be ready to talk about hospice care. How do you proceed?*
  Using the steps for consultation in Box 7–5, you determine the family's needs. Through mutual problem solving, you determine if and when the family is ready to meet with the hospice nurse. At that time, you contact her for the family and arrange for her to visit.

 **CONCLUSIONS**

Although case management is a role for nurses that is more than 100 years old, the model has evolved. Nurses on all levels are care managers for some parts of their jobs. Themes from the care manager role include establishing trust, giving control, helping families hold it all together, being advocates, taking care of the environment, and dealing with absent families. Interventions commonly used in case management are case finding, referral and follow-up, collaboration, consultation, and delegation. These interventions are particularly applicable in the changing managed care environment. The care manager in community-based settings always encourages self-care with a preventive focus that is provided within the context of the client's community while following the principles of collaboration to achieve continuity.

# What's on the Web

Case Management Society of America
8201 Cantrell Road, Suite 230
Little Rock, AR 72227
Telephone: (501) 225-2229
Fax: (501) 221-9068
**Internet address:** *http://www.cmsa.org*
This site offers educational opportunities, both CEU (continuing education units) and case management credential courses. It also provides extensive information on case management.

Case Management Resource Guide
**Internet address:** *http://www.cmrg.com/*
This site has a comprehensive, on-line directory of health care organizations. It also contains an extensive case manager resource guide.

National Council of State Boards of Nursing

Delegation Resource Folder
**Internet address:** *http://www.ncsbn.org*
The NCSBN has produced an excellent resource on delegation, which serves as the major reference for information on delegation. The council's material is contained in the delegation resource folder and can be downloaded from the council's Web site. Click on "nursing regulation" once on that page. Click on "delegation of VAP issues" under nursing regulation. There is great overlap between case management and continuity of care; Chapter 8 has additional resources.

## References and Bibliography

Advocacy in action. (1999). *RN, 62*(7), 262.

Allender, J. A., & Spradley, B. W. (2001). *Community health nursing: Concepts and practice* (5th ed.). Philadelphia: Lippincott, Williams & Wilkins.

American Nurses Association (ANA). (1999). *Scope of standards of home health nursing practice and standards of home health nursing practice.* Washington, DC: American Nurses Publishing.

American Nurses Association (ANA). (1988). *Nursing case management.* Kansas City, MO: Author.

Burke, S. (1999). Creating competency for home healthcare: Case management manual. *Home Healthcare Nurse Manager, 3*(6), 2–5.

Campinha-Bacote, J., & Campinha-Bacote, D. (1999). A framework for providing culturally competent health care services in managed care organizations. *Journal of Transcultural Nursing, 10*(4), 290–291.

Case Management Society of America. Center for Case Management Accountability (CCMA). (1998), available from http://www.cmsa.org

Chan, S., Mackenzie, A., Tin-Fu, D., Leung, J., & Ka-yi, B. (2000). An evaluation of the implementation of case management in the community psychiatric nursing service. *Journal of Advanced Nursing, 31*(1), 144–156.

Enguidanos, S. (2001). Integrating behavior change into geriatric case management practice. *Home Health Care Services Quarterly, 20*(1), 67–83.

Fletcher, I., & Coffman, S. (1999). Care management in the nursing curriculum. *Journal of Nursing Education, 38*(8), 371–372.

Howe, R. (1999). Case management in managed care: Past, present and future. *The Case Manager, 10*(5), 38–48.

Kersbergen, A. (2000). Managed care shifts health care from an altruistic model to a business framework. *Nursing and Health Care Perspectives, 21*(2), 81–83.

Kesby, S. (2002). Nursing care and collaborative practice. *Journal of Clinical Nursing, 11*(3), 357–366. Retrieved January 19, 2003, from the CINAHL database.

Lee, D., Mackenzie, A., Dudley-Brown, S., & Chin, T. (1998). Case management: A review of the definitions and practice. *Journal of Advanced Nursing, 27*, 933–939.

Ludwig-Beymer, P. (1999). Transcultural nursing's role in a managed care environment. *Journal of Transcultural Nursing, 10*(4), 286–287.

Lyon, J. (1993). Modules of nursing care delivery and case management: Clarification of terms. *Nursing Economics, 11*(3), 163–178.

McClaran, J., Franco, E., Lam, Z., & Snell, L. (1999). Can case management be taught in a multidisciplinary forum? *Journal of Continuing Education in the Health Professions, 19*(3), 181–191.

McKay, T. (1999). Managed care: A turning point for nursing. *Journal of Transcultural Nursing, 10*(4), 292.

McKenna, M. (1999). Let us try to keep culturally competent care in managed care. *Journal of Transcultural Nursing, 10*(3), 293–293.

Minnesota Department of Health, Section of Public Health Nursing. (2000). *Public health nursing interventions II.* Minneapolis: Author.

Mitchell, A., & Reaghard, D. (1996). Managed care and psychiatric–mental health nursing services: Implications for practice. *Issues in Mental Health Nursing, 17*(1), 1–9. Retrieved June 13, 2003 from the CINAHL database.

Moore, A. (1999). Hospitals shift responsibility for cross-continuum care. *RN, 62*(9), 28nm4–28nm6.

National Council of State Boards of Nursing. (1997). *The Delegation Resource Folder* [Data file]. Available from http://www.ncsbn.org/files/delegation.asp

Reed, B. (1999). Desperately seeking continuity. *The Practicing Midwife, 2*(9), 46.

Riegel, B., Carlson, B., Kopp, Z., LePetri, Glaser, D., & Unger, A. (2002). Effect of a standardized nurse case-management telephone intervention on resource use in patients with chronic heart failure. *Archives of Internal Medicine, 162*(6), 705–712.

Rodgers, B. (2000). Coordination of care: The lived experience of the visiting nurse. *Home Healthcare Nurse, 18*(5), 301–307.

Schmidt, S., Guo, L., Scheer, S., Boydston, J., Pelino, C., & Berger, S. (1999). Epidemiological determination of community-based nursing case management for stroke. *Journal of Nursing Administration, 29*(6), 40–47.

Sokol, D. (1999). John needed all I could give. *RN, 62*(11), 44–47.

*Standards of practice for case management.*[AQ] (1995). Little Rock, AR: Case Management Society of America (CMSA) Publications.

Tahan, H. (1998). Case management: A heritage more than a century old. *Nursing Case Management, 3*(2), 55–69.

Tholcken, M., Lehna, C., & Robinson, S. (1999). Children with disabilities: Teaching baccalaureate nursing students community-based case management. *Journal of Care Management, 5*(4), 32–39.

Walsh, K. (1999). ED case managers: One large teaching hospital's experience. *Journal of Emergency Nursing, 25*(10), 17–20.

Wayman, C. (1999). Hospital-based nursing case management: Role clarification. *Nursing Case Management, 4*(5), 236–241.

Wenat, D (1996). Building trust during the initial home visit. In: *Readings in community-based nursing* (p. 154–160). Philadelphia: Lippincott Williams & Wilkins.

What preparation do case managers really need? (1999). *Case Management Advisor, 10*(7), 112–113.

Zerull, L. (1999). Community nurse case management: Evolving over time to meet new demands. *Community Health, 22*(3), 12–29.

Zimmerman, P., & Pierce, B. (1998). Case managers. *Journal of Emergency Nursing, 24*(6), 589–591.

Zink, M. (2001). Case management is critical in PPS. *Home Healthcare Nurse, 19*(5), 283–288.

# LEARNING ACTIVITIES

## JOURNALING ACTIVITY 7-1

In your clinical journal, describe a situation you have observed in clinical where a client experienced difficulty caused by lack of effective case management. If you were the nurse in charge, what would you have done differently?

In your clinical journal, describe a situation you have observed in clinical where a client received effective case management. What made the care effective?

In your clinical journal, describe a situation where you observed or initiated two of the following intervention strategies. Discuss what happened.

Referral and follow-up
Consultation
Collaboration
Advocacy

### PRACTICAL APPLICATION: ACTIVITY 7–2

You are a home health care nurse responsible for the care of 15 clients. It's Monday morning, and you are reviewing your phone messages as well as looking over the charts of the clients you are scheduled to visit in the next 2 days. How will you rearrange home visits for the next 2 days based on the following information?

SCHEDULED VISITS FOR MONDAY AFTERNOON AND TUESDAY
MONDAY

1:00 Mr. Carmody—routine visit to monitor symptoms of congestive heart failure
2:30 Mrs. Gothie—routine follow-up visit after hip replacement and discharge from acute care last Wednesday, and your last visit was Friday
4:00 Mrs. Violet—monthly blood draw for lithium levels

TUESDAY

9:00 Mr. Heaney—scheduled to discharged from the hospital Monday night after open heart surgery; assessment visit and blood draw
10:30 Mr. Sund—follow-up visit for knee replacement surgery; discharged from the hospital last Thursday, and your last visit was Friday
1:00 Mr. Vang—reinforcement teaching for care of a leg wound
2:30 Mrs. O'Conner—follow-up visit for assessment after scheduled discharge from the hospital on Monday evening; administration of IV antibiotic medication

PHONE MESSAGES ON MONDAY AT 8:00 am

Mr. Vang called you this morning and said that he ran out of dressings on Friday. He was upset and stated that the sore on his leg looked redder, and there was some sticky green stuff dripping off of it.
Mrs. Sund called and said her husband had so much pain in his knee over the weekend that he could not sleep. She said he also has pain in the back of his calf, it is red, and it hurts if he flexes his foot.

### PRACTICAL APPLICATION: ACTIVITY 7–3

Describe a situation that you have observed or participated in where some of the steps of case management (Box 7–1) were followed. Which steps were used? What happened? What worked and didn't work? What do you think could have been done next time to improve the situation?

### PRACTICAL APPLICATION: ACTIVITY 7–4

Interview a nurse who is a case manager or has case management as a part of his or her role. Ask what he or she thinks are the essential components of care coordination related to the nurse–client relationship and the nurse's knowledge about the community. Then compare what the nurse says to the stages in Box 7–2. Ask the nurse to explain why the stages in the Box 7–2 apply to the work that she or he does or why not. Does he or she agree or disagree with Rodgers's essentials of care coordination? Which does he or she think are most important?

### CRITICAL THINKING: ACTIVITY 7–5

List at least three barriers you have observed in your clinical setting that hinder effective case management. Discuss what could be done differently to enhance case management and continuity in these situations.

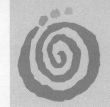

# Continuity of Care

Roberta Hunt

## THE NURSE SPEAKS

While working as a staff nurse in a children's hospital, I had the opportunity to care for a 13-year-old young man on his day of discharge. Josh was an "old pro" when it came to the hospital environment, as he had endured 12 reconstructive surgeries on his right ear since birth. When I entered his room, Josh was lying in bed with the head of the bed slightly elevated. He was alone in the room and had turned off the radio and TV. He had a large dressing over his right ear, and a bandage wrapped around his head to hold the dressing in place. On assessing his vital signs, I noted that he was afebrile; however, his blood pressure and pulse were slightly elevated. After assessing his vital signs, I asked Josh to rate his pain on a numeric scale of 0 to 10. Without hesitation, Josh replied a 9. I was quite concerned about his pain intensity level as the surgeons had already examined his ear and decided that he was ready to go home. In addition, they recommended over-the-counter analgesics for postoperative ear pain.

Before consulting with his physicians, I continued with my pain assessment. I asked Josh about the quality and duration of his pain, along with analgesic effectiveness. Then I asked Josh what the color of pain was, and he replied red. Lastly, I asked Josh to use my red pen to mark on a body outline pain tool the exact location of the pain. Much to my surprise, when Josh handed the pain tool back to me, there was a large red mark on his left leg, the donor site for his ear grafting!

When I inquired about the pain in his right ear, his replied, "What pain? My ear feels fine." Josh taught me an important lesson about the subjectivity of pain. Although the obvious site of pain was his right ear, as a nurse, I cannot assume the obvious. I needed to be holistic in my pain assessment and remember to assess the location(s) of pain. Based on the valuable information from Josh, I was able to consult with his physicians and arrange for an effective analgesic to cover the pain at his donor site that would allow him to have pain control once he was home.

— **Susan O'Conner-Von, DNSc, RNC**
Assistant Professor
School of Nursing
University of Minnesota, Minneapolis, Minnesota

Nurses have been involved in **continuity of care** since the late 1880s. In 1906, both Massachusetts General Hospital in Boston and Bellevue Hospital in New York City designated a nurse to tend to the needs of those patients about to be discharged. Recently, interest in discharge planning was renewed with the concern about escalating medical costs. Currently, nurses are involved with continuity of care more than ever as health care reform continues. Future reforms center around the use of inpatient facilities for briefer, more intense care; cost-containment efforts to deliver care at the lowest cost with more efficiency; expanded community-based care; and an emphasis on primary, preventive care delivered with a continuum of care. Nursing will focus on quality-of-care issues and development of skills in community-based care.

Ongoing health care planning and referral are described as a bridge between one health care setting and another environment. A comprehensive plan of care and effective referrals are essential elements for continuity of care. Collaboration is important for the multidisciplinary team, working together to promote quality health care. The team's goal is to optimize the client and family's functioning and self-care. The nurse is often the primary player in ascertaining the quality of the health plan.

Both discharge planning and continuity of care rely on community resources. A community with many resources can help support the client and family through a recovery period or can help families in their health promotion. The community with few resources will be inefficient in its support of citizens who require assistance with health care needs.

In this chapter, continuity of care is presented as facilitating entrance into, exit out of, and transfer within the health care system. Examples are given to show how coordination of services is used in continuity. The concepts of community resources and referral are discussed. Two types of resources are explained. Steps in the referral process are outlined, along with information about financing referrals. The chapter ends with a section on skills and competencies the nurse needs to improve continuity of care, a discussion of barriers to continuity, and examples of programs that have been successful in enhancing continuity.

## SIGNIFICANCE OF CONTINUITY OF CARE

**Continuity of care** has been described as the coordination of activities involving clients, providers, and payers to promote the delivery of health care. This is the process by which a client's ongoing health care needs are assessed, planned for, coordinated, and met without disruption. Some may view it as a method to control health care costs. Clients may view it as promoting their right to make choices about health care services.

Continuity of care is achieved when all appropriate care and treatment interventions are provided in a planned, coordinated, and consistent manner by staff working across professional/agency boundaries and through the required period of time. This should be integrated with informal care and agreed upon and experienced by clients or users, their caregivers, and their families (Kesby, 2002, p. 359).

Regardless of how it is perceived, continuity of care requires a strong organizational structure to prevent the client from getting "lost" in the system. Nurses must provide a leadership role in determining how and where the best care can be provided for a client and then ensuring that the client receives that care. The nurse accomplishes this by thoroughly assessing the client's needs, participating in multidisciplinary planning and intervention, and using appropriate resources, follow-up, and evaluation. Successful attainment of continuity of care is essential to ensure quality health care and is promoted through successful planning and effective referral. Nurses play a vital role in promoting continuity in community-based settings (see Box 8–1).

## ENTERING AND EXITING THE HEALTH CARE SYSTEM

Principles of continuity apply to transitions of care between any community settings. "Discharge from a community-based healthcare setting needs the same, or possibly greater, level of attention than from acute care facilities" (Craven & Hirnle, 2000, p. 344). If discharge instructions for a client in ambulatory surgery are clearly explained, then successful follow-up, fewer complications, and good re-

**RESEARCH IN COMMUNITY-BASED NURSING CARE**

**Box 8-1 ▶** Clinical Pathway Versus a Usual Plan of Care for Clients With Congestive Heart Failure

Congestive heart failure is the most frequent reason for hospitalization of persons 65 years of age and older and one of the most common diagnoses of home health clients. This study explored the question: Is the clinical pathway more effective than the usual plan of care? Client data were collected through retrospective chart reviews of home health records. Data collected included the admission form, Health Care Finance Administration Form 485, initial nurse visit, data discharge form, and the form documenting the clinical pathway (for those being cared for using a clinical pathway). Client data for those clients cared for using the usual plan of care were then compared to those clients cared for by following the clinical pathway. The number of clients who were a) discharged to home, b) rehospitalized, or c) had other dispositions (eg, nursing home, death, transfer) were compared across groups. The rehospitalization rate for the usual care group was 23% and 12.5% for the pathway group. This was a 45% reduction in the rehospitalization rate for the pathway group. The most significant contributors to the likelihood of rehospitalization were need for assistance with eating, number of days of home health care service, and previous hospitalizations. The author cited that this research suggests several implications for home care. Clinical pathways are effective in quality improvement efforts, providing data for continuous evaluation. This research highlights the importance of case management skills for the home health nurse.

Hoskins, I., Thiel, L., Walton-Moss, B., Clark, H., & Schroeder, M. (2001). What is the difference: Clinical pathway versus a usual plan of care for clients with congestive heart failure. *Home Healthcare Nurse 19*(3), 142–150.

covery are more likely. Likewise, if the nurse in the clinic provides the client with a clear, succinct explanation for care at home, recovery will be enhanced. If the home health care nurse of a pediatric client communicates with the school nurse about daily treatment needs, continuity will be enhanced and complications and added costs avoided.

Unlike the past, when clients typically went from an acute care setting to home, clients today enter the health care system in various ways. They may be referred from a clinic visit to home care, from school to a physician's office, from home care to an acute care setting, or from adult day care to an extended care facility. Figure 8–1 llustrates the flow of continuity of care.

Clients may be transferred several times from one community-based setting to another. For example, Juan falls in the bathroom in his home and breaks his hip. He enters the system through the emergency department and is transferred to the operating room and then to the orthopedic unit in the hospital. After discharge

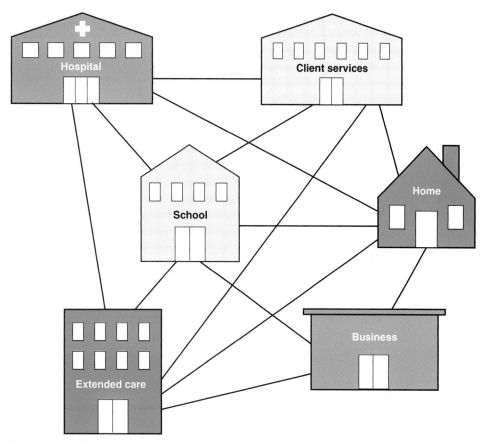

***Figure 8–1.*** ▶ Continuity of care in community-based nursing is like a web between and among settings.

from the hospital, he stays in a transitional facility for follow-up physical therapy and skilled nursing care. Then he is moved to assisted living for 4 months. After being transferred to three different services in the hospital and being discharged from four different agencies, he is back in his own home 6 months after the fall.

## Admission

Admission occurs when an individual enters the health care system. Each new setting involves a new admission, with continuity serving as a bridge between the new setting and the previous setting. No matter what the setting, the client and family enter with apprehension. Each new facility or agency presents strange surroundings and new people. Client and family anxiety levels may be high. In addition to concern over the client's present condition and the future outcome, the client and family may feel overwhelmed by new people and new equipment. What may be a routine admission to the nurse is seldom routine for a client. The nurse's confidence, competence, and concern are essential in putting the client and family at ease. The nurse's attitude may exert great influence on the course of care.

**TABLE 8-1** • Overview of Admission to Various Health Care Facilities

| Facility | Possible Admission Procedures |
| --- | --- |
| Acute care setting | Introduction; orientation to room and equipment; complete nursing history, vital signs, and other physical assessment |
| Emergency department | Introduction; ABCs (airway, breathing, and circulation); vital signs; focused assessment for acute problems; orientation to surroundings |
| Clinic or physician's office | Introduction; exploration of reason for seeking medical care and focused assessment of that problem; vital signs |
| Nursing home | Introduction; review of written or verbal report from transferring agency; nursing history and assessment focusing on functional abilities; orientation to new surroundings |
| Hospice | Introduction; review of referral; nursing history and assessment focusing on pain control, functional abilities, coping, and support; wishes concerning terminal care and death (eg, living will); orientation to procedures and care |
| Psychiatric facility | Introduction; mental health evaluation, including history, mood state, suicide risk, use of drugs, support system |
| Home visit | Introduction; review of referral and client's medical and nursing problems, home environment, caretaker and family support, community resources |

Source: Craven, R. F., & Hirnle, C. J. (2000). *Fundamentals of nursing: Human health and function* (3rd ed.). Philadelphia: Lippincott Williams & Wilkins.

Apprehension may be lessened by the following nursing actions:

▸ Establishing rapport
▸ Indicating sincere concern for the client and family
▸ Defining the purpose and expectations of this admission
▸ Aiding the client in understanding how to participate as fully as possible in care-related decisions
▸ Clarifying the nursing role in relation to the client's health care needs
▸ Including the family in explanations, unless the client indicates otherwise
▸ Explaining equipment and procedures
▸ Explaining equipment to be used when calling for assistance
▸ Documenting the procedure

Admission procedures for entering any system share similarities. Examples of admission procedures in various health care facilities are summarized in Table 8–1.

An admission form is always completed on entry into any health care service. Depending on the client's condition and the reason for admission, the form may be short or rather long. Insurance information, consent forms, and other forms are included in the admission paperwork.

During admission, it is reassuring if the nurse explains to the client and family members how they can participate in decision making and care planning. The nurse may say, "The nutritionist will be here to talk to you this afternoon. He will discuss your food preferences. Unless the physician or nurse tells you differently, you may also eat any food brought from home. Perhaps your spouse will want to cook your favorite dish."

Admission may be as anxiety provoking for the family as for the client. The nurse supports the family by giving the location of waiting rooms, rest rooms, public telephones, the nurse's station or offices, and other areas of interest, such as vending machines or cafeterias. If the client is being admitted for day surgery, the nurse may explain where the family can wait, who will bring a report, and when they can expect it. In many cases, comforting the family is as important as calming the client.

## Transferring

Sometimes the term *discharge* is used when client **transferring** is taking place. A client typically is transferred within the same institution, most often from the emergency department to the acute care setting or intensive care unit. Another type of transfer is when the client leaves the emergency department by ambulance to be transferred to another acute care facility or transitional hospital. For example, Nhu is an 80-year-old woman who is admitted to the emergency department after a fall at her daughter's home. After examination, it is discovered that she has shattered her hip and requires extensive surgery to repair the fractures. The physicians recommend transfer to a large medical center that specializes in orthopedic repair of complex hip fractures. Nhu is transferred by ambulance to the medical center. In community-based health care, clients may be transferred from one setting to another.

With transfer, specific information must accompany the client. In a general transfer, the packet includes the following:

▶ Physician transfer orders
▶ Chest radiograph (preferably within 39 days)
▶ Medical history and physical examination results
▶ Laboratory results
▶ Electrocardiogram (ECG) results
▶ Urinalysis results
▶ Preadmission screening (PAS) and preadmission screening and annual resident review (PASARR) forms
▶ Assessment from nursing, physical therapy, occupational therapy, and speech therapy (as needed)
▶ Social service assessment
▶ Do-not-resuscitate (DNR) forms (if appropriate), living wills, and medical power of attorney
▶ Copies of important information, such as results of computed tomography (CT) scans, echocardiograms, Dopplers, magnetic resonance imaging (MRI) scans, and miscellaneous cardiodiagnostic tests as appropriate (Powell, 2000, p. 404)

 ## Discharge Planning

**Discharge planning** is an accepted nursing intervention aimed at the prevention of problems after discharge. Discharge planning ensures continuity of care by a systematic process of coordinating various aspects of care at the time the client is discharged from a facility or program. This planning involves many individuals who make assessments, collaborate with the client and family, plan, and then communicate the critical information to the organization or individual who will assume responsibility for the client's health care needs after discharge. The process, when it works well, is dynamic, interactive, and client centered.

The inception of Medicare in 1966 promoted discharge planning as an essential component of client care. Social Security legislation in the 1960s and 1970s provided coverage for hospital, physician, and other health care costs. Discharge planning became a central event as a method to reduce costs, lower hospital readmission rates, and provide the client with posthospital care options. The concept of discharge planning, beginning with admission to a hospital or ambulatory care setting, became even more critical with the advent of the diagnosis-related group system.

Discharge planning is not limited to the physical transfer of the client, nor does it focus only on physical needs. It is much more. It is a process of early assessment of anticipated, individual client needs centered on concern for the total well-being of the client and family. It involves the client, family, and all caregivers in interactive communication during the entire planning process. It also requires ongoing interdisciplinary collaboration among many health care providers. This results in mutual agreement and appropriate options for meeting health care needs through a thorough and up-to-date review of all of the resource alternatives.

Ongoing nursing assessment of future client needs is mandated by accreditation agencies. The Joint Commission on the Accreditation of Healthcare Organizations (JCAHO) requires that the discharge plan should be initiated at admission as part of the nursing care plan.

Discharge planning creates bridges between settings, as shown in Figure 8–1. If the discharge plan is carefully thought out and based on collaboration among the nurse, physician, other health care providers, the client, and family, then the bridge will be strong and the transition between settings smooth. On the other hand, if the discharge plan is nonexistent or haphazardly thrown together, the transition will be bumpy with resulting complications, rehospitalizations, or unnecessary stress, all interrupting the client's recovery. Consequently, poor continuity of care has the potential to result in disaster for the client and increased cost for the health care system.

## The Discharge Planning Process

Discharge planning is similar to the nursing process. It begins with the initial assessment at the first encounter. The nurse needs to know the client's plans and expectations for managing care. Planning and setting goals focus on both client and family needs. Written and verbal instructions about the medication regimen, treatment, and follow-up must be provided to the client. The client also needs to be educated about any signs and symptoms that may indicate problems or complications with the condition and who to contact if these should occur. At this point, the client must have the opportunity to discuss any concerns or questions regarding care and recovery. The intervention phase of the nursing process involves identifying needed resources and making appropriate referrals. Important telephone numbers, names, and community services should be given in writing to the client and family and explained thoroughly. The steps of the discharge planning process follow.

### Identify Client Discharge Needs
The nurse is often the first link in the discharge planning process. In some settings, social workers may have the primary responsibility for discharge plan-

ning; however, nurses frequently coordinate and communicate the discharge plan. This may involve the nurse asking questions, making sure the client is satisfied with the information given, and questioning any inconsistencies. Without clear verbal and written communication among all participants, the plan may be unsuccessful.

The nurse must concentrate on careful assessment of the client, identifying needs as early as possible. As soon as a client is admitted, the nurse assesses him or her for discharge needs. With each client encounter, the nurse discusses the discharge and asks the following questions: "When you are discharged . . ."

> How are you going to manage at home?
>
> Considering the treatments ordered for you, what are you going to need to manage at home?
>
> What help will you need?
>
> What help do you have at home now?

The nurse is in the best possible position to clearly identify the client's needs. The nurse provides direct care and treatment for the client, which allows for the observation of responses to care. Nurses have contact around the clock in an acute care setting. The information gained about the client's ability to provide self-care after discharge is critical to planning for discharge. Assessing needs, communicating with others, and involving the client and family on an ongoing basis contribute to a realistic strategy.

### Anticipate Changes in Client Needs and Plan How They Will Be Met

Nurses have an ongoing relationship with the client, family, and caregivers. Frequent communication with the client gives the nurse the opportunity to learn about client and family interactions and communication. If the client has special care needs after discharge, the trusting relationship established between nurse and client is essential to the next step of client and family teaching. The nurse can also anticipate the needs of the client and family at home because the nurse has observed their interactions in the acute care setting—and sometimes even in the home. The nurse can provide answers to the following questions:

> Will the family need changes in routine?
>
> Will the family be able to provide all of the care needed?
>
> Do they need home health care assistance?
>
> What are the family's resources and limitations?

### Ensure Continuity of Care and Progress Toward Health and Quality of Life

Once client needs are identified and plans are made to meet these needs, nurses promote continuity of care through coordination of services for the client and communication among health care team members. A discharge plan is not complete without considering community resources and subsequent referrals based on client needs and resources. Today, because of the costs of health care, the discharge plan is driven more often by resources than by needs. Referrals must consider client resources (eg, insurance coverage, financial status) as well as community resources. The availability of services within the geographic area can also limit access to resources. For instance, there may or may not be a hospital, nursing home, or home health care agency in the client's community.

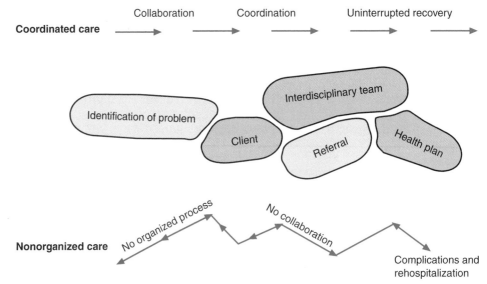

*Figure 8–2.* ▶ There are major differences between coordinated care and nonorganized care.

## Coordination of Services

Successful continuity of care depends on the coordination of interdisciplinary sources of care and support. **Coordinated care** includes assisting with financial arrangements, contacting vendors and arranging for equipment, making referrals to home health care agencies, making appointments with health care providers, conducting predischarge teaching, and following up with arrangements for additional referrals as indicated. Figure 8–2 illustrates differences between coordinated care and unorganized care.

Appropriate use of resources and effective referrals promote continuity of care. Resources are defined as the available means for accomplishing a task, including staff and budget as well as physical space and equipment. Referrals are the actual exchange of information and constitute the formal links between the client, the health care setting, and the community or home. The information exchanged is the sum of assessment, nursing diagnosis, and planning. The intervention phase of the nursing process includes identifying resources and making referrals.

### Client and Community Resources

Because of current health care costs, the health plan is often driven by the client's financial resources rather than by need. An example is a client who needs home visits for assistance with activities of daily living (ADL), meal preparation, household chores, transportation, and physical therapy. The client's insurance pays only for physical therapy. This requires that the nurse, client, and client's support person, physician, and multidisciplinary team (eg, social worker, physical therapist) set priorities based on what the client can afford and explore alternative ways to meet the additional needs. Alternatives might be Meals On Wheels, volun-

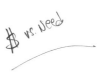

teer transportation, family participation, or church visitation. Referrals must consider the client's resources as well as the community's resources.

To facilitate continuity of care when referring clients to an acute care setting, home, or community, the nurse must be aware of the various types of individuals and organizations available as community resources. Box 8–2 lists resources that can be used for the ill or older population of the community. Resources include physicians, hospital centers, clinics and nursing centers, specialized care centers, and long-term care facilities. School nurses and occupational nurses are resources, as are various agencies and organizations. Resources may include a range of health-related services, from drug and alcohol treatment programs to safety education to prevent roller-blading injuries. Each resource exists to provide services to meet particular needs. The nurse must know what these resources are and their eligibility requirements.

Community resources can be characterized as either health care providers or supportive care providers. Health care providers include all health care settings, health departments, community service agencies, and private practice physicians. Support care providers include psychologic services, churches, and self-help groups.

### Health Care Providers

Health maintenance, health promotion, and illness prevention are universal needs. Health care providers include, but are not limited to, physicians, dentists, ophthalmologists, therapists (such as occupational and physical), alternative care practitioners (such as chiropractors and acupuncturists), home health care agencies, outpatient clinics, diagnostic screening programs, and health education programs. Such diverse providers and programs may be funded by the government and may include private offices, neighborhood centers, and schools, to name only a few. Table 8–2 gives examples of the roles of some health care providers. Community services share one thing in common—they provide services to the public to meet the health care needs of clients and families in the community.

### Supportive Care Providers

Supportive care providers, or support services, are services that help people avoid problems or solve problems that interfere with their self-care and well-being. The primary service offered is not necessarily health related. This category of service may be more difficult to find and identify than services directly related to health care needs. Other resources on the health care team may be able to assist with a support need. The hospital social worker, for example, will be knowledgeable about financial aid, legal services, recreation programs, housing programs, protective services, day care, peer support groups, community education, and food services. Support services are not always obvious to clients or their families, but acquiring information about them is an important piece of continuing care.

When the nurse looks for information before making a referral to an agency or service with which he or she is not familiar, the nurse should ask specific questions related to the services required:

> Can you adequately serve this client? Do you work with individuals? Families? Is your agency culturally competent and sensitive to diversity?
>
> What are the eligibility requirements for your services? How does a client or family contact you? When can my client get an appointment?

> ▶ **Box 8–2**   Community Resources for Elderly and Ill Clients ◀

**Transportation Difficulty**
- Provisions for older people offered by states and city services through reduced bus fares, taxi vouchers, and van services
- Volunteer organizations: Red Cross, Salvation Army, senior citizen centers and nonprofits, church organizations for emergency or occasional transportation

**Prevention of Home Injuries**
- Telephone checkup services through local hospitals, local services or friends, neighbors, or relatives
- Postal alert: register with local senior center; sticker on mailbox alerts letter carrier to check for accumulation of mail
- Private services paid for hourly
- Aide services by the Visiting Nurse Association
- Medicaid and Medicare provisions for home aides, which are limited to strict eligibility requirements
- Student help (inexpensive helpers) solicited by posting notices on bulletin boards at colleges and allied health schools
- Home sharing with another person who is willing to provide this kind of assistance in exchange for room and board

**Nursing Care or Physical Therapy**
- Visiting nurse services provided through Medicare, Medicaid, or other health insurance (must be ordered by a physician)
- Home health services through private providers listed in the phone book; also nonprofit providers, Medicare and Medicaid reimbursement for authorized services

**Shopping, Cooking, and Meal Planning**
- Home-delivered meals delivered by Meals On Wheels or church organizations once a week, with sliding fees
- Meals served at senior centers, churches, schools, and other locations
- Cooperative arrangements with neighbors to exchange a service for meals, food shopping, and other tasks

**Social Isolation**
- Senior centers or community education programs that provide social opportunities, classes, volunteer opportunities, and outings
- Church-sponsored clubs with social activities, volunteer opportunities, and outings
- Support groups for widows, stroke victims, and general support
- Adult day care with social interaction, classes, discussion groups, outings, and exercise

*(continued)*

▶ Box 8–2   Community Resources for Elderly ◀
and Ill Clients *(Continued)*

**Need for Assistance With Home Management**
- Homemaker services for those meeting income eligibility criteria
- Service exchanges with neighbors and friends (eg, baby-sitting exchanged for housework help)
- Home helpers hired through agencies or through employment listings at senior centers, schools, etc.
- Help with housework in exchange for home sharing by renting out a room or portion of the home for reduced rent

**Financial Issues**
- Power of attorney given to a friend or relative for handling financial matters
- Joint checking account with friend or relative to facilitate paying bills
- Financial assistance available from the American Red Cross, Salvation Army, church groups, senior centers, or other organizations

**Legal Assistance**
- AARP legal services
- Legal aid or other lawyer referral services offered by the county or state bar association
- Other city/county aging services, hot lines for information and assistance in phone book

What is the cost of the service? What financial arrangements can be made? Do you accept payment from the client's third-party payer?

Where are you located? Are you near public transportation? Is parking available? What about accessibility for the disabled? Do you travel to the area where the client lives?

What else do I need to know about your agency?

## Referrals

The purpose of a **referral** to another organization or provider is to ensure that appropriate and timely information is communicated so that the client's needs are met and care is coordinated effectively. During the referral, information about the client's medical condition, care needs, and social environment is exchanged, and a formal relationship is established between the discharging and care-providing organizations. The acute care nurse will refer primarily to health care resources. The community-based nurse will not only initiate referrals to other support services, but will also receive referrals from other community providers.

Characteristics of an effective referral include the following:

▶ *Merit and reliability are evident.* A careful assessment of the client's needs and resources will reveal if the referral has merit; similarly, follow-up evaluations of the community resources determine the reliability of the referral.

### TABLE 8–2 • Health Care Providers Used in Discharge Referrals

| Health Care Provider | Role |
| --- | --- |
| Home health nurse | Provides assessments, direct care, client teaching and support; coordinates services; evaluates outcomes |
| Home health aide | Provides hygiene care, cooking, supervision, and companionship |
| Social worker | Assists in finding and connecting with community resources or financial resources; provides counseling and support |
| Physical therapist | Assists with restoring mobility, strengthens muscle groups, teaches ambulation with new devices |
| Occupational therapist | Helps clients adjust to limitations by teaching new vocational skills or better ways to perform activities of daily living |
| Nutritionist | Teaches clients about meal planning and diet restrictions |
| Speech therapist | Assists clients to communicate better and works with clients who have swallowing problems |
| Respiratory therapist | Provides home follow-up for clients with respiratory problems including assessment, oxygen administration, and home ventilator care |

Craven, R. F., & Hirnle, C. J. (2000). *Fundamentals of nursing: Human health and function* (3rd ed., p. 348). Philadelphia: Lippincott Williams & Wilkins.

▶ *The referral is practical and timely.* A nurse making a referral must consider the client's ability to pay, the client's time and personal responsibilities, and whether the client is willing and able to address a health care need.

▶ *The referral is individualized.* What works for one client may not work for another. Differences in individual needs, resources, family, culture, and support systems must be recognized, respected, and communicated to ensure appropriate planning and intervention.

▶ *The referral is coordinated and mutually agreed on by all involved.* Are services being duplicated? Have the client and family been involved in initiating the referral? Is the referral clear and mutually agreed on by all involved?

*Client participation*
*Preference*

All of these are essential elements for success of the plan of care and the client's return to the optimum level of health. Keep in mind that clients have the right to say no to any referral or recommendation about their health care.

The ideal circumstance is to have the client and family participate in the referral process so they are involved in decision making and can choose the providers or organizations they prefer. The nurse, however, may be in the best position to determine needs. For example, Suzie, a juvenile diabetic, is having trouble regulating her glucose levels. She asks you, "What *can* I eat?" Her mother says, "Sometimes I'm confused about what she can eat." Her father states, "We've been having problems with our car lately. We can't drive all the way across town to talk to someone about this." The nurse makes a referral to a dietitian located near the family's home to help determine the source of the glucose level variances and to initiate nutritional planning with Suzie and her family. Often there are multiple referrals to make for a client, and the nurse acts as coordinator among members of this expanding team.

Sometimes it is necessary to have different service providers collaborate and coordinate treatment for a client's care to continue uninterrupted. For example, physical therapy for an older client with arthritis may be most effective in the afternoon, when the nurse is scheduled to visit. After discussing this with the client and the physical therapist, the nurse changes her visits for medication instruction to the morning so the client's need can be met.

### Steps in the Referral Process

The following are the steps in making an effective referral. They provide a simple framework applicable to most community settings and client situations.

#### THE HEALTH CARE TEAM AND THE CLIENT AND FAMILY ESTABLISH THE NEED

The need is identified based on the clinical assessment by the physician, information provided or questions asked by the client, and a thorough assessment by all team members, including the nurse.

#### THE NURSE, CLIENT, AND FAMILY SET OBJECTIVES FOR THE REFERRAL

The client or family's needs from community resources are identified as the nurse assists the client to understand what is needed and the available resource options. The nurse does not assume that the client knows what he or she wants because the client may not know the range of options. By establishing a trusting relationship with the client and family, the nurse will be better able to identify the objectives.

#### THE NURSE CONTINUOUSLY EXPLORES AVAILABLE RESOURCES

Appropriate continuing care relies on nurses having detailed, current knowledge about the community's resources. The nurse should collect data over time concerning community organizations and agencies. Reference books on community resources are available through organizations such as the United Way. It is important to know what these service organizations can provide, as well as each one's specific services, location, telephone number, contact person, eligibility requirements, and referral procedures. Current and reliable knowledge about resources that exist in the community is essential to assist the client or family in learning about and identifying appropriate organizations to provide care.

#### THE CLIENT MAKES THE DECISION ABOUT THE REFERRAL

The nurse acts as a teacher to facilitate a decision by the client and family. This involves helping the client identify a need and accept help. The nurse's manner should reassure the client that the client is in control and making decisions and that these decisions will be respected. The client's feelings about the need for the referral will invariably affect the outcome.

#### THE NURSE MAKES THE REFERRAL TO THE SELECTED SERVICE

A variety of formats can be used when making a referral. Not all standard forms are suited for every need and every client. The nurse can adapt or modify a form to communicate complete, appropriate information.

#### THE NURSE SUPPLIES THE AGENCY WITH NEEDED INFORMATION

Basic client information must be communicated along with health care needs: medical diagnosis, nursing problems, limitations or barriers to health, special procedures or treatments, continuing care objectives, a client's perception of the prognosis, and attitudes toward continuing care. The personal information that needs to be communicated is the client's level of knowledge about the medical condition and prognosis; the client's emotional and physical response to treatment; attitudes, beliefs, and values that affect care; level of support from family; and important features of the living situation.

**THE NURSE SUPPORTS THE CLIENT AND FAMILY IN PURSUING THE REFERRAL**

In the following situation, the nurse listens carefully to the family and client to determine their priorities and identifies a community-based service for referral. As a result of the nurse following the steps of the referral process, Amy, a young teen recently diagnosed with diabetes, is able to take charge of managing her chronic condition early in the disease process.

## CLIENT SITUATIONS IN PRACTICE

### ▶ Supporting the Client and Family in the Referral Process

Amy is a 14-year-old Native-American girl admitted to the acute care setting with type 1 diabetes mellitus. She is afraid and does not want to face the realities of her new diagnosis. She tells the physician, "I don't want anything to do with this diet and stuff! I just want to go home, hang out with my friends, and eat what I want." The physician asks the nurse to explore this statement and Amy's general feelings about her diagnosis. Amy, her mother and father, and the nurse sit down in the conference area. As the discussion proceeds, the nurse discovers that Amy is afraid that she won't ever be able to eat out with her friends. Amy's mother says, "She loves fry bread, but she can't ever eat that again, right? What am I supposed to cook for her, anyway?"

At this point, the nurse suggests the diabetes education classes at the hospital clinic. Amy's father responds, "I don't want to go back to that clinic where there are only White people." The nurse makes several telephone calls, trying to identify a resource for a teenager with a new diagnosis of diabetes who follows a traditional Native-American diet and whose family prefers a caretaker who is Native American. The nurse identifies the International Diabetes Clinic, which has a clientele and staff of many different nationalities. He also learns that there is a support group for Native-American teens with diabetes at the American Indian Center near the family's home.

The nurse visits Amy's home. He gives Amy and her parents a pamphlet about managing diabetes and discusses setting an appointment with the International Diabetes Clinic. The nurse tells Amy about the support group at the neighborhood American Indian Center. He gives Amy the name of the nurse at the American Indian Center and encourages her to call and check out the support group.

### *Financing Referrals*

Because of rising health care costs, health care organizations must now find additional funds in the form of voluntary donations and state and federal programs. The same is true for many individuals who join Health Maintenance Organizations (HMOs) or rely on government-funded health care such as Medicare and Medicaid. Insurance plans, HMOs, and governmental-funded programs provide a variety of coverage plans. Many do not cover preventive care, psychiatric treatment, outpatient support services, and medications. Most limit the amount of service for which payment is made (eg, the number of home health care visits).

Nurses must assist clients in learning about their insurance coverage and in creating a plan of care that the payer will cover. Most health care plans employ case managers who understand health care needs and subsequently make decisions, based on diagnosis and need, about services that will be authorized for payment. Sometimes the authorization or denial of authorization conflicts with decisions made by the health care team. This may require the interdisciplinary team to revise the plan, based not necessarily on what is felt to be best for the client but on what the client's financial resources and insurance coverage will pay. For example, insurance companies will not pay for home health care that consists solely of a home health aide making daily visits for the client's personal care. The client must need the skilled services of an RN or physical or occupational therapist before the payer will pay for personal care needs. If the client cannot pay out of pocket for personal care, the team must reevaluate the client to determine if there are skilled nursing needs that could qualify the client for authorization of payment by the insurance carrier. The nurse is an important player when resource availability is dictated not necessarily by need but by payment source.

## NURSING SKILLS AND COMPETENCIES IN CONTINUITY OF CARE

To enhance continuity, the nurse must develop nursing expertise in anticipating the needs of clients and their families. Continuity of care also requires collaboration skills such as knowledge of the workings of other departments within the system (eg, physical therapy, social services, transportation, pharmacy, home health care). Discharge planning is the primary role for nurses related to continuity of care in community-based care. In some areas of the country, this person is titled continuity-of-care nurse, discharge-planning nurse, or case manager. Primary competencies include those of a manager, teacher, and communicator. There is no universal level of educational preparation required for any of these roles.

A significant correlation exists between the degree of structure provided in the plan and the client's return to health. Success is more likely if the discharge plan is viewed as a methodical placing of building blocks, as illustrated in Figure 8–3.

## CLIENT SITUATIONS IN PRACTICE

### ▶ Building-Block Phases in Client Care

Margret Carolan is a 72-year-old retired woman who lives alone and has no family, but she has supportive friends from her church. She does not drive because of her poor vision. She has a history of type 2 diabetes mellitus and congestive heart failure. Currently, she takes insulin, ASA, propranolol, K-Dur, and Lasix every day. Three months ago, Ms. Carolan was seen in the emergency department for a transient ischemic attack. She is in the acute phase of recovery (see Fig. 8–4) when she is admitted to ambulatory surgery for arthroscopic surgery on her left knee under general anesthesia. She is instructed not to bear weight on her operative knee for 24 hours and to arrange for physical therapy twice a week for 1 month.

Ms. Carolan's Blaylock Discharge Planning Risk Assessment score is 11 (see Fig. 8–5). She is alert and oriented and depends on assistance for her transportation needs. Her history indicates that because she has complex problems, careful dis-

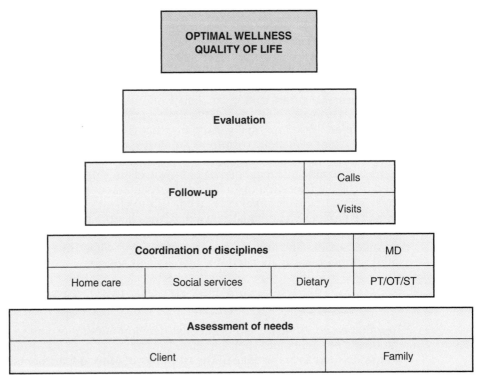

*Figure 8–3.* ▶ Building blocks of a well-organized discharge planning process.

charge planning is required. The team collects further data on her health, her personal situation including her environment, any teaching she may require for ongoing care, her financial status, and support needs she may require at home.

Ms. Carolan enters the transitional phase of recovery. Her discharge plan includes teaching her the following: weight-bearing instructions for the first 24 hours, signs and symptoms of infection, wound care, analgesic use, dosage of insulin, and possible increased or decreased dosage need. Referrals for postdischarge physical therapy are made, and transportation to and from the outpatient therapy clinic is arranged. No identified needs for home health care are apparent at this time. If complications arise, a home health care agency will be contacted.

When Ms. Carolan leaves the surgery center, she is in the continuing care phase of her recovery. At this point, the nurse may lose contact with the client. Other members of the multidisciplinary team assume responsibility for the client's ongoing needs and implementation of the discharge plan.

When Mrs. Carolan returns to the orthopedic clinic a month after surgery, she is assessed by a physician and nurse practitioner. They find her completely recovered from her surgery and refer her back to her primary clinic. No more specialist visits are necessary. The orthopedic surgeon sends a report to her primary provider stating all goals were met.

When using the nursing process to ensure continuity, the nurse follows the same steps as any clinical situation. In discharge planning, nursing process paral-

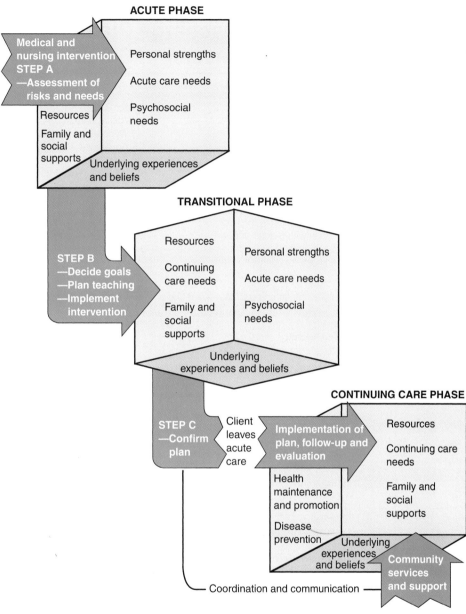

**ACUTE PHASE**

Medical and nursing intervention
STEP A
—Assessment of risks and needs

Personal strengths

Acute care needs

Psychosocial needs

Resources

Family and social supports

Underlying experiences and beliefs

**TRANSITIONAL PHASE**

STEP B
—Decide goals
—Plan teaching
—Implement intervention

Resources

Continuing care needs

Family and social supports

Personal strengths

Acute care needs

Psychosocial needs

Underlying experiences and beliefs

**CONTINUING CARE PHASE**

STEP C
—Confirm plan

Client leaves acute care

Implementation of plan, follow-up and evaluation

Resources

Continuing care needs

Health maintenance and promotion

Disease prevention

Family and social supports

Underlying experiences and beliefs

Community services and support

Coordination and communication

***Figure 8–4.*** ▶ Rorden and Taft's model of the phases of the discharge planning process. Rordan, J. W., & Taft, E. (1990). *Discharge planning guide for nurses* (p. 26). Philadelphia: Saunders.

lels defined phases. Although the nurse is a key player in determining continuity of care in transitions from one setting to another, a comprehensive plan must involve the entire multidisciplinary team, including the client and the family. A health care plan is not complete without considering community resources and referrals to meet the client's needs.

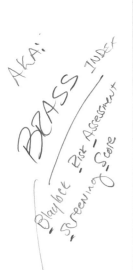

# Blaylock Discharge Planning Risk Assessment Screen

Circle all that apply and total. Refer to the Risk Factor Index*

**Age**
0 = 55 years or less
1 = 56 to 64 years
(2) = 65 to 79 years
3 = 80 + years

**Living Situation/Social Support**
0 = Lives only with spouse
1 = Lives with family
2 = Lives alone with family support
(3) = Lives alone with friends' support
4 = Lives alone with no support
5 = Nursing home/residential care

**Functional Status**
0 = Independent in activities of daily living and instrumental activities of daily living
Dependent in:
1 = Eating/feeding
1 = Bathing/grooming
1 = Toileting
1 = Transferring
1 = Incontinent of bowel function
1 = Incontinent of bladder function
1 = Meal preparation
1 = Responsible for own medication administration
1 = Handling own finances
1 = Grocery shopping
(1) = Transportation

**Cognition**
(0) = Oriented
1 = Disoriented to some spheres some of the time†
2 = Disoriented to some spheres all of the time
3 = Disoriented to all spheres some of the time
4 = Disoriented to all spheres all of the time
5 = Comatose

**Behavior Pattern**
(0) = Appropriate
1 = Wandering
1 = Agitated
1 = Confused
1 = Other

**Mobility**
0 = Ambulatory
(1) = Ambulatory with mechanical assistance
2 = Ambulatory with human assistance
3 = Nonambulatory

**Sensory Deficits**
0 = None
(1) = Visual or hearing deficits
2 = Visual and hearing deficits

**Number of Previous Admissions/Emergency Room Visits**
0 = None in the last 3 months
(1) = One in the last 3 months
2 = Two in the last 3 months
3 = More than two in the last 3 months

**Number of Active Medical Problems**
(0) = Three medical problems
1 = Three to five medical problems
2 = More than five medical problems

**Number of Drugs**
0 = Fewer than three drugs
1 = Three to five drugs
(2) = More than five drugs

Total Score: __11__

*Risk Factor Index: Score of 10 = at risk for home care resources; score of 11 to 19 = at risk for extended discharge planning; score greater than 20 = at risk for placement other than home. If the patient's score is 10 or greater, refer the patient to the discharge planning coordinator or discharge planning team.
†Sphere = person, place, time, and self.
Copyright 1991 Ann Blaylock

*Figure 8–5.* ▶ Sample of the Blaylock Discharge Planning Risk Assessment Screen.

## Assessment

Assessment of client needs must begin on admission to the facility or shortly thereafter. It can also begin at a preadmission point. The nurse uses his or her skills to identify and anticipate the client's specific needs and the services that will be needed after discharge. Assessments may be conducted by different disciplines (eg, the nurse, someone from the financial department, a physician, and a social worker) when the client enters the health care environment. The initial assessment identifies acute problems and needs. It must include a discussion with the client and family about what they perceive their health care needs to be.

Discharge planning assessment begins at admission. Ongoing assessment monitors the client's response to treatment; seeks the client and family's input regarding their desires, needs, and resources; and initiates the coordination of the multidisciplinary team. The essential elements of a discharge planning assessment for a client include the following:

▶ Health data
▶ Client and family knowledge
▶ Personal data
▶ Financial and support needs
▶ Environmental data

Increasingly, the benefit of screening populations who are at high risk for rehospitalization has been recognized. Because elderly clients are more likely to return to inpatient care than any other category of clients, many of the tools designed for this type of assessment are intended for them. Further, because of the shift in demographics with an increasing percentage of the population being over age 60, the cost–benefit value of this type of assessment is being investigated (Brody, 2002; Desai, Bogardus, Williams, Vitagliano, & Inouye, 2002).

One such tool is the Blaylock Risk Assessment Screening Score (BRASS) index. This may be used by the nurse at the bedside to gather comprehensive initial and ongoing data. The aim of the BRASS index is to identify, after hospital admission, elderly clients who are at risk for a prolonged hospital stay. Early identification of people who will have intense discharge needs may prevent or reduce postdischarge problems.

The index is shown in Figure 8–5. It contains 10 items, each judged by a nurse, using normal diagnostic procedures and questions at admission. The nurse goes through the questions, giving the client a score for every section. The Risk Factor Index at the bottom of the page indicates the client's need for discharge planning and resource planning. Box 8–3 presents recent research on the BRASS index.

A second assessment tool designed to enhance continuity of care is the Nursing Continuing Care Needs (NCCN) assessment tool. This form is a valid, sensitive, specific, and feasible tool first developed by the Health Care Financing Administration. A revised version is used extensively at Mayo Clinics. The NCCN Assessment serves a valuable purpose before a client is discharged in enhancing communication between hospital nurses and any receiving care providers. Further, it contributes to efficient assessment and communication of discharge planning needs. An outline of the NCCN tool is shown in Box 8–4.

Assessments also are used to determine continuing care needs. When assessing the need for ongoing care, the client, family, culture, and environment are all viewed as a unit of care. The nurse cannot collect all of the data. Information about the client's home environment may require a home visit by social services, for example. The interdisciplinary team collects information about the client's health,

## RESEARCH IN COMMUNITY-BASED NURSING CARE

**Box 8–3** ▶ Predictive Validity of the
Blaylock Risk Assessment Screening Score

Discharge planning is one of the most important nursing interventions related to ensuring continuity. The Blaylock Risk Assessment Screening Score (BRASS) index is a risk screening instrument that can be used at admission to identify clients in need of discharge planning. This research tested the predictive validity of the BRASS index in screening clients with postdischarge problems.

Five hundred and three elderly clients were screened at admission with the BRASS index. It was found that the higher the BRASS scores, the greater the difficulty after discharge in all domains. This study found that the BRASS index is a good predictor for identifying clients who are not candidates for discharge to home. It also accurately predicts clients who will have problems after discharge.

Mistiaen, P., Duijnhouwer, E., Prins-Hoekstra, A., Ros, W., & Blaylock, A. (1999). Predictive validity of the BRASS index in screening clients with post-discharge problems. *Journal of Advanced Nursing, 30*(5), 1050–1056.

personal circumstances, home, community, environment, and background, as well as current conditions and any financial or support services. The elements of health planning are valuable in providing a general source of information about the client, family, and environment. Some clients are at higher risk and need immediate intervention by specific supportive services.

A thorough collection of information is needed to plan effectively for continuity of care, but it is not always easily obtained. The client's successful recovery and return to optimal health often depend on collecting the right information during the assessment phase of planning. Nurses need to have multiple skills to facilitate this collection of information and plan adequately.

### Nursing Diagnosis

The nurse needs to be skillful in identifying the client's strengths and needs so that efficient care may be given. Nursing diagnoses will help other nurses streamline their care. For instance, if the visiting nurse sees that the previous visiting nurse has noted Parental Role Conflict, the second nurse will be ready to pick up on communications occurring within the home. Risk for Loneliness would be a clue the clinic nurse could state to direct follow-up. In an ongoing manner, this information is shared with all pertinent members of the health care team.

### Planning

The goal of health planning is to assist the client and family in the achievement of an optimal level of wellness (Fig. 8–6) The key to successful planning is the exchange of information between the client, present caregivers (eg, nurse, physician,

## ASSESSMENT TOOLS

**Box 8–4   Domains and Subcategories of the Nursing Continuing Care Needs (NCCN) Assessment Instrument**

### Cognitive/Behavioral/Emotional Status

Anticipated level of consciousness on discharge
Cognition
Comprehension
Expression
Usual mode of communication
Emotional/behavioral factors

### Health Status

Perception of prognosis
Current health problems
Risk factors

### Functional Status

Activities of daily living
Instrumental activities of daily living

### Finances

Resources

### Environmental Factors in Postdischarge Care

Barriers
Need for assistive devices

### Anticipated Skilled Care Requirements for Discharge

Skin: pressure ulcer
Skin: wound care
Nutrition
Hydration
Respiration
Cardiovascular function
Elimination
Neuromusculoskeletal function
Speech and language
Counseling
Client/family education
Administration of medications
Coordination of care needed

### Continuing Care Needs

Summary of continuing care needs
Resource availability
Resource provider

Adapted from Holland, D., Hansen, D., Matt-Hensrud, M., Severson, M., & Wenninger, C. (1999). Continuity of care: A nursing needs assessment instrument. *Geriatric Nursing, 19*(6), 331–334.

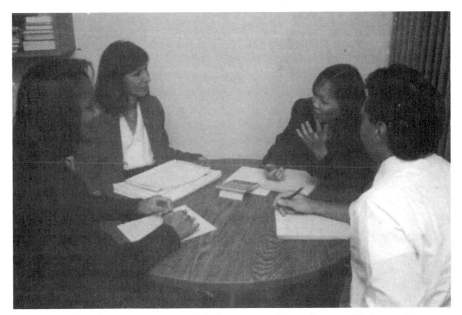

***Figure 8–6.*** ▶ The key to successful planning is the exchange of information among those concerned about the client's care.

social worker, respiratory therapist, physical therapist, occupational therapist, nutritionist, psychologist, speech therapist), and those responsible for the continuing care (eg, family, support services, and caregivers). Planning for the client involves the following:

> ▶ Recognizing and using the resources of the family
> ▶ Educating family members about the options available and encouraging their participation in the decision-making process
> ▶ Assisting the client and family to feel they have control over their own welfare and to identify resources that could help them in this process

Sociocultural factors can influence the planning phase. It is important for the nurse to identify and acknowledge issues that may influence the plan. These may include beliefs about the causes of illness and death and dying, language, nutrition practices, healing practices, and sexual orientation.

During the planning phase, the client and the multidisciplinary team develop realistic expected outcomes. Frequent communication and coordination among the multidisciplinary team, client, and client's family facilitates reaching realistic expected outcomes in a well-designed discharge plan. This is accomplished through these actions:

> ▶ Consulting between the physician and the social worker or discharge planner
> ▶ Determining the client's prognosis
> ▶ Setting priorities
> ▶ Designing realistic time frames
> ▶ Determining responsibility
> ▶ Analyzing alternative resources for appropriateness and availability

▶ Exploring financial resources and burdens
▶ Involving and educating the family
▶ Setting appropriate and realistic expected outcomes
▶ Coordinating community resources

Expected outcomes help the multidisciplinary team know what is expected of the client. When these outcomes have been agreed on by the client and family, all participants know the goals and can evaluate whether they have been met.

## Implementation

Nursing interventions focus on assisting the client to achieve the highest possible level of functioning and wellness. Interventions involve coordinating multidisciplinary plans, teaching the client and family, using appropriate community resources through referrals, performing case management, and dispelling the client or family's apprehension about continuing care needs.

Discharge plan interventions such as providing health education, making referrals to community resources, and ordering equipment for the home depend on the nurse to competently assess the client's ability to manage daily activities in the home, judge the client and family's compliance with the therapeutic regimen, assess the client's knowledge of self-care, and coordinate the team members.

Because the plan involves a multidisciplinary team, it is critical for the plan to be structured and organized. However, it must also be flexible enough to allow for change as the client progresses toward health. The team begins activities that lead toward the achievement of expected outcomes. Revisions to the plan must be made as indicated.

As the client moves from one care setting or care provider to another, the team must plan intervention strategies carefully, considering how the changes affect the client and the family. Clients and family members will probably feel anxious about the change. This is especially true if they have been hurried through an acute care setting or if discharge plans were discussed only on admission when the client's acute condition prohibited them from fully participating. From the time of admission on, the nurse will need to work with the client and family to reinforce the importance of early discharge planning for the client to achieve the maximum quality of health. Being sensitive to the client's needs while planning care will help to reduce anxiety and increase the client's participation and acceptance of care transitions.

A variety of intervention skills promote recovery and increase the effectiveness of the plan of care. Teaching skills are important and may include both prevention and promotion strategies (Fig. 8–7). Teaching and demonstrations are integral to some types of ongoing care. They may need to be repeated because of the client and family's anxiety or inability to learn quickly. The nurse must use effective interpersonal skills when communicating with other organizations or individuals who will provide continuing care to the client. Proper implementation of the plan ensures that duplication of services does not occur and that confusion or conflicts that arise are promptly handled.

## Evaluation

Evaluation is the measurement of the outcomes or results of implementing the plan for continuity. This involves gathering data on the client's response to interventions. Data can be collected from the client, family, physician, and referral

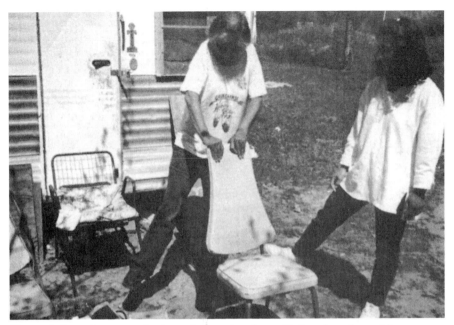

***Figure 8–7.*** ▶ A community-based nurse teaches a Native American elder range-of-motion exercises outside his rural home. She is providing prevention and promotion strategies in her continuity of care of her client.

sources. The major purpose of evaluation is to see if expected outcomes were reached. Evaluation is ongoing; reviews are made to determine if needs were met, if problems were resolved, and if the plan needs to be revised. Evaluation continues as the client moves from one setting to another.

In evaluating the effectiveness of continuity of care, it is essential to consider these points:

▶ Whether health planning was initiated when the client first obtained health care services
▶ If discharge planning was discussed with the client and family at the beginning of care
▶ Whether the client and family participated in early planning for ongoing care
▶ If there was interdisciplinary planning with all involved professionals
▶ If the care being provided to the client was empathic, based on mutual trust and cultural sensitivity
▶ If the client and family believe they had all the information they needed
▶ Whether the client felt prepared for self-care at home
▶ Whether the client and family believe they had the resources needed for self-care
▶ If there is new information that suggests the plan should be revised

The nurse is responsible for monitoring and documenting the client's response to care. Evaluation is effective only if there is a plan with expected outcomes or goals established by the interdisciplinary team. The evaluation process is more meaningful if the expected outcomes are written in a clear, measurable way.

Judgment skills are necessary when comparing real outcomes with expected outcomes. If the client's behavior matches the desired outcomes, the goal has been met. If the goals are not met, then the nurse must examine the reasons for the shortfall.

Unmet goals may be caused by inadequate data collection, incorrect identification of need, unrealistic planning, or poor implementation. The client's living situation or physical condition may have changed. New, previously unidentified needs may require additional care or services. Some services may no longer be necessary, or the client may be ready for discharge. Whatever the conclusion, after evaluation, the appropriate members of the interdisciplinary team must reassess and plan for the continuing needs of the client.

## Documentation

The nurse is always responsible for documenting the client's response to care. Concise and reliable documentation that reflects both progress and response to treatment builds a clear outline for subsequent evaluation. Documentation of all teaching performed is critical to team communication. What was taught, what return demonstrations were completed, and what written materials were given to the client should be included.

A written discharge plan is one method used for communication and coordination among team members. Collection and evaluation of data for the purpose of discharge planning are done in varying degrees of formality (eg, interviews, physical examinations, questionnaires), but communication is better served if the recording of such data is kept formal and organized. Use of well-constructed and consistently used discharge planning documents becomes vital to the success of coordination of disciplines and, therefore, to effective planning. Essential for successful implementation of the discharge plan is documentation that includes the client's response to interventions in the plan, continued assessment for changes in client needs, the client's desires and goals, and evidence of continued collaboration among all involved disciplines.

Documentation has a valuable role in the evaluation of discharge planning, using record audits as in quality improvement programs. The retrospective review of client records to determine compliance with standards of quality care has an advantage in that an audit deals with "hard" data. A client record either has a discharge plan documented or it does not; either discharge teaching was documented, or it was not. A review of records is the most straightforward way of determining whether procedures have been done.

 ## BARRIERS TO SUCCESSFUL CONTINUITY OF CARE

Each client situation is unique. The nurse must be aware of barriers that may adversely affect continuity. These blocks may result from social factors, resource limitations, family matters, communication difficulties, or cultural differences. For example, a center for diabetic education may have materials printed in English only, thereby creating a communication and cultural barrier. When individuals cannot fully understand the material, a communication barrier is created. The health care system itself poses many barriers to continuity of care.

## Social Barriers

### Attitude of the Health Care Worker

The health care worker's attitudes and biases can affect whether the client and family will use available resources. Clients are quick to sense bias and judgment. For example, a prenatal clinic for low-income women may have no place for small children to wait while their mothers are examined. In fact, the mothers are discouraged from bringing their children to the clinic when they have appointments. The women sense this judgment, but most of them cannot afford child care. Consequently, they do not follow through on essential prenatal care, resulting in interrupted continuity.

### Client Motivation

The client may not follow through on a suggested referral if there are more pressing matters at hand. When people are ill, they are often concerned only with meeting basic needs and not with meeting more involved goals, such as belonging or self-esteem. Consequently, when clients are asked to make decisions about their higher needs, their motivation may be diminished because all their energy is going toward getting their basic health care needs met. Client priorities can explain why preventive health care services, for instance, may not be considered a priority when the client has difficulty just feeding and clothing the family. The nurse must be aware of the client's priorities. The nurse must first assist with meeting the needs the client sees as a priority before progressing.

### Lack of Knowledge

When clients do not understand the need for a service, they may avoid using that service. Understanding the reason for a referral to an outside organization, as well as understanding the consequences of not following through, increases the likelihood of clients using the service. This can be true in the case of prenatal care for the adolescent who is pregnant for the first time. She may know she "should" go to the clinic for checkups during pregnancy, but she may not know why. If the adolescent understands the purpose of prenatal care and the consequences of not receiving care, she is more likely to follow up with a referral to the antenatal clinic.

## Family Barriers

Both being involved in decisions about care after discharge and receiving relevant self-care information are rated as very important to clients and families being discharged from one setting to another (Clare & Hofmeyer, 1999). Family involvement may either enhance or interrupt continuity. Whatever the contributing factor affecting family involvement, be it family stress, family functioning, or financial resources, it is up to the nurse to address these issues with input from the family.

### Family Stress

Coping can be especially difficult for the client and family in the acute care phase of treatment when they are asked to begin planning for posthospital care. They may be just beginning to recognize and respond to the severity of the condition and subsequent need for treatment. The client and family are in the throes of a health crisis, while the health care team is attempting to educate, assess, and plan for continuing care needs. The nurse must assess the client's level of stress before involving that client and family in discharge planning, and then the nurse must proceed accordingly.

### Family Functioning

Sometimes care is delayed at the request of the family because of work schedule, other responsibilities, or illness. For example, a test or procedure may be delayed or scheduled on a day when a family member is able to be present. The nurse should evaluate, as much as possible, the home environment and relationships among family members. This can be accomplished by talking to the client, building a level of trust, and then assessing the level of family functioning. Every family operates differently; consequently, every family handles situations in different ways. It is up to the nurse to be aware of the client's needs and choices and to be prepared to advocate for the client when conflict arises.

A supportive family provides an environment conducive to healing and is more likely to help the client recover. An unsupportive family, on the other hand, can be an obstacle. For example, suppose a gay man who is positive for human immunodeficiency syndrome (HIV) has a family that is ashamed of and judgmental about his lifestyle. This conflict of values may stop him from seeking out and using appropriate community resources because he may feel that everyone will make the same judgments.

### Financial Resources

Health care services are costly in the United States, and not everyone has health insurance. Consequently, many people do not seek health care services because they cannot afford them. This is often the case with the "working poor" who are underinsured or uninsured or those who are on medical assistance and may not qualify for needed services. The nurse must be aware of the client's financial and insurance resources before making a referral. Financial reality creates a challenge for the nurse. At times it is difficult to find services in the community that will fill a client's needs when financial resources are inadequate.

## Communication Barriers

Poor communication about recovery information is often attributed to language problems and hearing limitations. In general, health care providers expect client compliance, respect, and cooperation. Communication barriers can occur when the client does not speak English. They also occur when there is a cultural difference significant enough to prohibit communication (eg, reading and comprehension) or to create misunderstandings because of, for example, the age of the client, sexual orientation, or use of nonverbal communication. A client may be offended and not listen to instructions or refuse referrals to community providers if the nurse does not practice culturally sensitive communication techniques (Box 8–5). Increasing age brings hearing limitations, impaired eyesight, and memory loss, which can interfere with communication and retention of information.

## Cross-Cultural Barriers

The biggest barrier, although not the most obvious, is the cross-cultural barrier that may exist between the provider and client. It may be difficult for the nurse to withhold judgment and accept the client or family of another culture. In the opin-

### COMMUNITY-BASED NURSING CARE GUIDELINES

**Box 8–5** ▶ Strategies to Reduce Cultural Barriers
in Discharge Planning

- Encourage nurses and health care workers to speak the language or provide competent interpreters for the population being served.
- Encourage health care workers to be sensitive to the background and previous health care experiences of the target group.
- Listen attentively; be aware of any impairment to communication.
- Elicit information about preferences and health care beliefs and include them in the plan of care.
- Actively inquire about significant others and available support.
- Inquire about the home environment.

ion of the nurse, clients from a different culture may ask "too many" questions, exhibit defensive behavior, lack deference to the recognized authority figure (eg, nurses and other health care providers), or have different perceptions of their role in the discharge planning and referral process.

Health care providers may have different cultural backgrounds, ethnicity, race, age, sexual orientation, gender, and experience in health care practices. The use of culture-specific behaviors positively influences the health care provided and, subsequently, the outcomes. The nurse learns culture-specific behaviors by building knowledge about cultural beliefs related to causes of illness and treatment of disease.

Ethnic and cultural values are pervasive in a person's life, and it is important for the nurse to identify them as they relate to health care practices. Chapter 3 focuses on cultural care and the necessary transcultural nursing skills and competencies required of nurses in community settings.

## Health Care System Barriers

### Reimbursement

Because health care policy is driven by cost, client-centered choices and quality of care are often denied. Rules for health care reimbursement and qualifications for access to and use of services often create a lopsided service system with gaps in care. In some instances, the lack of payment for services creates a barrier to the health care system itself, which purportedly is the client's advocate. The health care worker may be left feeling apathetic toward planning and referral when services are available only when there is a source of payment. Problem solving must occur to remove or work with these constraints.

### Failed Systems

Sometimes systems within the health care setting create barriers to successful continuity. The primary health care team may unintentionally interrupt continuity in several different ways. First, insufficient staff may create delays. Lack of time to address continuity needs is another barrier to continuity (Pichitpornchai, Street, & Boontong, 1999). Third, if staff communication is poor, delays may result.

Caregivers and services outside of the primary health care team may create delays. For example, laboratory test results may not be ready on time, or transport may not be provided during prescribed time lines. These delays are often not within the control of the primary health care team. Sometimes a lack of services may create lack of continuity (Pichitpornchai et al., 1999).

### Lack of Discharge Planning

Other barriers to continuity relate to discharge planning, such as failure to obtain skilled nursing care or to visit nurse service placement for approval in time for discharge. Sometimes delays arise from the nurse's inability to locate family members responsible for discharge (Perlmutter, Suico, Krauss, & Auld, 1998).

Medical equipment essential for home monitoring must be ordered in a timely fashion to avoid delays. There are often policies regarding discharge of a client who is dependent on high-technology monitoring devices. For example, an infant discharged with an apnea–bradycardia monitor may have to be free of apnea and bradycardia episodes for 48 hours before the infant can be discharged (Perlmutter et al., 1998).

## Barriers to Using Community Resources

### Previous Experiences

If a client has not had a good experience with a referral in the past, he or she may be hesitant to use this type of service again. The same is true for a client's perception of a particular agency or organization. The nurse must acknowledge the client's feelings and opinions about past experiences. Talking with and listening to the client will help the nurse work with the client to get the best results from a referral to a community provider. The nurse may find that the client lacked information about the organization and a different approach is all that is necessary. Perhaps the client's complaints about the organization are justified, in which case it may be in the client's best interest to find an alternative provider.

### Accessibility

A major barrier to using health care services is accessibility. Many communities do not have public transportation. Hospitals, clinics, and other health care services are closing, especially in rural areas, and many rural communities are left with no local health care services. This loss requires clients to travel long distances to reach health care services. Conversely, a city-dwelling client who may not own a car might have difficulty getting to a suburban clinic. The nurse must get information from the client about access to transportation before making a referral. This is especially important with low-income clients, urban clients, and those living in rural areas.

## ELEMENTS OF SUCCESSFUL CONTINUITY OF CARE

As with all nursing care, it is always best to begin with the simplest interventions. These include building a trusting relationship and using therapeutic communication as the client and family are interviewed. All of the interventions discussed in Chapter 7 apply: care coordination, collaboration, delegation, and referral and follow-up. Much can be learned from successful programs designed to enhance continuity. Some simple interventions emerge.

Several current studies show that clients benefit from nursing follow-up after discharge from the hospital. One study found that when nurse practitioners (NPs) provided follow-up care with clients with hypercholesterolemia who had undergone coronary artery bypass grafting or percutaneous coronary surgical intervention, their cholesterol level was lower and their diet and exercise improved when compared to clients who did not receive follow-up nursing care. The NPs spent an average of 4.5 hours per client over the year. After one year, 65% of those receiving nurse follow-up had reduced their cholesterol to desirable levels, compared with 35% of clients who did not receive nurse follow-up (Allen et al., 2002). Nursing follow-up also proved effective for women with abusive partners to take protective measures against future abuse. In a randomized case-control study, the group with the nursing intervention adopted substantially more safety behaviors than those in the control group as measured 6 months after the intervention (McFarlane et al., 2002).

A home-based program enhances successful continuity of care for clients with chronic congestive heart failure (CHF), according to a study by Stewart, Marley, and Horowitz (1999). Because hospital admissions among clients with CHF are a major contributor to health care costs, this study investigated the impact of a comprehensive home assessment by a cardiac nurse on CHF readmission rates over a 6-month period. Both study groups received the usual discharge planning, but only one group received a home visit during which the visiting cardiac nurse completed a comprehensive assessment 7 to 10 days after discharge. Another home visit was made only if the client had two or more unplanned readmissions within the 6-month period. Overall, there were fewer exacerbations of the condition and unplanned hospital readmissions with the group receiving the home visit.

Hip fractures represent a major health problem with the older population. This condition frequently results in care in several settings (eg, the hospital, transitional/subacute hospital, and assisted living or long-term care facility). Robinson (1999) studied factors that promote function and enable a successful transition to home for elderly clients recovering from a hip fracture. Several things can be learned from this study. First, discharge planning and follow-up should receive greater attention, with identification of resources at admission. Second, telephone reminders from the physical therapist after discharge result in the client continuing to exercise. This study reinforces the importance of nurse involvement, even with the simplest intervention of a follow-up telephone call to enhance self-care. Box 8–6 offers another example of a successful program to enhance continuity of care.

## CONCLUSIONS

This chapter has taken a broad look at continuity of care. Essential to quality health care is a strong, ongoing health care plan that includes appropriate use of resources and effective referrals. Discharge planning has been described as a significant process that ensures continuity of care by coordinating various aspects of a client's care beginning with admission through transition from one health care setting to another. Planning for discharge begins with entrance into the health care system. Coordination of activities involving the clients,

## RESEARCH IN COMMUNITY-BASED NURSING CARE

**Box 8–6** ▶ Information Needs of Elderly Postsurgical Cancer Clients During the Transition From Hospital to Home

The purpose of this study is to describe information needs of elderly postsurgical cancer clients. The 148 clients surgically treated for a new diagnosis of cancer were randomly assigned to the treatment group, and their responses were compared to a similar control group. The experimental group received a home care intervention consisting of three home visits and five telephone contacts from an advanced practice nurse.

Both groups received information during hospitalization and discharge with written instruction. It was found that the experimental group still needed information on multiple topics. The teaching needs identified as important by the clients and families included the topics of outlining the clinical course of the illness, community resources, events to report, and pain management.

The study concluded that the learning needs of elderly postsurgical cancer clients during the transition from hospital to home are complex and cannot be adequately addressed during hospitalization. Despite the teaching and written information received during usual discharge planning, these clients needed ongoing contact with nurses. Further, a nurse case manager model using a combination of home and telephone contacts may be a cost-effective option for providing continuity. Forty percent of the teaching completed in this study was done on the telephone. Further research is needed to determine the best methods for enhancing continuity between hospital and home for postsurgical clients.

Hughes, L., Hodgson, N., Muller, P., Robinson, L., & McCorkle, R. (2000). Information needs of elderly postsurgical cancer patients during the transition from hospital to home. *Journal of Nursing Scholarship, 32*(1), 25–30.

providers, and payers is essential in providing continued care. Identification of current and future needs leads to implementation of the referral process and continued care. The discharge planning process resembles the nursing process; therefore, the nurse is in an advantageous position to manage effective planning and continued care. Barriers to effective discharge planning include social, family, communication, health care system, and community resources issues. In evaluating the effectiveness of continuity of care, one must consider whether planning was initiated when the client entered the system, whether the client and family were part of the planning, and whether the plan was well coordinated with all members of the team.

# What's on the Web

American Association for Continuity of
Care
P.O. Box 532
Dunedin, Florida 34697
1-800-816-1575 Fax 1-727-738-8099

**Internet address:**
*http://www.continuityofcare.com*
This site has extensive information about
the organization and pertinent issues. It also
provides many links to other professional
organizations related to continuity care.
See Chapter 7 for additional resources.

## References and Bibliography

Allen, J. K., Blumenthal, R., Margolis, S., Young, D., Miller, R., & Kelly, K. (2002). Nurse case management of hypercholesterolemia in patients with coronary heart disease: Results of a randomized clinical trial. *American Heart Journal, 144*(4), 678–686.

Blaylock, A., & Cason, C. L. (1992). Discharge planning: Predicting patient's needs. *Journal of Gerontological Nursing, 18*(7), 5–10.

Brody, K., Johnson, R., Reid, D., Carder, P., & Perrin, N., (2002). A comparison of two methods for identifying frail Medicare-aged persons. *Journal of the American Geriatrics Society, 50*(3), 562–569.

Clare, J., & Hofmeyer, A. (1999). Discharge planning continuity of care for aged people; Indicators of satisfaction and implications for practice. *Australian Journal of Advanced Nursing, 16*(1), 7–13.

Craven, R. F., & Hirnle, C. J. (2000). *Fundamentals of nursing: Human health and function* (3rd ed.). Philadelphia: Lippincott Williams & Wilkins.

Desai, M., Bogardus, S., Williams, C., Vitagliano, G., & Inouye, S. (2002). Development and validation of a risk-adjustment index for older patients: The high-risk diagnoses for the elderly scale. *Journal of the American Geriatrics Society, 50*(3), 475–481.

Hall, M., & Lawrence, L. (1998). *Ambulatory surgery in the United States, 1996. Advance data* (p. 300). Washington, DC: U.S. Department of Health and Human Services.

Holland, D., Hansen, D., Matt-Hensrud, M., Severson, M., & Wenninger, C. (1999). Continuity of care: A nursing needs assessment instrument. *Geriatric Nursing, 19*(6), 331–334.

Hoskins, I., Thiel, L., Walton-Moss, B., Clark, H., & Schroeder, M. (2001). What is the difference: Clinical pathway versus a usual plan of care for patients with congestive heart failure. *Home Healthcare Nurse 19*(3), 142–150.

Hughes, L., Hodgson, N., Muller, P., Robinson, L., & McCorkle, R. (2000). Information needs of elderly postsurgical cancer patients during the transition from hospital to home. *Journal of Nursing Scholarship, 32*(1), 25–30.

Joint Commission on Accreditation of Healthcare Organizations. (1996). *Accreditation manual for hospitals.* Chicago: Author.

Kesby, S. (2002). Nursing care and collaborative practice. *Journal of Clinical Nursing, 11*(3), 357–366. Retrieved January 19, 2003, from the CINAHL database.

McFarlane, J., Malecha, A., Gist, J., Watson, K., Batten, E., Hall, I., & Smith, S. (2002). An intervention to increase safety behaviors of abused women: Results of a randomized clinical trial. *Nursing Research, 51*(6), 347–354.

Mistiaen, P., Duijnhouwer, E., Prins-Hoekstra, A., Ros, W., & Blaylock, A. (1999). Predictive validity of the BRASS index in screening patients with post-discharge problems. *Journal of Advanced Nursing, 30*(5), 1050–1056.

Pearson, B., Skelly, R., Wileman, D., & Masud, R. (2002). Unplanned readmission to hospital: A comparison of the views of general practitioners and hospital staff. *Age and Ageing*, 31, 141–143.

Perlmutter, D., Suico, C., Krauss, A., & Auld, P. (1998). A program to reduce discharge delays in a neonatal intensive care unit. *American Journal of Managed Care, 4*(4), 548–552.

Pichitpornchai, W., Street, A., & Boontong, T. (1999). Discharge planning and transitional care: Issues in Thai nursing. *International Journal of Nursing Studies, 36*(5), 355–362.

Powell, S. (2000). *Case management: A practical guide to success in managed care* (2nd ed.). Philadelphia: Lippincott Williams & Wilkins.

Robinson, S. (1999). Transitions in the lives of elderly women who have sustained hip fractures. *Journal of Advanced Nursing, 30*(6), 1341–1348.

Sparbel, K., & Anderson, M. (2000). Integrated literature review of continuity of care: Part 1, conceptual issues. *Journal of Nursing Scholarship, 32*(1), 17–24.

Stewart, S., Marley, J., & Horowitz, J. (1999). Effects of multidisciplinary, home-based intervention on unplanned readmission and survival among patients with chronic congestive heart failure; a randomized controlled study. *Lancet, 354*(9184), 1077–1083.

Ware, N., Tugenberg, T., Dickey, B., & McHorney, C. (1999). An ethnographic study of the meaning of continuity of care in mental health services. *Psychiatric Services, 50*(3), 395–400.

# LEARNING ACTIVITIES

## JOURNALING: ACTIVITY 8–1

In your clinical journal, describe a situation you observed in which a client or family experienced difficulty because of poor continuity. If you were the nurse in charge, what would you have done differently?

In your clinical journal, relate a situation in which you observed a client who received effective continuity of care. What made the care effective?

List any barriers you have noticed that have interrupted continuity for a client you have cared for in clinical. Discuss what happened and what you would do differently. Identify any systems issues that you think did not address the barriers (eg, chart forms such as discharge forms, admission forms, unit policies).

## CLIENT CARE: ACTIVITY 8–2

Mr. Heaney, a 66-year-old man, is admitted for a total knee replacement. He has had continuous pain in his left knee for the past 2 years secondary to osteoarthritis. His wife of 45 years died just 2 months ago, and he has remained alone in their two-story home. Only one of their six children lives in the metropolitan area. On postoperative day 1 he begins physical therapy. His left leg is in a continuous passive motion device when he is in bed. The plan is to discharge him on postoperative day 2 with outpatient physical therapy, the use of the continuous passive motion device at home, and continuation of oral analgesics for pain. He appears to be slightly confused during the discharge planning conference when the discussion about his continuing care is discussed.

1. Describe your role as the primary nurse in Mr. Heaney's discharge planning.
2. Explain why you are in an effective position to coordinate continuity of care.

3. Identify the risks Mr. Heaney may have after discharge. Use the Blaylock Discharge Planning Risk Assessment Screen (Fig. 8–5) to assess for risks.
4. Propose recommendations for his living situation and home care.
5. List agencies, facilities, or individuals you would recommend for Mr. Heaney's continuing care and give your reasons.

### PRACTICAL APPLICATION: ACTIVITY 8–3

Observe a nurse doing routine discharge planning with a client in the hospital. How did the nurse assess the following with the client or the client's family? (This could be done either through questions on the discharge form or additional questions the nurse asks.)

- How are you going to manage at home?
- Considering the treatments ordered for you, what are you going to need to manage at home?
- What help do you need?
- What help do you have at home now?
- Will family members need to change their routines?
- Will family members be able to provide all of the care needed?
- Do they need home health care assistance?
- What are the family's resources and limitations?

If you were the nurse, what would you have done differently from or in addition to the activities of the nurse you observed?

### CRITICAL THINKING: ACTIVITY 8–4

Explore methods to enhance continuity in the settings where you do clinical work. Identify areas where continuity is weak and determine strategies for improvement.

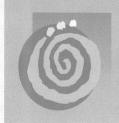

# COMMUNITY-BASED NURSING ACROSS THE LIFE SPAN

In Chapter 2, you learned that although the U.S. health care system is the most expensive in the world, the United States lags behind other nations in key health indicators. This unit uses the recommendations from *Healthy People 2010* to outline the role that the nurse must play in improving the nation's health.

Each chapter begins with a discussion of the goals of *Healthy People 2010*, as well as the major causes of mortality and morbidity for each age group. Nursing assessments and interventions follow. Chapter 9 discusses health promotion and disease prevention for maternal/infant, child, and adolescent populations. Chapter 10 outlines health promotion and disease prevention for adults, and Chapter 11 focuses on elderly adults.

The content of each chapter is organized around the leading causes of mortality for each group. Disease prevention and health promotion strategies that address these causes are highlighted. Based on numerous sources, these strategies are intended for the practicing nurse to use to teach clients about health promotion and disease prevention. Unit III also contains numerous Web site and organization addresses, as well as resources related to health promotion and disease prevention for clients across the life span.

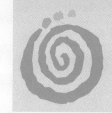

## CHAPTER 9

# Health Promotion and Disease Prevention for Maternal/Infant, Child, and Adolescent Populations

### Roberta Hunt

## KEY TERMS

Denver Developmental Screening Test (DDST)
fetal alcohol syndrome (FAS)
infant mortality rate
lead poisoning
low birth weight (LBW)

morbidity
mortality
neural tube defects (NTDs)
sudden infant death
   syndrome (SIDS)

## THE NURSE SPEAKS

For over 10 years, I worked as a school nurse at a large high school in a small Midwestern town. One day, a 15-year-old student named Jennifer came into my office. She was obviously pregnant. She told me that she was going to the doctor the next day to find out if she was pregnant. She didn't think that she was, but wanted to find out for sure. I asked her if she could feel any kicking, and she said she could. I asked her if she could feel kicking when she held her hand on her stomach, and she said she could. When she left my office she said that she would let me know what the doctor said.

Several days later, she returned to see me and said that she had had an exam and was indeed pregnant and due in 1 month. I asked about the possibility of finding a prenatal class for her, but she wasn't interested. Although I saw her several times before her baby was born, she remained detached and uninterested in the baby or learning about the impending delivery. I was very concerned about Jennifer and her baby. I wondered if she would attach to the baby and thought that this family was at risk for lack of early bonding and attachment. I knew that babies born to young teen moms were at higher risk for child abuse and neglect than infants born to older women.

A month after her baby was born, I called Jennifer and asked if I could come to see her. She was living with her parents. She agreed to a home visit the next week. When I entered the home, Jennifer was holding her daughter and sitting at the kitchen table with her father. I sat down and explained that I was the school nurse and did home visits with some of the students from the high school. I kept things casual and at first we talked about general things. Then Jennifer began to talk about when she would be returning to school, when she hoped to graduate, and the classes she would be taking. Jennifer's mother came in as we were talking and stated, "The baby is sleeping all night now. Jennifer is a great mom. I am working the evening shift now, so I will take care of the baby when Jennifer is in school."

All the time we were talking, I was quietly observing Jennifer with her baby daughter. She was holding her close but with a relaxed posture. She frequently looked at the baby, and when the baby woke up Jennifer looked into her sleepy eyes and said softly said, "Hi Tiffany. Did you have a good nap?" Then she fed Tiffany a bottle. As she was feeding her, Jennifer was watching Tiffany's face. As soon as the baby started to act like she wanted to stop feeding, Jennifer would take the bottle out of her mouth. She said, "Tiffany likes to just drink a little and then be burped and rest."

I left Jennifer's home confident that with the support of her parents, Tiffany would be well cared for and Jennifer would be able to finish high school. My concern about her nonchalance about being pregnant and the birth of her baby did not appear to have interfered with her attaching to her baby. I was relieved that despite the lack of prenatal care and preparation, this family had all the basics to care for this newborn.

**— Ashley Moore RN, PHN**
St Paul, Minnesota

## SIGNIFICANCE OF HEALTH PROMOTION AND DISEASE PREVENTION

Crucial issues of health and health care are different today from what they were in the early part of the 20th century. Public health efforts have increased the life span of the average person, thanks to the development of effective medications, particularly antibiotics, and universal access to clean water, sanitation, and immunization. Our focus as health care providers has changed from combating infectious diseases to addressing chronic conditions and unintentional injuries.

Health promotion is typically defined as a primary disease prevention strategy. It is commonly interchanged with terms such as health education and disease prevention. Often health promotion is discussed as the epitome of empowerment in that it is a process that enables people to use health as a resource for their lives. Health promotion is most often discussed as a strategy for an already healthy individual or population, but it applies to those with health conditions as well. Disease prevention is just as it states: preventing a disease from occurring. It also includes injury prevention, which will be discussed a great deal in this and the following two chapters.

Recommendations from *Healthy People 2010* form the foundation for all health promotion and disease prevention nursing actions. These recommendations are based on the primary causes of death, or **mortality,** rates and the rates of illness or injury, or **morbidity,** rates. The *Healthy People 2010* report is based on mortality and morbidity statistics that represent the primary causes of death and illnesses and injuries experienced by the people living in the United States.

Most diseases and deaths result from preventable causes. The negative impact of many conditions can be minimized by early identification and intervention. This chapter addresses health promotion and disease prevention for pregnant women, infants, children, and adolescents.

## ELIMINATING DISPARITY IN HEALTH CARE

Another central goal of *Healthy People 2010* is to eliminate health disparities. Health disparities exist by gender, race or ethnicity, education, income, disability, rural living localities, and sexual orientation. A good example is infant mortality, which was 7.1 per 1,000 live births for all infants in the United States in 1999. In the same year, the infant mortality rate among African-American infants was 14.1, whereas that of White infants was 5.8, making the rate of death for Black infants more than double that of White infants. Infant mortality rates have declined within all racial groups, yet the proportional discrepancy between African Americans and Whites remains largely unchanged (U.S. Department of Health and Human Services [DHHS], 2002; Federal Interagency Forum on Child and Family Statistics, 2002). Comparisons between races and infant mortality rates can be seen in Figure 9–1.

Disparity by ethnicity is believed to result from complex interactions among genetic variations, environmental factors, and specific health behaviors.

Income and education underlie many health disparities in the United States. Income and education are intrinsically related; people with the worst health status are among those with the highest poverty rates and least education. Income inequality in the United States has increased over the past 3 decades.

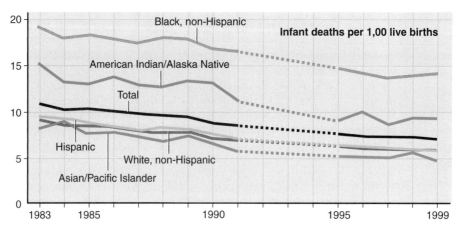

NOTE: Data are available for 1983-91 and 1995-99.[48] Infant deaths are deaths before the child's first birthday.
SOURCE: Centers for Disease Control and Prevention, National Center for Health Statistics, National Linked File of Live Births and Infant Deaths.

**Figure 9–1.** ▶ Infant Mortality Rate by Race. Source: Federal Interagency Forum on Child and Family Statistics. (2002). *America's children: Key national indicators of well-being, 2002.* Federal Interagency Forum on Child and Family Statistics. Washington, DC: U.S. Government Printing Office (p 31).

 ## MATERNAL/INFANT POPULATIONS

Florence Nightingale wrote in 1894 that "money would be better spent in maintaining health in infancy and childhood than in building hospitals to cure disease" (Monteiro, 1985, p. 185). The same philosophy holds true today. The health of infants and children has farther-reaching implications than that of other population groups. "The health of mothers, infants and children is of critical importance, both as a reflection of the current health status of a large segment of the U.S. population and as a predictor of the health of the next generations" (DHHS, 2000b, p. 16–23). Box 9–1 lists the *Healthy People 2010* objectives for maternal and infant health.

Infant death is a critical indicator of the health of a population because it reflects the overall state of maternal health, as well as the quality and access of primary health available to pregnant women and infants. The **infant mortality rate** is the number of infants (ages birth to 1 year) who die out of every 1,000 live births. Although the 1980s and 1990s saw steady declines in the infant mortality rate in the United States, 27th among industrialized nations, it remains among the highest in the industrialized world (DHHS, 2002).

### Prenatal Care

The United States is the only industrialized nation in which not all pregnant women receive prenatal care. In the United States, the percentage of mothers receiving early prenatal care (in the first trimester of pregnancy) varies substantially among racial and ethnic groups, from 74% for Black and Hispanic mothers to 88%

## HEALTHY PEOPLE 2010

### Box 9–1   Objectives for Maternal and Infant Health

Reduce fetal and infant deaths.

Increase proportion of pregnant women who receive early and adequate prenatal care.

Increase the proportion of pregnant women who attend a series of prepared childbirth classes.

Reduce preterm births.

Reduce the occurrence of spina bifida and other neural tube defects.

Increase abstinence from alcohol, cigarettes, and illicit drugs among pregnant women.

Increase the percentage of healthy full-term infants who are put down to sleep on their backs.

Increase the proportion of mothers who breast-feed their babies.

———

U.S. Department of Health and Human Services. (2000b). Maternal, infant, and child health. In *Healthy people 2010. National health promotion and disease prevention objectives.* Washington, DC: U.S. Government Printing Office.

---

for White mothers. Of mothers in their teens, 33% received no early prenatal care in 2000 (Infant Mortality, 2002).

Every nurse in every setting should encourage pregnant women to begin prenatal care in the first trimester. One effective intervention is home visitation, where nurses can provide prenatal care and lower the probability of low-birth-weight infants, thus helping to lower the infant mortality rate (Kitzman et al., 2000). Healthy Start uses home visits as one strategy to expand the availability and accessibility of prenatal health care in more than 100 communities nationwide with higher-than–average infant mortality rates. Designed to meet community needs, the projects include outreach, case management, health education, and community consortia. More information about Healthy Start can be found at http://www.healthy-start.com/. Some of the topics that are important for the nurse to assess and intervene accordingly in home visits to pregnant women are those that *Healthy People 2010* has deemed the leading causes of infant mortality: low birth weight, birth, and congenital anomalies.

### Low Birth Weight

**Low birth weight (LBW)**, or weight less than 2,500 g or 5.5 lb, is the leading cause of preventable neonatal death. This is included under disorders related to premature birth in Table 9–1. Approximately 7.5% of babies are LBW infants (Centers for Disease Control and Prevention [CDC], National Center on Birth Defects and Developmental Disability [NCBDDD], 2000). This figure continues to rise. LBW is associated with long-term disabilities, such as cerebral palsy, autism, mental retardation, vision and hearing impairment, and other developmental disabilities. LBW is also the main reason premature infants require care in neonatal intensive care units. It does not take a complicated cost analysis to conclude that it is much more

| TABLE 9–1 • Leading Causes of Death by Age Group, United States, 1997 | | |
|---|---|---|
| **Age** | **Cause of Death** | **Number of Deaths** |
| Younger than 1 y | Birth defects | 5,473 |
| | Disorders related to premature birth | 4,392 |
| | Sudden infant death syndrome | 2,646 |
| 1–4 y | Unintentional injuries | 1,898 |
| | Birth defects | 549 |
| | Cancer | 418 |
| 5–9 y | Unintentional injuries | 1,459 |
| | Cancer | 509 |
| | Homicide | 207 |
| 10–14 y | Unintentional injuries | 1,636 |
| | Cancer | 503 |
| | Homicide | 246 |
| 15–24 y | Unintentional injuries | 13,656 |
| | Homicide | 4,998 |
| | Suicide | 3,901 |

U.S. Department of Health and Human Services. (2000b). Maternal, infant, and child health. In *Healthy people 2010. National health promotion and disease prevention objectives.* Washington, DC: U.S. Government Printing Office.

expensive to care for a newborn in an intensive care unit than it would have been to provide prenatal care for the infant's mother. In 1995, the cost of a normal, healthy delivery averaged $2,842, whereas hospital costs for LBW infants averaged $21,000 (Healthy Start, 1996). The primary intervention to prevent LBW is early initiation of prenatal care.

### Neural Tube Defects

Approximately 50% of all **neural tube defects (NTDs)** may be prevented with adequate consumption of folic acid in the first trimester of pregnancy. Currently, the U.S. Public Health Service recommends that all women of childbearing age consume 400 μg of folic acid daily. For women who are planning a pregnancy, 4,000 μg is recommended.

### Cigarette Smoking

A pregnant woman who smokes is 1.5 to 3.5 times more likely to have a LBW infant, 1.8 times more likely to have an ectopic pregnancy, and 1.6 times more likely to have a spontaneous abortion than a nonsmoker (CDC, 2002). Between 20% and 33% of women smoke during pregnancy. Up to 25% of women who smoke before pregnancy stop before their first antenatal visit. However, the rest continue to smoke throughout the pregnancy (DHHS, 2000b). In approximately 14% of all births, the mother reports smoking during the pregnancy. Smoking cessation programs have been shown to be effective in reducing smoking rates. Nurses are often the best health care providers to promote smoking cessation programs to help their clients quit, especially when the client is pregnant (Todd, LaSala, & Neil-Urban, 2001). Smoking cessation programs can be found on the Internet through Healthfinder (http://www.healthfinder.gov/).

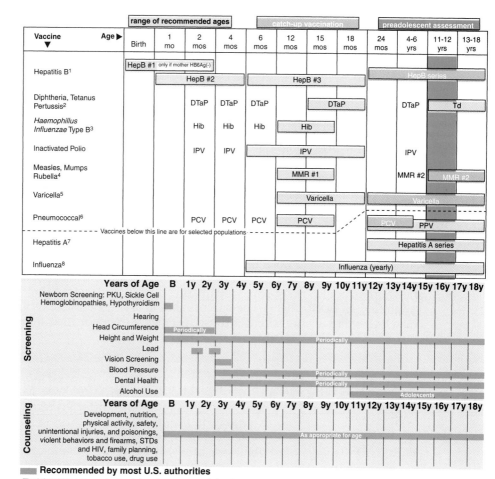

**Figure 9–2.** ▶ Clinical preventive services for normal-risk children. Source: Agency for Healthcare Research and Quality. (2000). *Child health guide: Put prevention into practice.* Rockville, MD. Available at http://www.ahcpr.gov/ppip/ppchild.htm. Note: immunization schedule may change yearly. Check it at: *http://www.ecbt.org/immsche.htm* or call the hot line at 1-800-232-2522 English, or 1-800-232-0233 Spanish.

### Alcohol and Drug Use

Moderate to heavy alcohol use by women during pregnancy has been associated with many severe adverse effects, including **fetal alcohol syndrome (FAS)** and other developmental delays. FAS is recognized as the leading cause of mental retardation. Infants and children with FAS have characteristic facial and associated physical features attributed to excessive ingestion of alcohol by the mother during pregnancy. It is the nurse's responsibility to discuss alcohol and drug use with the client in an open and nonjudgmental manner. Currently, it is recommended that women do not consume any alcohol during pregnancy.

## Newborn Care

The *Child Health Guide: Put Prevention into Practice* (Agency for Healthcare Research and Quality, 2000) is an excellent tool for monitoring infant and child health. It is available on-line at http://www.ahcpr.gov/ppip/ppchild.htm, or a free copy can be ordered by calling (800) 358-9295. It provides parents with explanations of child preventive care and a convenient place to keep records of health care visits, growth, and immunizations. It recommends checkups at 3 weeks; 2, 4, 6, 9, 12, 15, and 18 months; and 2, 3, 4, 5, 6, 8, 10, 12, 14, 16, and 18 years with a pediatric nurse practitioner or physician. *Bright Futures: Guidelines for Health Supervision for Infants, Children, and Adolescents*, 2nd edition (DHHS, 2000a), can be downloaded from the Bright Futures Web site (http://www.brightfutures.org/). It contains health supervision guidelines and information, including developmental charts for children, ages newborn through adolescence.

Box 9–2 presents an example of research relating to newborn care.

### Screening

All newborns should have blood tests in the hospital for phenylketonuria (PKU), thyroid disease, and sickle cell disease. The current recommendation is that all newborns should be screened for hearing impairment before they leave the hospital (CDC NCBDDD, 2000). The parents should ask the nurse practitioner or physician if they are unsure whether these tests were done for their infant.

---

**RESEARCH IN COMMUNITY-BASED NURSING CARE**

**Box 9–2** ▸ Massage as an Intervention for Preterm, Low-Birth-Weight Infants

Infant massage has been associated with improved sleep and contentment with both preterm and term infants. This integrative review discussed studies over the past 10 years that examined the impact of massage on preterm infants. One study compared preterm, LBW infants who received massage interventions to a comparable group who did not receive massage. It found that the group receiving massage gained more weight per day than control infants. Massage interventions decreased length of stay by 4.6 days. Those infants in the massage group improved performance slightly on the Brazelton scale for habituation, motor maturity, and range of state. No evidence was found of an effect of gentle, still touch on neonatal morbidity score, days on oxygen, blood transfusions, activity, or behavioral distress cues. No adverse effects of touch or massage were reported in any study.

The nursing literature strongly advocates massage interventions in the care of preterm, LBW infants.

Vickers, A., Ohlsson, A., Lacy, J. B., & Horsley, A. (1999). Massage for promoting growth and development of preterm and/or low birthweight infants. Cochrane Database System Review, 2, CD000390.

All infants' growth should be monitored and plotted on a growth chart outlining the developmental status of the infant. Charts are available from the DHHS in French and Spanish at http://www.cdc.gov/growthcharts. To reduce mortality and morbidity, both the parent and the nurse must be diligent in following preventive measures for normal-risk infants. In all community-based settings, the nurse can assist the parent in following basic prevention recommendations for children. Figure 9–2 outlines current recommendations for clinical preventive services for normal-risk children.

### Immunizations

Fifty years ago, many children died from what today are preventable childhood diseases. Smallpox has been eradicated, poliomyelitis has been eliminated from the Western hemisphere, and cases of measles and chickenpox in the United States are at a record low. All of this progress has been made possible by immunizations. However, only if the number of vaccinated children and adults remains high will immunization programs continue to be effective.

Immunizations are considered primary prevention because they prevent the occurrence of a disease. It is imperative that all children be immunized according to recommended standards. Immunizations should begin at birth and continue as recommended in Figure 9–3 Once a year, consult Every Child by Two at (800-232-2522 in English or 800-232-0233 in Spanish) or (http://www.ecbt.org/) for updates.

### Nutrition

Breast milk is widely acknowledged to be the most complete form of nutrition for infants (see Box 9-3). The range of benefits includes health, growth, immunity, and de-

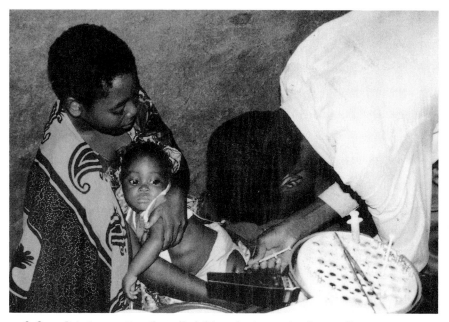

*Figure 9–3.* ▶ It is imperative that all children be immunized according to recommended standards.

velopment. Breast-fed infants have decreased rates of diarrhea, respiratory infections, and ear infections (Wright, Bauer, Naylor, Sutcliffe, & Clark, 1998). Breast-feeding improves maternal health by reducing postpartum bleeding, promoting return to prepregnancy weight, and reducing the risks of breast cancer and osteoporosis long after the postpartum period. The American Academy of Pediatrics (AAP) considers breast-feeding to be the ideal method of feeding and nurturing infants.

As with any teaching, consider the developmental stage, cognitive abilities, and culture of the client when initiating breast-feeding teaching. Teenage mothers are more interested in knowing that breast-feeding is easy, saves time, and will enhance weight loss so they can fit into their prepregnancy clothes sooner. Older mothers are typically more interested in the long-term benefits to their babies. The La Leche League is a wonderful resource for information on breast-feeding http://www.lalecheleague.org). Encouraging new mothers to breast-feed is a simple intervention that can have a strong and lasting effect on the health of the mother and baby, second only to early prenatal care.

## COMMUNITY-BASED TEACHING

**Box 9–3** ▸ Guidelines for a Healthy Diet for the Infant to 2-Year-Old Child

- Breast milk is the single best food for infants from birth to 6 months of age. It provides good nutrition and protects against infection.
- Breast-feeding should continue for at least the first year, if possible.
- If breast-feeding is not possible or not desired, iron-enriched formula (not cow's milk) should be used during the first 12 months of life. Whole cow's milk can be used to replace formula or breast milk after 12 months of age.
- Breast-fed babies (particularly dark-skinned infants) who do not get regular exposure to sunlight may need to receive vitamin D supplements.
- Suitable solid foods should be introduced at 4 to 6 months of age. Most experts recommend iron-enriched infant rice cereal as the first food.
- Start new foods one at a time to make it easier to identify problem foods. For example, wait 1 week before adding each new cereal, vegetable, or other food.
- Use iron-rich foods, such as iron-enriched cereals, other grains, and meats.
- Do not give honey to infants during the first 12 months of life.
- Do not limit fat during the first 2 years of life.

Agency for Healthcare Research and Quality. (2000). *Child health guide: Put prevention into practice.* Rockville, MD. Retrieved on May 15, 2002 from http://www.ahcpr.gov/ppip/ppchild.htm

## COMMUNITY-BASED TEACHING

### Box 9–4 ▶ Safety Guidelines for Infants and Young Children

- Use a car safety seat at all times until your child weighs at least 40 lb.
- Car seats must be properly secured in the back seat, preferably in the middle.
- Keep medication, cleaning solutions, and other dangerous substances in childproof containers, locked up, and out of reach of children.
- Use safety gates across stairways (top and bottom) and guards on windows above the first floor.
- Keep hot-water heater temperatures below 120°F.
- Keep unused electrical outlets covered with plastic guards.
- Provide constant supervision for babies using baby walkers. Block the access to stairways and to objects that can fall (such as lamps) or cause burns (such as stoves).
- Keep objects and foods that cause choking away from your child, such as coins, balloons, small toy parts, hot dogs (unmashed), peanuts, and hard candies.
- Use fences that go all the way around pools and keep gates to pools locked.

Agency for Healthcare Research and Quality. (2000). *Child health guide: Put prevention into practice.* Rockville, MD. Available at: *http://www.ahcpr.gov/ppip/ppchild.htm.*

*Safety*

Because more children die of unintentional injuries than any other cause, it is important to counsel parents on home safety (see Box 9–4). The primary issue related to safety of the infant is sleeping positioning. Parents should put newborns to sleep on their backs. This position dramatically reduces deaths from **sudden infant death syndrome (SIDS)**, a leading cause of death in infants. More information for parents on reducing the risk of SIDS is available from the National Institute of Child Health and Human Development, at http://www.nichd.nih.gov/sids/.

## PRESCHOOL-AGE CHILDREN

*Healthy People 2010* objectives for child health are listed in Box 9–5. The leading cause of death in children of all ages is injury. Among children ages 1 to 4 years, the leading injury-related causes of death are motor vehicle crashes, drowning, and fires and burns. These deaths are, for the most part, preventable.

> ### HEALTHY PEOPLE 2010
>
> **Box 9–5 Objectives for Child Health**
>
> Reduce the rate of child deaths (ages 1–4 years).
>
> Reduce or eliminate indigenous cases of vaccine-preventable disease.
>
> Reduce iron deficiency among young children and females of childbearing age.
>
> Increase the proportion of persons ages 2 years and older who consume at least two daily servings of fruit.
>
> Increase the proportion of persons ages 2 years and older who consume at least three daily servings of vegetables.
>
> Reduce the proportion of children and adolescents who have dental caries in their primary or permanent teeth.
>
> Increase the proportion of children and adolescents who view television 2 hours or less per day.
>
> Increase the proportion of the nation's public and private schools that provide access to their physical activity spaces and facilities for all persons outside of normal school hours (before and after the school day, on weekends, and during summer and other vacations).
>
> Increase the proportion of preschool children ages 5 years and under who receive vision and hearing screening.
>
> ---
>
> Sources: U.S. Department of Health and Human Services. (2000b). Maternal, infant, and child health. In *Healthy people 2010. National health promotion and disease prevention objectives.* Washington, DC: U.S. Government Printing Office.
>
> U.S. Department of Health and Human Services. (2002). *Preventing infant mortality* [Fact sheet]. Retrieved January 21, 2003, from *http://hhs.gov/news/pres/2002pres/infant.html*

## Screening

In all community-based settings, the nurse can assist the parent in following basic prevention recommendations for children to reduce mortality and morbidity. Figure 9–2 outlines current recommendations for clinical preventive services for normal-risk children. All young children's growth should be monitored and plotted on a growth chart.

Periodic screening benefits all children. Most screening programs are developed and run by nurses in community-based settings. Preschool screening, which typically includes vision, hearing, height and weight, immunization status, and developmental screening, is an important preventive intervention. The cost of preschool screening is minimal when compared with the cost of undetected deficits that result in hardship and monetary costs to the child, parents, and society. The earlier a condition is identified, the greater the chances of lessening or eliminating the long-term effects.

The most widely used tool to assess development is the **Denver Developmental Screening Test (DDST)**. It is used to screen children from 1 month to 6 years, covering the topics of gross motor skills, fine motor skills, language development, and personal/social development. This easy-to-administer screening tool has the potential to identify developmental issues early for prompt intervention. The AAP states that early identification leads to more effective therapy for children with developmental disabilities (AAP, 1995). The DDST is an excellent example of secondary prevention.

### Lead Screening

Lead has been present in our environment since industrialization. Children are particularly sensitive to the toxic effects of lead. Most often, **lead poisoning** is silent, with the individual having no symptoms until systemic damage has occurred. Decreased stature or growth, decreased intelligence, impaired neurobehavioral development, and adverse effects on the central nervous system, kidneys, and hematopoietic system are some of the common consequences of lead poisoning.

Lead poisoning is widespread. It was estimated that almost 1 million children in the United States, 22% of which are Black children and 13% of which are Mexican children, had lead blood levels above safe levels in 2002. More than half of occupied, privately owned housing built before 1980 contains lead-based paint. In general, screening and assessment for lead poisoning should focus on children younger than 24 months and should begin at 12 months because these ages are the most vulnerable (CDC, 2002). Assessment of high-dose lead exposure should take place at birth.

### Vision and Hearing Screening

Vision and hearing screening should be performed at 3 or 4 years of age and repeated once a year. New recommendations are to screen newborns for hearing right after birth (CDC NCBDDD, 2000). Screening should be done earlier or more frequently than recommended if any of the following warning signs of visual or hearing impairment is present:

▶ Inward- or outward-turning eyes
▶ Squinting
▶ Headaches
▶ Schoolwork not as good as before
▶ Blurred or double vision
▶ Poor response to noise or voice
▶ Slow language and speech development
▶ Abnormal sounding speech (Agency for Healthcare Research and Quality, 2000)

## Immunizations

Immunizations are important preventive health measures for the preschool child. The current recommended immunization schedule for children and adolescents is found in Figure 9–2.

## Nutrition

Nutritional status should be assessed. Infants and toddlers should be tested for anemia starting at 9 months of age. Hematocrit and hemoglobin screening should take place by 9 months if any of the following factors are present:

## COMMUNITY-BASED TEACHING

**Box 9–6** ▶ Safety Guidelines for Parents of
Children of All Ages

- Use smoke detectors in your home. Change the batteries every year and check once a month to see that they work.
- If you have a gun in your home, make sure that the gun and ammunition are locked up separately and kept out of children's reach.
- Never drive after drinking alcohol.
- Use car safety belts at all times.
- Teach your child traffic safety. Children under 9 years of age need supervision when crossing streets.
- Teach your children how and when to call 911.
- Learn basic lifesaving skills (cardiopulmonary resuscitation [CPR]).
- Post the telephone number of the poison control center near your telephone. Also, be sure to check the expiration date on the bottle of ipecac to make sure it is still good.

Agency for Healthcare Research and Quality. (2000). *Child health guide: Put prevention into practice.* Rockville, MD. Retrieved on May 18, 2003 at: *http://www.ahcpr.gov/ppip/ppchild.htm*

---

▶ Low socioeconomic status
▶ Birth weight less than 1,500 g
▶ Whole milk given before 6 months of age (not recommended)
▶ Low-iron formula given (not recommended)
▶ Low intake of iron-rich foods (not recommended)

## Safety

Injury is the leading cause of death in young children. Many of the dangers for young children are in the home (see Box 9–6).

Automobile crashes cause the most deaths in this population ("Motor-Vehicle Occupant," 2001). In most states, the law requires that infants and children be restrained in a safety seat when riding in a car, and parents who are not compliant may be fined. Figure 9–4 shows the proper method of using a car seat by the child's age and weight, and Table 9–2 displays a proper child safety seat use chart. The AAP recommends that infants ride in rear-facing safety seats until they weigh at least 20 lb and are 1 year old. They should never be placed in the front seat of a vehicle with a passenger-side air bag. Children older than 1 year who weigh between 20 and 40 lb should ride in a forward-facing child safety seat as long as the seat fits well (National Highway Traffic Safety Administration [NHTSA], 2003).

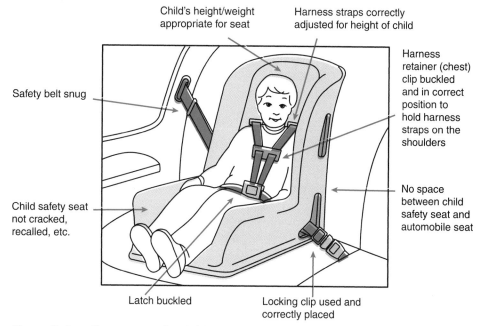

*Figure 9–4.* ▸ Correct use of a child safety seat. Source: Centers for Disease Control and Prevention. (1998). Improper use of child safety seats—Kentucky, 1996. *MMWR Morbidity and Mortality Weekly Report 47*(26), 541-543.

## Other Preventive Health Measures

Child abuse is a serious concern in the United States, where more than 903,000 children were victims of abuse and neglect in 2001. Of these, approximately 1,200 fatalities resulted from child abuse or neglect, with 85% of the victims younger than 6 years old and 44% younger than 1 year old (National Clearing House on Child Abuse, 2003). Even when an adult's account of how a child is injured seems plausible, it is imperative that the nurse reassess the situation for possible child abuse (Koschel, 2003). See Box 9–7 for ways to prevent child abuse.

Infants and children of all ages should be protected from the harmful effects of the sun. The number of skin cancer cases has increased in the United States, with more than 1.3 million new cases diagnosed in 2000. Anyone can get skin cancer, but individuals with certain risk factors are particularly vulnerable. Some risks for skin cancer are the following (CDC, National Center for Chronic Disease Prevention and Health Promotion [NCCDPHP], 2002a):

▸ Lighter natural skin color
▸ Skin that burns, freckles, gets red easily, or becomes painful in the sun
▸ Blue or green eyes
▸ Blond or red hair
▸ Certain types of and a large number of moles
▸ Family history of skin cancer
▸ Personal history of skin cancer
▸ Constant exposure to the sun through work and play
▸ A history of sunburns early in life

**TABLE 9–2 • Proper Child Safety Seat Use Chart**

|  | Infants | Toddlers | Young Children |
|---|---|---|---|
| Weight | Birth to 1 year at least 20–22 lbs. | Over 1 year and over 20 lbs.–40 lbs. | Ages 4–8, unless 4'9" over 40 lbs. |
| Type of Seat | Infant only or rear-facing convertible | Convertible/forward-facing | Belt positioning booster seat |
| Seat Position | Rear-facing only | Forward-facing | Forward-facing |
| Always Make Sure: | Children to 1 year and at least 20 lbs. in rear-facing seats | Harness straps should be at or above shoulders | Belt positioning booster seats must be used with both lap and shoulder belt |
|  | Harness straps at or below shoulder level | Most seats require top slot for forward-facing | Make sure that the lap belt fits low and tight across the lap/upper thigh area and the shoulder belt fits snug crossing the chest and shoulder to avoid abdominal injuries |
| Warning | All children age 12 and under should ride in the back seat | All children age 12 and under should ride in the back seat | All children age 12 and under should ride in the back seat |

Source: National Highway Transportation Safety Administration, U.S. Department of Transportation.

Poor nutrition and dental hygiene contribute to dental caries. Dental caries represent the single most common chronic disease of childhood, occurring five to eight times as frequently as asthma, the second most common chronic condition among children. Unless identified and addressed early, caries are irreversible (DHHS, 2000b).

Hand washing is a simple and effective disease-prevention measure (Fig. 9–5). It is important to teach children hand-washing skills. *Those Mean Nasty Dirty Downright Disgusting but . . . Invisible Germs,* a children's book by Judith Rice, is a good resource for educating children and is also available in Spanish and Hmong. (See Web site listed at the end of the chapter.)

As with all assessment, the effectiveness lies in the strength of the questions asked. General interview and developmental surveillance questions for children of all ages and their parents can be found at http://www.brightfutures.org/.

## SCHOOL-AGE CHILDREN

The leading cause of death for all children between ages 5 and 14 years is motor vehicle accidents. Factors that contribute to these fatalities include drunk drivers and unrestrained children. Pedestrian deaths account for 25% of all motor vehicle-related deaths sustained by children (CDC, 1999).

Middle childhood is when the foundations of a healthy lifestyle are formed and when health promotion programs are likely to have the greatest impact (Polivka & Ryan-Wenger, 1999). A survey of elementary school-age children examined health and lifestyle behaviors. This research found that 68% did not always sleep 8 hours a night, only 50% brushed their teeth daily, and fewer than 50% reported having annual dental visits. The youngest children reported eating unhealthy snacks and not eating vegetables on a daily basis. Only 50% of the children followed bicycle

**COMMUNITY-BASED TEACHING**

**Box 9–7** ▸ Ways to Prevent Child Abuse

- Teach your child not to let anyone touch his or her private parts.
- Tell your child to say "No!" and run away from sexual touches.
- Take any reports by your child of physical or sexual touches seriously.
- Report any abuse to your local or state child protection agency.
- If you feel angry or out of control, leave the room, take a walk, take deep breaths, or count to 100. Don't drink alcohol or take drugs. These can make your anger harder to control.
- If you are afraid you might harm your child, get help *now*. Call someone and ask for help. Talk with a friend or relative, other parents, your clergy, or your health care provider. Take time for yourself. Share child care between parents, trade baby-sitting with friends, or use day care. Call a hot line. The National Child Abuse Hot Line number is (800) 422-4453.

Agency for Healthcare Research and Quality. (2000). *Child health guide: Put prevention into practice.* Rockville, MD. Retrieved on May 20, 2003 from: *http://www.ahcpr.gov/ppip/ppchild.htm.*

safety rules consistently, and fewer than 30% always wore a bicycle helmet. Only 60% of the children reported always used a seat belt. Fewer than 50% of the students reported that they always swim with a buddy.

Box 9–8 presents *Healthy People 2010* objectives for middle childhood.

## Screening

The growth rate of children slows somewhat in the middle childhood years. Children's readiness for school depends on their experiences in the first 5 years of life. Nurses should assess the achievement of the child and provide guidance to the family on anticipated tasks. See the Bright Futures Web site for information on developmental tasks.

At age 5, screening should include vision and hearing, blood pressure, risk for lead exposure (with blood draw if deemed necessary), blood cholesterol, and developmental screening. Weight and height should also be assessed.

## Safety

The most important topic to cover with all families with children is safety, and the one intervention that prevents the most loss of life and injury is using appropriate restraints when riding in an automobile. In 2000, about 62% of all children who died in motor vehicle crashes were unrestrained (CDC, National Center for Injury Prevention and Control [NCIPC], 1999a).

Seat-belt laws vary from state to state. In some states, children are required to be in a booster seat until they are over 70 lb, while other states require them to ride in a booster seat until they are 80 lb. Contact your jurisdiction's department of motor

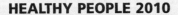

## HEALTHY PEOPLE 2010

**BOX 9–8** **Objectives for School-Age Children and Adolescents**

Reduce the rate of child (ages 5–9 years), adolescent, and young adult deaths.

Reduce coronary heart disease deaths.

Reduce or eliminate indigenous cases of vaccine-preventable disease.

Reduce the suicide rate.

Reduce iron deficiency among young children and females of child-bearing age.

Reduce the proportion of children and adolescents who are overweight or obese.

Increase the proportion of persons ages 2 years and older who consume at least two daily servings of fruit.

Increase the proportion of persons ages 2 years and older who consume at least three daily servings of vegetables.

Reduce the proportion of children and adolescents who have had dental caries in their primary or permanent teeth.

Increase the proportion of adolescents who engage in moderate physical activity for at least 30 minutes on 5 or more of the previous 7 days.

Increase the proportion of adolescents who engage in vigorous physical activity that promotes cardiorespiratory fitness 3 or more days per week for 20 or more minutes per occasion.

Increase the proportion of children and adolescents who view television 2 hours or less per day.

Increase the proportion of the nation's public and private schools that provide access to their physical activity spaces and facilities for all persons outside of normal school hours (before and after the school day, on weekends, and during summer and other vacations).

Reduce the proportion of adolescents and young adults with *Chlamydia trachomatis* infections.

Reduce tobacco use by adolescents.

U.S. Department of Health and Human Services. (2000b). Maternal, infant, and child health. In *Healthy people 2010. National health promotion and disease prevention objectives*. Washington, DC: U.S. Government Printing Office.

vehicles for the seat-belt law in your state. At this time, air bags are not safe for children younger than 13 years and can cause fatalities. Until passenger vehicles are equipped with air bags that are safe and effective for children, those younger than 13 years should not ride in a front passenger seat that is equipped with an air bag.

Another important safety intervention is the use of a bike helmet. Bicycling is a popular activity in the United States. About half a million people are injured in bike

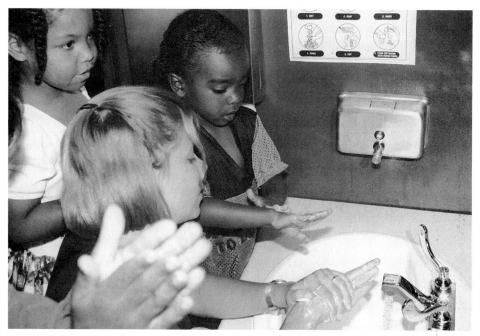

***Figure 9–5.*** ▶ Good handwashing skills have been associated with a decrease in colds and influenza.

mishaps each year. Of these injuries, head injury is the most common cause of death and serious disability. The use of a bike helmet is effective in preventing head injury. Community programs to increase bike helmet use can reduce the incidence of head injury among bicycle riders. All people should wear a helmet when riding a bike (Bicycle Helmet Safety Institute, 2003).

## Prevention of Chronic Conditions

As the child enters middle childhood, even more emphasis should be placed on secondary prevention, which allows early intervention for health conditions that may develop into chronic conditions in adulthood. The primary contributors to chronic conditions that can be addressed are weight, nutrition, and physical activity level.

### Nutrition and Weight

Overweight and obesity are increasing among children and adolescents in the United States. The rate of overweight among children ages 6 to 17 years has more than doubled in the past 30 years, with most of the increase since the late 1970s. Eleven percent of those between 6 and 17 are seriously overweight. Obesity puts individuals at risk for elevated blood cholesterol and high blood pressure, which are in turn associated with heart disease and stroke, two leading causes of death in adulthood. Being overweight in childhood and adolescence has been associated with increased adult morbidity (CDC, NCCDPHP, 2002a). Disease prevention and health promotion activities that decrease the incidence of obesity are directed at improving nutrition and increasing physical activity levels.

Reviewing basic information about the recommended intake by food groups with parent and child is an important intervention in helping families improve their nutrition and avoid overweight and obesity.

### Physical Activity

Many states have eliminated physical education programs and after-school sports programs. Physical education programs are determined by state, but only one state follows the American Heart Association recommendation of daily physical education from kindergarten through 12th grade. These changes have had an impact on the daily reported activity of children. Further, children participate in more sedentary activities after school, such as watching television and playing computer games, than children did 10 years ago. *Healthy People 2010* recommends children watch less than 2 hours of television a day.

Discussing the need for daily physical activity is an important strategy for nurses in community-based settings. Children should be encouraged to participate in activities that provide an aerobic component, such as riding bikes every day (wearing a helmet, of course), walking instead of riding in a car from place to place, and playing outside everyday. Swimming, playing organized or unorganized sports, or doing physical activities as a family are other ways to increase a child's activity level.

Pointing out the benefits of exercise may also help parents encourage children to be more physically active. Helping parents understand the relationship between activity and normal weight, future health, and the threat of developing chronic disease are a few of the strategies the nurse can use to help parents understand the importance of structuring family life and the child's life to include physical activity.

 **ADOLESCENCE**

Adolescence is one of the most dynamic stages of human development. It is accompanied by dramatic physical, cognitive, social, and emotional changes that present both opportunities and challenges for the adolescent, the family, and the broader community. Nurses must be sensitive to the dynamic nature of this stage as well as the increasing need for independence balanced with dependence. Further, as adolescents progress through the teen years, they become increasingly able to make their own health care decisions, and they want to make these choices.

Half of all deaths among adolescents age 15–19 are from unintentional injuries. The majority (78%) of the total mortality in this age group can be attributed to preventable causes (CDC, 2001).

Teens are far less likely to use seat belts than any other age group (CDC, NCIPC, 1999b). Alcohol is involved in about 35% of adolescent fatalities and 40% of all adolescent drownings. Suicide is the third leading cause of death among those ages 15 to 24. As with the 15- to 19-year-old group, 76% of the deaths in this age group can be attributed to preventable causes. At this time, most of the new human immunodeficiency virus (HIV) infections occur each year among those between ages 13 and 21 years.

One comprehensive survey of high school students in 1999 found that 85% rode bicycles without a helmet, 17% carried a weapon, and 8% had attempted suicide in the 12 months preceding the survey. Thirty-five percent smoked cigarettes, 50%

**COMMUNITY-BASED TEACHING**

**Box 9-9** ▶  What You(th) Should Know About Tobacco

**Tobacco and Athletic Performance**
- Smoking can trap you. Nicotine in cigarettes, cigars, and spit tobacco is addictive.
- Nicotine narrows your blood vessels and puts added strain on your heart.
- Smoking can wreck lungs and reduce oxygen available for muscles used during sports.
- Smokers suffer shortness of breath (gasp!) almost three times more often than nonsmokers.
- Smokers run slower and can't run as far, affecting overall athletic performance.
- Cigars and spit tobacco are *not* safe alternatives.

**Tobacco and Personal Appearance**
- Yuck! Tobacco smoke can make hair and clothes stink.
- Tobacco stains teeth and causes bad breath.
- Short-term use of spit tobacco can cause cracked lips, white spots, sores, and bleeding in the mouth.
- Surgery to remove oral cancers caused by tobacco use can lead to serious changes in the face. Sean Marcee, a high school star athlete who used spit tobacco, died of oral cancer when he was 19 years old.

**So . . .**
- Know the truth. Despite all the tobacco use on TV and in movies, music videos, billboards, and magazines, most teens, adults, and athletes *don't* use tobacco.
- Make friends, develop athletic skills, control weight, be independent, be cool . . . play sports.
- Don't waste (burn) money on tobacco. Spend it on CDs, clothes, computer games, and movies.
- *Get involved*: Make your team, school, and home tobacco-free; teach others; join community efforts to prevent tobacco use.

Source: http://www.cdc.gov/tobacco/edumat.htm (click on youth; click on what you should know)

had at least one drink of alcohol, and 32% had 5 or more drinks of alcohol on at least one occasion during the 30 days preceding the survey (CDC, NCIPC, 1999b).

A survey in 2001 found that of the 33% of teens who had had sexual intercourse during the previous 3 months, 51% used a condom during the last intercourse. This figure is down from 58% response in 1999 (CDC, NCIPC, 1999b; Brener, Lowry, Kann, Kolbe, & Jaffe, 2002). As far as dietary behaviors, 10% were overweight, 24%

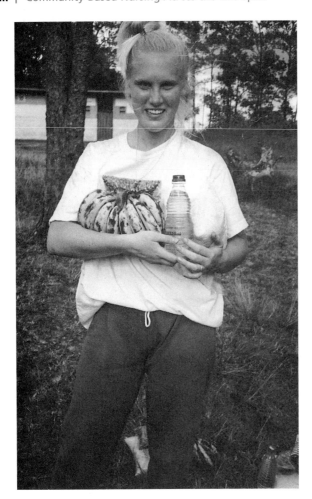

***Figure 9–6.*** ▶ Suggestions for teaching adolescents about nutrition include instilling a sense of pride in identifying and choosing healthy meals and snacks.

ate five or more servings of fruits and vegetables during the 7 days preceding the survey, and 5% took laxatives or vomited to lose weight during the 30 days preceding the survey. Related to physical activity, 65% did vigorous physical activity, 27% did moderate physical activity for at least 20 minutes on 3 or more of the 7 days preceding the survey, and 56% were enrolled in physical education class with 29% attending physical education class daily (CDC, NCCDPHP, 1999). These results compare to other surveys, which show that nearly half of American youths ages 12 to 21 years are not vigorously active on a regular basis (CDC, NCCDPHP, 1999).

When results from 1999 were compared with results from 1991 and 1995, the percentage of students who felt unsafe going to school increased from 6% to 26%. Students were smoking more cigarettes in 1999, with an increase of 1% to 11% in those smoking more than 10 cigarettes per day. There was also an increase in those having sexual intercourse before 13 years of age, from 3% to 16%. The percentage of students attending physical education class increased from 6% to 16%.

*Healthy People 2010* objectives for school-age children and adolescents are shown in Box 9–8.

## Screening

Recommendations for screening in early and later adolescence are found in the Bright Futures guidelines. Some other areas for screening adolescent clients include questions concerning smoking, alcohol and drug use, sexual activity, and injury prevention behaviors. Teens' behaviors often place them at risk for serious injury, sexually transmitted diseases (STDs), and chronic diseases. Bright Futures provides excellent developmental surveillance questions that address these issues. It is also important to keep developmental tasks in mind when assessing health issues and planning health promotion and disease prevention activities.

Because such a large proportion of deaths in this age group are preventable, safety should be the number one priority for health promotion and injury prevention. However, because of the nature of the adolescent client, this is a formidable challenge.

## Prevention of Chronic Conditions

### Smoking Cessation

Several excellent resources on the Internet address smoking cessation. Some are very colorful, specifically designed by teens for teens. One site is http://www.cdc.gov/tobacco/sgr/sgr4kids/6facts.htm. See Box 9–9 for community-based teaching strategies for adolescents who want to know more about the dangers of tobacco.

### Nutrition

Teaching teens about nutrition is challenging (Fig. 9–6). *Bright Futures in Practice: Nutrition* is an excellent resource for nutrition information for infancy through adolescence. This resource is available through http://www.brightfutures.org/.

### Physical Activity

Nearly half of American youths ages 12–21 years are not vigorously active on a regular basis. Adolescents and young adults benefit from physical activity, particularly considering 14% of all adolescents are overweight. Moderate amounts of daily physical activity are recommended for people of all ages (CDC, NCCDPHP, 2002b). This amount can be obtained in longer sessions of moderately intense activities, such as brisk walking for 30 minutes, or in shorter sessions of more intense activities, such as jogging or playing soccer or basketball for 15 to 20 minutes. Physical activity helps build and maintain healthy bones, muscles, and joints; controls weight; builds lean muscle; and reduces fat. Most importantly, physical activity prevents or delays the development of high blood pressure, helps reduce blood pressure in some adolescents with hypertension, and prevents the development of type 2 diabetes.

## Health Promotion

### Sexual Health Promotion

The incidence of STDs has skyrocketed, and most new HIV infections occur in people between 13 and 21 years of age. Teens are at high behavioral risk for acquiring most STDs. Teenagers and young adults are more likely than other age groups to have multiple sex partners, to engage in unprotected sex, and (for young women) to choose sexual partners older than themselves (CDC, 2001). As part of holistic

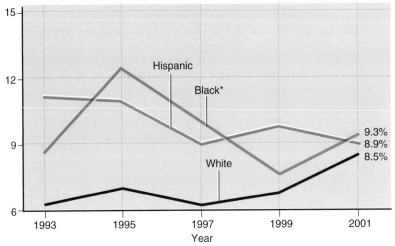

***Figure 9–7.*** ▶ Percentage of High School Students Who Were Threatened or Injured with Weapons on School Property, by Race: 1993-2001. Source: U.S. Department of Health and Human Services. (2002). Health Resources and Services Administration. Maternal and Child Health Bureau. *Child Health USA 2002.* Government Printing Office: Washington, DC. (p. 41).

care, nurses in community-based settings should always assess sexuality. When assessing and teaching teens in this area, an open, frank, direct, and nonjudgmental approach is best. Talking openly and frankly with young teens about the benefits and risks of being sexually active may allow teens, especially girls, to understand that being sexually active is a choice. Early age of first coitus is a well-established risk factor for STDs because there is greater opportunity for exposure to pathogens. Early coitus is also associated with later high-risk cognitive, affective, and behavioral choices. Opportunities to interact with caring adults outside of their families, self-esteem building, and empowerment activities contribute to delay of first intercourse (Klerman, 2002).

Other primary prevention strategies to promote sexual health include comprehensive sex education beginning in primary school. Abstinence is a highly positive choice for both sexes until they are ready to deal with the responsibility of being sexually active. However, it is not realistic as a sole strategy. The emphasis must be that sexual health promotion is for life and that contraception is useless if not practiced consistently.

Some sexuality health promotion programs use a more dramatic approach, with speakers who are HIV positive or have acquired immunodeficiency syndrome (AIDS). These speakers tell their stories to teen groups, often with great success. Nurses can develop audiovisual aids (eg, diagrams, pictures, computer-assisted instruction, PowerPoint presentations, and videos) to make sex education unforgettable. Nurses can explore with teens the differences between the facts of physiology and untrue but fervently held beliefs. Helping teens understand the relationship between substance abuse and STDs is another important issue to address. Peer education is a program model that is highly successful and inexpensive to implement.

Nurses can play a critical role in the improvement of sexual health counseling by using a direct and frank approach in interactions with individual teens, parents, groups, and peers. Nurses in community-based settings can have enormous impact on sexual health promotion by acting as a positive role model for sexual health and being involved in issues related to sexual health.

### Suicide and Violence Prevention

Suicide is a complex problem that can, in some cases, be prevented by early recognition and treatment of mental disorders. At least 90% of people who kill themselves have mental or substance abuse disorders (DHHS, 2000b). Thus, early identification and treatment of these disorders is paramount in the prevention of suicide.

Violence is a critical public health issue in the United States. In 2001, homicide was the fourth leading cause of death for U.S. children ages 1 to 9, the third leading cause of death for children ages 10 to 14, and the second leading cause of death for youth. Violence among adolescents is a critical public health issue in the United States. Most of these deaths are from guns. Figure 9–7 depicts the percentage of high school students who were threatened or injured with a weapon on school property.

### Health Prevention and Disease Prevention Activities With Teens

When teaching teens about health, it is particularly important to base the teaching on what the teen already knows about the subject. Cognitively, many teens are not able to conceptualize or hypothesize. This, coupled with the fact that teens tend to be egocentric, complicates determining the best teaching modalities to reach the teen population. Successful disease prevention and health promotion activities for teens incorporate these considerations. Thus, it is most effective when teaching teens about physical activity or nutrition to talk about the immediate, particular, personal impacts in areas of importance to them.

For instance, a teenage girl who is overweight may respond to information on nutrition with the incentive of losing weight so she can wear the latest clothing styles. A boy may respond to the suggestion to increase physical activity in his daily life if the nurse talks about the benefits of belonging to a team or being a sports hero. When taught about smoking cessation, teens respond to the idea that if they smoke, they are less desirable to kiss, or that their hands, clothes, and hair will smell, but not to the notion that smoking increases the chances of developing lung cancer. Nor do teens respond to the idea that if they are not physically fit and well nourished there is an increased chance that they will develop heart disease, diabetes, stroke, and cancer. They are developmentally unable to value such notions.

## CONCLUSIONS

The primary issues involved in health promotion and disease prevention, based on *Healthy People 2010,* have been discussed from infancy through adolescence. Providing early prenatal care would eliminate many health conditions for newborn babies, save precious health care dollars, and improve the quality of life for countless infants. During infancy and childhood, periodic screening allows for early identification and intervention of common and preventable conditions. Helping young children and teens value and adopt healthy lifestyle choices by improving nutrition, increasing physical activity, and following basic safety recommendations is an important contribution nurses in community-based settings can make. Advocating and participating in activities related to these issues in their own communities is another way nurses can contribute to the health of children. Lastly, being vocal and involved in public policy issues such as gun control and allocation of health care dollars for public health, as well as supporting political candidates who value public health, are all ways that nurses can improve the health of the nation's children.

# What's on the Web

American Social Health Association (ASHA)
P.O. Box 13827
Research Triangle Park, NC 27709
**Internet address:** *http://www. iwannaknow.org*
This site is a part of the American Social Health Association. It is designed for teens and provides answers to questions about teen sexual health and STDs.

Bright Futures
**Internet address:**
*http://www.brightfutures.org*
This Web site provides information about preventive and health promotion needs of infants, children, adolescents, families, and communities. A number of publications, including handouts in Spanish, can be downloaded or ordered through the site.

*CDC Tobacco Information and Prevention Source*
Tips4Youth Web page
**Internet address:**
*http://www.cdc.gov/tobacco/tips4youth.htm*
This page compiles sites listing smoking cessation programs geared toward children and teens.

*Child Health Guide: Put Prevention into Practice*
**Internet address:**
*http://www.ahcpr.gov/ppip/ppchild.htm*
This on-line consumer guide from the Agency for Healthcare Research and Quality explains children's preventive care.

Print copies, available free of charge, can be requested by calling (800) 358-9295. The guide is also available in Spanish.

Healthfinder
**Internet address:**
*http://www.healthfinder.gov*
Healthfinder is a search engine for consumer health education material, maintained by the U.S. Department of Health and Human Services.

*Healthy People 2010*
**Internet address:**
*http://www.health.gov/healthypeople*
This document outlines the nationwide health promotion and disease prevention initiative designed to improve health for all people in the United States.

La Leche League
1400 North Meacham Road
Schaumburg, IL 60173-4808
Telephone: (847) 519-7730
**Internet address:**
*http://www.lalecheleague.org*
This Web site provides information on breast-feeding, on-line discussion groups, and listings of local groups.

National Asthma Control Program
**Internet Address:**
*http://www.cdc.gov/nceh/airpollution/ asthma/children.htm*
Asthma is a serious and growing health problem with the asthma rate rising more rapidly in preschool-age children than in any other group. Client education is imperative for effective management of asthma.

This is one of many Web sites offering health education about asthma. On the last page of this Web site you will find a comprehensive list of organizations offering information on pediatric asthma.

National Immunization Program/Six Common Misconceptions About Vaccinations and How to Respond to Them
**Internet Address:**
*http://www.cdc.gov/nip/publications/6mishome.htm*
Parents often have questions about vaccinations. Unfortunately, information is sometimes published that is inaccurate or can be misleading when taken out of context. This site helps provide accurate information about immunizations.

National Institute of Child Health and Human Development
**Internet address:** *http://www.nichd.nih.gov*
This site is an excellent resource for health education information for nurses to use with parents and families. It includes research about the health status of children.

WHY HOW WHEN to Wash Hands: A Handwashing Curriculum
**Internet address:**
*http://www.co.ramsey.mn.us/ph/hi/hdwsh.asp*

Studies have found that caregivers who teach and model good hand washing can reduce illness by 50%. A creative and engaging curriculum to teach children why, when, and how to wash their hands can be ordered through this site. This resource, available as a video, curriculum booklet, and book, provides an easy, entertaining way to teach preschoolers the importance of hand washing. All materials are available in Spanish, Hmong, and English.

The Women, Infants, and Children (WIC) Program
**Internet Address:**
*http://www.fns.usda.gov/wic/*
The WIC Program saves lives and improves the health of nutritional at-risk women, infants, and children. Numerous studies prove that the WIC Program is one of the nation's most successful and cost-effective nutrition intervention programs. Since its beginning in 1974, the WIC Program has earned the reputation of being one of the most successful federally funded nutrition programs in the United States. All nurses working in community-based settings benefit from knowing about the WIC Program and sharing that information with the clients they serve.

## References and Bibliography

Agency for Healthcare Research and Quality. (2000). *Child health guide: Put prevention into practice.* Rockville, MD. Retrieved May 18, 2003. http://www.ahcpr.gov/ppip/ppchild.htm

American Academy of Pediatrics, Committee on Practice and Ambulatory Medicine. (1995). Recommendations for pediatric health care. *Pediatrics, 96*(2) 373–374.

Beitz, J. (1998). Sexual health promotion in adolescents and young adults: Primary prevention strategies. *Holistic Nursing Practice, 12*(2), 27–38.

Bicycle Helmet Safety Institute. (2003). *A compendium of statistics from various sources.* Retrieved on February 3, 2003, from http://www.helmets.org/stats.htm

Brener, N., Lowry, R., Kann, L., Kolbe, L., & Jaffe, H., (2002). Trends in sexual risk behavior among high school students: 1991–2001. *Morbidity and Mortality Weekly Report (MMWR), 5*(38), 856–859.

Centers for Disease Control and Prevention. (2000). *Pedestrian injury prevention.* Retrieved on February 3, 2003, from http://www.cdc.gov/ncipc/factsheets/.htm

Centers for Disease Control and Prevention. (2001). Tracking the hidden epidemic: Trends in STDs in the U.S. in 2000. Retrieved on March 18, 2003, at http://www.cdc.gov/nchstp/dstd

Centers for Disease Control and Prevention. (2002). *Health & economic impact: Smoking cessation for pregnant women.* Washington, DC: U.S. Government Printing Office.

Centers for Disease Control and Prevention, National Center for Chronic Disease Prevention and Health Promotion. (1999).

Adolescents and young adults. In *Physical Activity and health: A report of the surgeon general.* Retrieved May 15, 2003 from http://www.cdc.gov/nccdphp/sgr/adoles.htm

Centers for Disease Control and Prevention, National Center for Chronic Disease Prevention and Health Promotion. (2002a). *Physical activity and health: A report of the surgeon general.* Retrieved on February 3, 2003, from http://www.cdc.gov/nccdphp/sgr/adoles.htm

Centers for Disease Control and Prevention, National Center for Chronic Disease Prevention and Health Promotion. (2002b). *The surgeon general's call to action to prevent and decrease overweight and obesity, 2002.* Retrieved on February 3, 2003, at http://www.cdc.gov/nccdphp/dnpa/obesity/recommendations.htm.

Centers for Disease Control and Prevention, National Center for Chronic Disease Prevention and Health Promotion, Division of Cancer Prevention and Control. (2000). *Facts and statistics about skin cancer.* Retrieved January 20, 2003 from http://www.cdc.gov/chooseyourcover/skin.htm

Centers for Disease Control and Prevention, National Center for Injury Prevention and Control. (1999a). *Child passenger safety* [Fact sheet]. Retrieved January 29, 2003 from http://www.cdc.gov/ncipc/factsheets/childpas.htm

Centers for Disease Control and Prevention, National Center for Injury Prevention and Control. (1999b). *Facts on adolescent injury* [Fact sheet]. Retrieved January 29, 2003 from http://www.cdc.gov/ncipc/factsheets/adoles.htm

Centers for Disease Control and Prevention, National Center on Birth Defects and Developmental Disability. (2000). *Early hearing detection and intervention program.* Retrieved January 30, 2003 from http://www.cdc.gov/ncbddd/ehdi/ehdi.htm

Every child by two. (2003). Retrieved on May 13, 2003 from www.ccbr.org

Federal Interagency Forum on Child and Family Statistics. (2002). *America's children: Key national indicators of well-being, 2002.* Washington, DC: U.S. Government Printing Office.

Green, P. M., & Adderley-Kelly, B. (1999). Partnership for health promotion in an urban community. *Nursing and Health Care Perspectives, 20*(2), 76–81.

Healthy Start. (2003). Infant mortality and low weight births policy discussion. Retrieved January 21, 2003, from http://trfn.clpgh.org/hspgh/infant%20%20low%20birth%20weight.html

Infant mortality and low birth weight among black and white infants. United States, 1980–2000. (2002). *MMWR, 51*(27), 589–592.

Kitzman, H., Olds, D., Sidora, K., Henderson, C., Hanks, C., Cole, R., Luckey, D., Bondy, J., Cole, K., & Glazner, J. (2000). Enduring effects of nurse home visitation on maternal life course. *JAMA, 283*(15), 1983–1999.

Klerman, L. (2002). Adolescent pregnancy in the United States. *International Journal of Adolescent Medicine & Health, 14*(2), 91–96.

Koschel, M. (2003). Is it child abuse? *American Journal of Nursing, 102*(4), 45–46.

Minnesota Department of Health, Division of Family Health, Minnesota Healthy Beginnings. (1999). *Promoting Minnesota healthy beginnings: Findings from focus groups with expecting moms and new parents.* Minneapolis: Minnesota Department of Health.

Monteiro, L. (1985). Florence Nightingale on public health nursing. *American Journal of Public Health, 75*(2), 181–185.

Motor-vehicle occupant injury: Strategies for increasing use of child safety seats, increasing use of safety belts, and reducing alcohol-impaired driving. (2001). *MMWR, 50*(RR–07), 1–13.

National Clearing House on Child Abuse. (2002). *Summary from findings calendar year 2000.* Retrieved on March 6, 2004 from www.calib.com/nccanch/pubs/factsheets/canstats.

National Highway Traffic Safety Administration (U.S.) Department of Transportation. *Buckle up America: Child passenger safety week.* Washington, DC: NHTSA.

Polivka, B., & Ryan-Wenger, N. (1999). Health promotions and injury prevention behaviors of elementary school children. *Pediatric Nursing, 25*(2), 127.

Todd, S., LaSala, K., & Neil-Urban, S. (2001). An integrated approach to prenatal smoking cessation interventions. *MCN, American Journal of Maternal/Child Nursing, 26*(4), 185–191.

U.S. Department of Health and Human Services, National Center for Education in Maternal Child Health, Maternal and Child Health Bureau. (2000a). *Bright futures: Guidelines for health supervision for infants, children, and adolescents* (2nd ed., rev.). Arlington, VA. Retrieved January 18, 2003 from http://www.brightfutures.org

U.S. Department of Health and Human Services. (2000b). Maternal, infant, and child health. In *Healthy people 2010. National health promotion and disease prevention objectives.* Washington, DC: U.S. Government Printing Office.

U.S. Department of Health and Human Services (2002). *Preventing infant mortality factsheet.* Retrieved on May 18, 2003 from http: //www.hhs.gov/news

U.S. Department of Health and Human Services. (2000c). *Project to promote health education among children wins top prize in HHS secretary's award for health innovation.* Washington, DC: U.S. Government Printing Office.

U.S. Department of Health and Human Services, Administration on Children, Youth, and Families, Children's Bureau. (2003). *National Child Abuse and Neglect Data System (NCANDS): Summary of key findings from calendar year 2001.* Washington, DC. Retrieved May 19, 2003, from http://www.calib.com/naccanch/pubs/factsheets/canstats.cfm

U.S. Department of Health and Human Services, Health Resources and Services Administration, Maternal and Child Health Bureau. (2002). *Child health USA 2002.* Washington, DC: Government Printing Office.

Wright, A., Bauer, N., Naylor, A., Sutcliffe, E., & Clark, L. (1998). Increasing breastfeeding rates to reduce infant illness at community level. *Pediatrics. 101*(5). 837–844.

Vickers, A., Ohlsson, A., Lacy, J. B., & Horsley, A. (1999). Massage for promoting growth and development of preterm and/or low birthweight infants. *Cochrane Database System Review, 2,* CD000390.

## LEARNING ACTIVITIES

### JOURNALING: ACTIVITY 9–1

1. In your clinical journal, describe a situation you have encountered when screening and doing health promotion activities.
   - *What did you learn from this experience?*
   - *How will you practice differently based on this experience?*
2. In your clinical journal, describe a situation in which you have observed infants or children not receiving the health care that they needed.
   - *How could or would you like to advocate for this issue when you begin to practice as an RN?*
   - *What could you do now?*

### CLIENT CARE: ACTIVITY 9–2

You are working as a community-based nurse making home visits to pregnant teens through the clinic where you are employed. The school nurse calls the clinic and requests that a home visit be made to Shantrell, who has shared with the school nurse that she is pregnant. She has been to your clinic for health care but has not had prenatal care. All you know is that Shantrell is 16 years old and pregnant and is no longer going to school.

When you drive to the client's home, you notice that the house is very old, with old cars and debris in the yard.

*What else do you assess as you drive through the neighborhood?*

You knock on the door. You notice that the paint is peeling on the outside of the house, and it looks like it hasn't been painted in a long time. Your client, Shantrell, comes to the door. You greet her, tell her your name, the name of the clinic you work for, and why you are visiting. During the first part of the visit, you spend some time getting to know Shantrell.

*What could you use for a guide for interview questions?*

You learn that Shantrell found out she was pregnant 1 month ago, and she is now 3 months' pregnant. She has not come in to the clinic because she thought that she only needed to see the doctor the month before the baby was born.

*What would you want to screen for?*
*What topics would you want to address during the rest of the visit?*
*What other questions would you ask?*
*What will be your number-one priority?*
*What do you hope to screen for and teach about in the next visit?*

## CLIENT CARE: ACTIVITY 9–3

Shantrell has given birth to a baby girl weighing 7 lb., 6 oz. She named the baby Precious. Both mom and baby did well during and after delivery. The baby is crying when you arrive for the visit. Shantrell picks up the baby, holds her close, and quietly talks to her.

*What does this tell you about Shantrell's ability to comfort the newborn?*
*What do you do at this point?*

Shantrell says she is breast-feeding Precious because "You told me that if I breast-feed my baby, I will lose my big tummy and look slimmer faster." You ask how the feeding is going, and she states, "Good. When I am at school, my mom gives her a bottle of milk."

*What screening would you do at every visit?*
*What special risks may this infant have?*
*What would your priority be at this visit?*

## PRACTICAL APPLICATION: ACTIVITY 9–4

Contact the director of a day care center in a community where there is a high rate of poverty or that serves low-income families. (These are the families who are likely to have limited access to well child care and health care.) Talk to the day care director about the health teaching that he or she sees as important to the kids and parents they serve. Develop a class or classes according to the director's request. One idea is to use the hand-washing curricula listed in What's on the Web. (This curriculum is in Spanish and Hmong as well as English.) Another approach is to develop a teaching sheet according to the topics that the day care staff members identify as important for them.

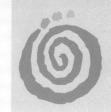

## CHAPTER 10

# Health Promotion and Disease Prevention for Adults

Roberta Hunt

1. Identify the leading causes of death for adults.
2. Discuss the major diseases and threats to health for adults.
3. Summarize the primary health issues for adults.
4. Identify nursing roles for each level of prevention for primary health issues for adults.
5. Compose a list of nursing interventions for the primary health issues for adults.
6. Determine health needs for adults for which a nurse could be an advocate.

## KEY TERMS

health indicator
moderate physical activity
obese
overweight

## CHAPTER TOPICS

- **Health Status of Adults**
- **Eliminating Disparity in Health Care**
- **Health Screening for Adults**
- **Interventions for Leading Health Indicators**
- **Conclusions**

My first job working as a staff nurse was on the oncology unit for a large teaching hospital in New York. Many of our patients did not have insurance. One day I floated to a general medical–surgical unit, where I took care of a 50-year-old woman named Linda who was admitted for cholecystitis. It was a quiet day on the unit, so as I was doing my morning assessment, I took some time to talk to her. She told me that her husband was disabled and that they had four children. Although she worked full time as a nurse's aide, to get family insurance, she had to pay $800 a month, and they could not afford to pay such a large premium. Consequently, no one in her family was insured except her husband. Her younger sister passed away the year before from breast cancer. She told me "that it was my third sister who has died of breast cancer. Two of my mother's sisters and my grandma died of breast cancer." We talked about the importance of yearly mammography for women over 50, particularly if they have a family history of breast cancer. She said she was aware of the need for the screening but had never had mammography because she could not afford to pay $900 for the test. I told her about the National Breast and Cervical Cancer Early Detection Program and gave her the number to call. She told me she would contact them and make an appointment.

Three months later I saw Linda on the oncology unit. She had contacted the NBC-CEDP and had mammography. She was in the hospital for surgery for early-stage breast cancer. I never appreciated the importance of early screening and detection so much as I did that day.

**—Susan Larson, RN**
Oncology Nurse
St. Paul Minnesota

# HEALTH STATUS OF ADULTS

The major causes of death in the United States (Table 10–1) often result from behaviors and lifestyle choices that contribute to injury, violence, and illness. Environmental factors, such as lack of access to quality health services, also contribute to the major causes of death. For the nurse, this underscores the importance of understanding and monitoring health behaviors, environmental factors, and community health systems. This chapter will assist the nurse to understand and learn to monitor health behaviors that affect health and contribute to the major causes of death and disability.

Because the average person is living longer, more attention is now focused on preserving quality of life rather than simply extending length of life. Chief among the factors involving preserving quality of life is the prevention and treatment of musculoskeletal conditions. Demographic trends also indicate that people will need to continue to work to an older age. Nurses will increasingly be involved in efforts to decrease the adverse social and economic consequence of high rates of activity limitation and disability of older persons.

| Age (y) | Cause of Death | Number |
|---|---|---|
| 25–44 | Unintentional injuries | 27,129 |
| | Cancer | 21,706 |
| | Heart disease | 16,513 |
| 45–65 | Cancer | 131,743 |
| | Heart disease | 101,235 |
| | Unintentional injuries | 17,521 |

**TABLE 10–1** •Leading Causes of Death in Adults, United States, 1997

Source: U.S. Department of Health and Human Services. (2000). *Healthy people 2010. National health promotion and disease prevention objectives.* Washington, DC: U.S. Government Printing Office.

Leading **health indicators** are shown in Box 10–1. These illuminate individual behavioral, physical, social, and environmental factors and health systems issues that affect the health of individuals. "The health indicators are intended to help everyone more easily understand the importance of health promotion and disease prevention and to encourage wide participation in improving health in the next decade" (U.S. Department of Health and Human Services [DHHS], 2000, p. 25).

## ELIMINATING DISPARITY IN HEALTH CARE

The central goals of *Healthy People 2010* (DHHS, 2000) are to increase quality and years of healthy life and to eliminate health disparities. Health disparities exist by gender, race or ethnicity, education, income, disability, rural living areas, and sexual orientation. Men have a life expectancy that is 6 years less than women's, and they have a higher rate of death for each of the 10 leading causes of death. Women have had an increasing rate of death from lung cancer in the past 20 years, whereas the men's rate has decreased.

Disparity by ethnicity is believed to result from complex interactions among genetic variations, environmental factors, and specific health behaviors. Heart disease death rates are more than 40% higher for African Americans than for Whites. Hispanics living in the United States are almost twice as likely to die from diabetes than are non-Hispanic Whites. Native Americans and Alaska Natives have twice the rate of diabetes than do Whites and disproportionately high rates of death from unintentional injuries and suicide. Asians and Pacific Islanders, on average,

### HEALTHY PEOPLE 2010

**Box 10–1  Leading Health Indicators**

1. Physical activity
2. Overweight and obesity
3. Tobacco use
4. Substance abuse
5. Responsible sexual behavior
6. Mental health
7. Injury violence
8. Environmental quality
9. Immunization
10. Access to health care

have health indicators that suggest they are one of the healthiest population groups in the United States.

Income and education underlie many health disparities in the United States. Income and education are intrinsically related; people with the worst health status are among those with the highest poverty rates and least education. Income inequality in the United States has increased over the past 3 decades. About 30% of Hispanic and 20% of Black Americans lack a usual source of health care, compared with less than 16% of Whites. African Americans and Hispanic Americans are far more likely to rely on hospitals or clinics for their usual source of care than are White Americans (16% and 13% versus 8%). African Americans are 13% less likely to undergo coronary angioplasty and one third less likely to undergo bypass surgery than are Whites. The length of time between an abnormal screening mammogram and the follow-up diagnostic test to determine whether a woman has breast cancer is more than twice as long in Asian American, Black, and Hispanic women as in White women (Agency for Healthcare Research and Quality [AHRQ], 2000).

People with disabilities are identified as people who have activity limitations, people who need assistive devices, or people who perceive themselves as having a disability. Roughly 21% of the population reports some level of disability. Many people with disabilities lack access to health services and medical care.

Rural localities are home to 25% of Americans. Those living in rural areas are less likely to use preventive screening services, exercise regularly, or wear seat belts, and they are more likely to be uninsured.

Gay men and lesbians have health problems unique to their populations. Gay men are more likely than heterosexual men to have human immunodeficiency virus (HIV) and other sexually transmitted diseases (STDs), and they are at an increased risk for substance abuse, depression, and suicide. Some studies show that lesbian women have higher rates of smoking, obesity, alcohol abuse, and stress than heterosexual women (DHHS, 2000).

## HEALTH SCREENING FOR ADULTS

As with clients at other ages, health screening for adults is intended for primary, secondary, or tertiary prevention. Primary prevention to prevent the initial occurrence of a disease with an adult client could be immunization screening and recommendation of an annual flu shot. Secondary prevention could be screening for hypertension at a health fair or yearly mammography for women over 50 years of age. Tertiary prevention could be initiating an exercise program for an obese client who has type 2 diabetes. Screening is always intended to identify people who are at risk for developing a health condition so that appropriate intervention can be undertaken.

The nurse should encourage the client to actively practice prevention. One way to accomplish this is to use the *Personal Health Guide: Put Prevention into Practice*, available from AHRQ at http://www.ahcpr.gov/ppip/adguide or by calling (800) 358-9295. This guide makes it easier for clients to keep accurate information about their health, health treatments, and screenings and for the nurse to guide clients in identifying and planning health promotion and disease prevention activities. The guide contains information on screening as well as topics related to the leading health indicators. It also contains forms for record keeping essential for health promotion and disease prevention.

> ▶ **Box 10–2.** Recommended Immunizations for Adults ◀

- Tetanus–diphtheria: every 10 years
- Rubella: for women considering pregnancy
- Pneumococcal (pneumonia): at about age 65
- Influenza: Those who work with high-risk populations or live with some-one who works with high-risk populations, pregnant women after the first trimester, or anyone older than 65 years of age need one every year. People who have a chronic condition, such as lung, heart, or kidney disease; diabetes; HIV; or cancer, may need both influenza and pneumococcal immunizations.
- Hepatitis B: for people who have contact with human blood or body fluids, have unprotected sex, or share needles during intravenous drug use. Health professionals should also consider hepatitis B immunization.

Agency for Healthcare Research and Quality. (2000). *Personal health guide: Put preventonprevention into practice.* Rockville, MD. Retrieved from http://www.ahcpr.gov/ppip/adguide

## General Screening

Major areas of adult health screening covered in the *Personal Health Guide* include blood pressure, cholesterol, weight, and immunizations. Maintaining a normal blood pressure protects people from heart disease, stroke, and kidney problems. It is recommended that all adults have their blood pressure checked regularly. Those with high blood pressure should work with their health care provider to lower it by changing their diet, losing weight, exercising, and if prescribed, taking medication.

Cholesterol should be checked in men from ages 35 to 65 years and women from ages 45 to 65. Cholesterol can be lowered by changing diet, losing excess weight, and getting exercise. The client's knowledge about cholesterol and heart disease can be assessed by using quizzes available from the National Heart, Lung, and Blood Institute at http://www.nhlbi.nih.gov/health/public/heart/index.htm. Weighing too much or too little can lead to health problems. Healthy diet and regular exercise are factors that contribute to weight loss. Assessment should include the evaluation of body mass index (BMI), waist circumference, and overall medical risk.

Immunization is cited as one of the greatest achievements of public health in the 20th century. Box 10–2 shows immunizations needed by adults. It is important to continue to increase the proportion of children who receive all vaccines, as well as the proportion of adults who are vaccinated annually against the flu.

Oral health care is also important for overall general health. Not only will proper oral care preserve teeth for a lifetime, but also flossing every day contributes to a longer life (Box 10–3).

## Cancer Screening

Colorectal cancer is the second leading cause of death from cancer. The risk of developing colorectal cancer increases with advancing age. Risk factors include inflammatory bowel disease and a family or personal history of colorectal cancer or polyps. Lack of regular physical activity, low fruit and vegetable intake, a low-fiber

**COMMUNITY-BASED TEACHING**

**Box 10–3** ▶ Basic Principles of Oral Health

- Visit your dentist regularly for checkups.
- Brush after meals.
- Use dental floss daily.
- Limit the intake of sweets, especially between meals.
- Do not smoke or chew tobacco products.

diet, obesity, and alcohol consumption are other contributing factors. Reducing the number of deaths from colorectal cancer chiefly depends on detecting and removing precancerous colorectal polyps, as well as detecting and treating the cancer in its early stages. People 50 years and older should been screened regularly with a fecal occult blood test yearly and sigmoidoscopy every 5 to 10 years (Centers for Disease Control and Prevention [CDC], 2002a).

Regular mammography screening for women age 50 and older has been shown to reduce deaths from breast cancer (CDC, 2002b). Some women may need to begin mammograms earlier, depending on their health history. All women should have an annual Pap smear at age 18 or when they become sexually active. Those who have three or more normal annual tests may be tested less frequently, at the discretion of the nurse practitioner or physician.

The CDC National Breast and Cervical Cancer Early Detection Program provides free screening exams for all women throughout the United States. Consult the Web site at http://www.cdc.gov/cancer/nbccedp/law106-354.htm for more information or to find out where your client can get a free or low-cost mammogram and Pap test in your area.

Prostate cancer is the most commonly diagnosed form of cancer, second to skin cancer, and is second to lung cancer as a cause of cancer-related death among men. The CDC does not recommend routine screening for prostate cancer because there is no scientific consensus on whether screening and treatment of early stage prostate cancer reduces mortality. The CDC does, however, support a man's right to discuss the pros and cons of prostate cancer screening and treatment with his doctor and his right to make his own decision about screening (CDC, 2003). The two common methods for detecting prostate cancer are digital rectal examination and prostate-specific antigen testing.

Skin cancer is the most common form of cancer in the United States. More than 1 million new cases of skin cancer will be diagnosed in 2002. Exposure to the sun's ultraviolet rays appears to be the most important environmental factor in the development of skin cancer. Skin cancer can be prevented by following consistent sun-protective practices. Risk factors include the following:

▶ Light skin color, hair color, and eye color
▶ Family history of skin cancer
▶ Personal history of skin cancer
▶ Chronic exposure to the sun
▶ History of sunburns early in life
▶ Certain types and a large number of moles
▶ Freckles, which indicate sun sensitivity and sun damage

Numerous resources can be found at this Web site: http://www.cdc.gov/chooseyourcover.

## Screening for High-Risk Groups

Overall, African Americans are more likely to develop cancer than persons of any other racial or ethnic group (CDC, 2002d). In addition, the following conditions may require additional screening. If the client falls into any of these categories, he or she should discuss potential screening with a nurse practitioner or physician.

- Has diabetes, or is older than 40 and African American, or is older than 60 years of age—requires additional eye exams
- Has had intercourse without condoms, has had multiple partners, or has had an STD—may require screening for STDs
- Has injected illegal drugs or had a blood transfusion between 1978 and 1985—may need an HIV or hepatitis test
- Has a family member with diabetes, is overweight, or has had diabetes during pregnancy—may need a glucose test
- Is over age 65—needs a hearing test
- Now or in the past, has consumed a lot of alcohol, smoked, or chewed tobacco—may need a mouth exam
- Is male and over age 50—needs a prostate exam
- Male between ages 14 and 35 years, particularly if a testicle is abnormally small or not in the normal position—may need a testicular exam
- Has had a family member with skin cancer or has had a lot of sun exposure—may need a skin exam
- Has had radiation treatments of the upper body—may need a thyroid exam
- Has been exposed to tuberculosis; has recently moved from Asia, Africa, Central or South America, or the Pacific Islands; has kidney failure, diabetes, HIV, or alcoholism; or uses illegal drugs—may need a tuberculosis (purified protein derivative [PPD]) test

(*Personal Health Guide: Put Prevention into Practice,* April 1998. Publication No. APPIP 98-0027. AHRQ, Rockville, MD. Available at http://www.ahrq.gov/ppip/adguide)

## INTERVENTIONS FOR LEADING HEALTH INDICATORS

Evidence exists that some of the leading causes of death and disability in the United States, such as heart disease, cancer, stroke, some respiratory diseases, unintentional injuries, HIV, and acquired immunodeficiency syndrome (AIDS), can often be prevented by making lifestyle changes. About two thirds of all mortalities and a great amount of morbidity, suffering, and rising health care costs among adults result from three causes. Heart disease causes 34% of all deaths. Cancer causes 25%, and stroke causes 7%. Only three categories of behavior contribute enormously to these causes: tobacco use, dietary patterns, and physical inactivity (CDC, 2002c). Staying physically active, eating right, and not smoking (or quitting if you do smoke) are the three most important strategies to better health (Fig. 10–1).

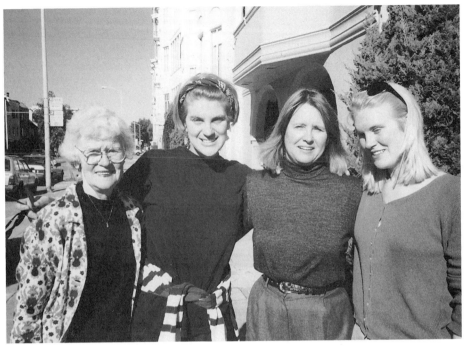

***Figure 10–1.*** ▶ A healthy lifestyle incorporating physical activity, good nutrition, social support, and avoidance of activities that are detrimental to health can improve quality of life for adults of all ages.

## Physical Activity

Engaging in regular physical activity on most days of the week reduces the risk of developing or dying from some of the leading causes of illness and death. Box 10–4 presents an overview of the relationship between physical activity and morbidity and mortality.

More than 60% of adults in the United States do not engage in recommended amounts of physical activity. Physical inactivity is more common among women than men, African-American and Hispanic adults than White adults, older adults than younger adults, and less affluent people than more affluent people.

"How much activity?" and "How do I start?" are two common questions clients ask regarding physical activity. Clients who have been sedentary or are obese may want to start by reducing sedentary time and gradually building physical activity into each day. A client may begin by gradually increasing daily activities such as taking the stairs or walking or swimming at a slow pace.

The need to avoid injury during physical activity is a high priority. Walking is an ideal activity to increase physical activity because it is safe and accessible to most people. For those who have been physically inactive, a starting point can be walking 10 minutes, 3 days a week, building to 30 to 45 minutes of more intense walking and gradually increasing to most if not all days. **Moderate physical activity** for 30 to 45 minutes, 3 to 5 days per week, is a reasonable initial goal. Most adults should be encouraged to set a long-term goal of 30 minutes or more of moderate-intensity physical activity on most, preferably all, days of the week. Table 10–2

> ▶ **Box 10–4.** The Effects of Physical Activity on Health ◀

Regular physical activity reduces the risk of the following:
- Dying prematurely
- Dying prematurely from heart disease
- Developing diabetes
- Developing high blood pressure
- Developing colon cancer

Regular physical activity helps in the following ways:
- Reduces blood pressure in those with hypertension
- Reduces feelings of depression and anxiety
- Controls weight
- Builds and maintains healthy bones, muscles, and joints
- Promotes psychologic well-being

These health burdens could be reduced through regular physical activity:
- 13.5 million people have coronary heart disease
- 1.5 million individuals have a myocardial infarction each year
- 8 million people have type 2 diabetes (adult onset)
- More than 60 million individuals (one third of the population) are overweight

Centers for Disease Control and Prevention. (1999). *The link between physical activity and morbidity and mortality. Physical activity and health: A report of the surgeon general.* Retrieved May 30, 2003 from: http//www.cdc.gov/nccdphp/sgr/mm.htm

shows examples of moderate amounts of physical activity achieved from both common chores and sporting activities.

With time, weight loss, and increased functional capacity, the client may want to engage in more strenuous activities. These include fitness walking, cycling, rowing, cross-country skiing, aerobic dancing, and jumping rope. If jogging is desired, the client's ability to jog must be assessed first. Competitive sports such as tennis, soccer, and volleyball provide enjoyable physical activity for some individuals, but again, care must be taken to avoid injury.

Individuals who are not physically active cite many reasons for their inactivity. In Appendix H of *The Practical Guide: Identification, Evaluation, and Treatment of Overweight and Obesity in Adults* by the National Institutes of Health (NIH), available on-line at http://www.nhlbi.nih.gov/guidelines/obesity/ob_home.htm, nurses can receive some pointers for helping the client overcome obstacles to regular activity. It also includes two sample exercise programs.

Social support from family and friends has been consistently and positively related to regular exercise. Nurses who work closely with clients in community-based settings have ample opportunity to encourage moderate physical activity for 30 minutes a day for all adults.

## Overweight and Obesity

Overweight and obesity are major contributors to many preventable causes of death, with a general rule that higher body weight is associated with higher death

**TABLE 10–2** • Examples of Moderate Amounts of Physical Activity*

| Common Chores | Sporting Activities | |
|---|---|---|
| Washing and waxing a car for 45–60 min | Playing volleyball for 45–60 min | Less Vigorous, More Time |
| Washing windows or floors for 45–60 min | Playing touch football for 45 min | |
| Gardening for 30–45 min | Walking 1¼ miles in 35 min (20 min/mile) | ↑ |
| Wheeling self in wheelchair for 30–40 min | Basketball (shooting baskets) for 30 min | |
| Pushing a stroller 1½ miles in 30 min | Bicycling 5 miles in 30 min | |
| Raking leaves for 30 min | Dancing fast (social) for 30 min | |
| Walking 2 miles in 30 min (15 min/mile) | Water aerobics for 30 min | |
| Shoveling snow for 15 min | Swimming laps for 20 min | ↓ |
| Stairwalking for 15 min | Basketball (playing a game) for 15–20 min | More Vigorous, Less Time |
| | Jumping rope for 15 min | |
| | Running 1½ miles in 15 min (10 min/mile) | |

*A moderate amount of physical activity is roughly equivalent to physical activity that uses approximately 150 calories of energy per day, or 1,000 calories per week.

Some activities can be performed at various intensities; the suggested durations correspond to expected intensity of effort.

National Institutes of Health. (1998). *The practical guide: Identification, evaluation, and treatment of overweight and obesity in adults.* National Heart, Lung and Blood Institute Obesity Education Initiative.

rates. The percent of the adult population that is overweight or obese has increased in the last 3 decades (Fig. 10–2). Being overweight or obese substantially raises the risk of illness from high blood pressure, high cholesterol, type 2 diabetes, heart disease and stroke, gallbladder disease, arthritis, sleep disturbances, and endometrial, breast, prostate, and colon cancers.

Women from lower income households are more likely to be overweight. Obesity is more common among African-American and Hispanic women than among White women. Eighty percent more African-American women than men are overweight (DHHS, 2000).

A person with a BMI between 25.0 and 29.9 is considered **overweight.** A person with a BMI of 30.0 or greater is considered **obese.** Box 10–5 shows how to calculate BMI and waist circumference. Table 10–3 provides a BMI estimation table.

Dietary therapy, physical activity, and behavioral therapy are the usual interventions for overweight and obesity. For the morbidly obese, pharmacotherapy and weight-loss surgery may be considered. A combination of diet modification, increased physical activity, and behavior therapy can be effective for most obese individuals. A guide to selecting appropriate treatment is found in the NIH *Practical Guide.*

Weight-loss therapy is not appropriate for some individuals, including most pregnant or lactating women, people with uncontrolled psychiatric illness, and with serious illnesses that might be exacerbated by caloric restriction. Clients with active substance abuse or a history of anorexia nervosa or bulimia nervosa should receive care by a specialist.

It is recommended that health care providers first complete a behavioral assessment to determine a client's readiness for weight loss. One example is found in the NIH *Practical Guide.* Appendix I of the NIH publication contains a guide to behavior change, which can be used to help the client plan a weight-loss program.

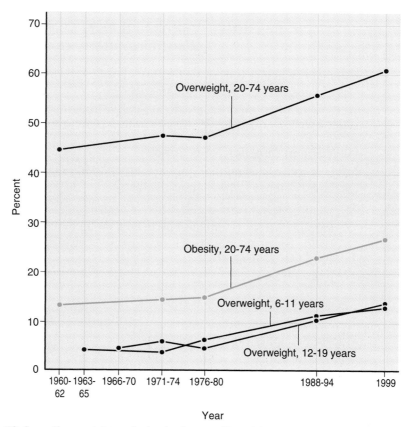

*Figure 10–2.* ▶ Overweight and obesity by age: United States, 1960-1999. Note: Percents for adults are age adjusted. Overweight for children is defined as a BMI at or above the sex- and age-specific 95th percentile BMI cut points from the 2000 CDC growth charts. Source: Chartbook on Trends in the Health of Americans Health. (2002). Centers for Disease Control and Prevention, National Center for Health Statistics, National Health Examination survey and National Health and Nutrition Examination Survey.

Next, a diet with a 500- to 1,000-calorie deficit should be planned. This usually means 1,000 to 1,200 calories for women and 1,200 to 1,600 calories for men. Sample diets for American, Asian, Southern, Mexican-American, and lacto-ovo vegetarian clients are found in the appendices of the NIH *Practical Guide,* along with tips for weight loss, including methods of food preparation and how to choose food when dining away from home.

The nurse and client can plan and monitor the weight-loss program by using a weight and goal record. The client can keep a record of food consumption and physical activity each week by using a diet and activity-tracking sheet. Samples of these resources are found in the appendices of the *Practical Guide,* along with additional resources for healthy eating and physical activity. Through health education, nurses can help reduce the proportion of adults who are obese.

> ▶ **Box 10–5.** Calculating Body Mass Index and ◀ Waist Circumference

You can calculate BMI as follows:
BMI = weight (kg) / height squared (m²)
If pounds and inches are used, do the following:
BMI = weight (lb) × IQ 703 height squared (inches²)

### Calculation Directions and Sample

Here is a shortcut method for calculating BMI. (Example: for a person who is 5 feet 5 inches tall weighing 180 lbs)

1. Multiply weight (in pounds) by 703: 180 × 703 = 126,540
2. Multiply height (in inches) by height (in inches): 65 × 65 = 4,225
3. Divide the answer in step 1 by the answer in step 2 to get the BMI:
   126,540/4,225 = 29.9
   BMI = 29.9

### Waist Circumference Measurement

To measure waist circumference, locate the upper hip bone and the top of the right iliac crest. Place a measuring tape in a horizontal plane around the abdomen at the level of the iliac crest. Before reading the tape measure, ensure that the tape is snug, but does not compress the skin, and is parallel to the floor. The measurement is made at the end of a normal expiration.

### High-Risk Waist Circumference

Men: F > 40 in (> 102 cm)
Women: F > 35 in (> 88 cm)

National Institutes of Health, National Heart, Lung, and Blood Institute, Obesity Education Initiative. (1998). *The practical guide: Identification, evaluation, and treatment of overweight and obesity in adults.* Bethesda, MD: U.S. Department of Health and Human Services.

**Measuring-Tape Position for Waist (Abdominal) (Circumference in Adults)**

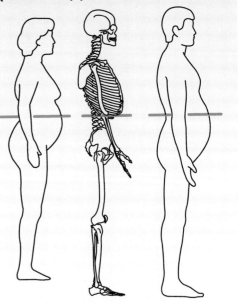

## Tobacco Use

Cigarette smoking, responsible for more than 430,000 deaths annually, continues to be the main preventable cause of disease and death in the United States ("Treating tobacco use," 2000). Smoking is a major risk factor for developing heart disease, stroke, lung cancer, and chronic lung disease. The percentage of adolescents who smoke has increased in the past decade, and each day, more than 3,000 children and adolescents start using tobacco ("Treating tobacco use," 2000). This trend is of great concern because most adult smokers tried their first cigarette before 18 years of age. Half of all adolescent smokers who continue to smoke in adulthood will die from smoking-related illness. Whites are more likely than African Americans and Hispanics to use tobacco (DHHS, 2000).

The financial costs of smoking and smoking-related disease, including lost earnings and productivity, approach $100 billion per year. It is estimated that a program to provide 75% of adult smokers with a smoking cessation intervention (nicotine replacement therapy, counseling, or a combination) would be cost effective in relation to other interventions, such as blood pressure screening and mammography. Currently, most medical schools do not require clinical training in techniques for smoking cessation ("Treating tobacco use," 2000).

An integrative literature review of 19 studies was conducted to determine the effectiveness of nursing-delivered smoking cessation interventions. It was found that smokers who were offered advice by nursing professionals had an increased likelihood of quitting compared to smokers without such nursing interventions. This result reflected a significantly positive effect for smoking cessation interventions by nurses. The challenge to nurses is to incorporate smoking cessation interventions as part of standard practice so that the nurse discusses tobacco use with all clients, gives advice to quit, and uses behavioral counseling. Nurses interface with clients in numerous settings, allowing them to play an important role in reducing cigarette smoking by adults (Rice & Stead, 1999).

The community-based nurse should screen for tobacco use and encourage cessation with every client. Current guidelines for clinicians assisting clients with smoking cessation are shown in Box 10–6.

## Alcohol and Substance Use and Abuse

There is a great deal of confusion about the benefits and detriments of alcohol consumption. In the last decade, some research suggested that moderate alcohol use might provide some protection from coronary artery disease. The most recent research reports that the pattern of drinking, or having a drink every day as opposed to drinking large quantities of alcohol at one sitting, is what determines the effects of alcohol on one's health (Mukamal, Conigrave, Mittleman, Carmergo, Stampfer, Willett, & Rimm, 2003). These findings are consistent with what we have known for some time—binge drinking creates health problems.

Many serious problems are associated with alcohol and illicit drug abuse. The financial costs of substance abuse are high, estimated at $276 billion per year (DHHS, 2000). Substance abuse is associated with child and spousal abuse, STDs, motor vehicle accidents, escalation of health care costs, low worker productivity, and homelessness. Alcohol abuse alone is associated with motor vehicle accidents, homicides, suicides, and drownings. Chronic alcohol use can lead to heart disease, cancer, liver disease, and pancreatitis (DHHS, 2000).

The rate of adult drinking and illicit drug use has been constant since 1980. Whites and Hispanics are more likely than African Americans to use alcohol. Whites are more likely than African Americans and Hispanics to use illicit drugs (DHHS, 2000).

Assessment and intervention with substance-related health issues is an important role for the nurse in community-based settings. The more direct, honest, and

**TABLE 10–2 •** Body Mass Index Estimation

| | Healthy Weight | | | | | | Overweight | | | | | | Obese | | | | | |
|---|---|---|---|---|---|---|---|---|---|---|---|---|---|---|---|---|---|---|
| BMI | 19 | 20 | 21 | 22 | 23 | 24 | 25 | 26 | 27 | 28 | 29 | 30 | 31 | 32 | 33 | 34 | 35 | |
| Height (inches) | | | | | | | | Body Weight (lbs.) | | | | | | | | | | |
| 58 | 91 | 96 | 100 | 105 | 110 | 115 | 119 | 124 | 129 | 134 | 138 | 143 | 148 | 153 | 158 | 162 | 167 | 172 |
| 59 | 94 | 99 | 104 | 109 | 114 | 119 | 124 | 128 | 133 | 138 | 143 | 148 | 153 | 158 | 163 | 168 | 173 | 178 |
| 60 | 97 | 102 | 107 | 112 | 118 | 123 | 128 | 133 | 138 | 143 | 148 | 153 | 158 | 163 | 168 | 174 | 179 | 184 |
| 61 | 100 | 106 | 111 | 116 | 122 | 127 | 132 | 137 | 143 | 148 | 153 | 158 | 164 | 169 | 174 | 180 | 185 | 190 |
| 62 | 104 | 109 | 115 | 120 | 126 | 131 | 136 | 142 | 147 | 153 | 158 | 164 | 169 | 175 | 180 | 186 | 191 | 196 |
| 63 | 107 | 113 | 118 | 124 | 130 | 135 | 141 | 146 | 152 | 158 | 163 | 169 | 175 | 180 | 186 | 191 | 197 | 203 |
| 64 | 110 | 116 | 122 | 128 | 134 | 140 | 145 | 151 | 157 | 163 | 169 | 174 | 180 | 186 | 192 | 197 | 204 | 209 |
| 65 | 114 | 120 | 126 | 132 | 138 | 144 | 150 | 156 | 162 | 168 | 174 | 180 | 186 | 192 | 198 | 204 | 210 | 216 |
| 66 | 118 | 124 | 130 | 136 | 142 | 148 | 155 | 161 | 167 | 173 | 179 | 186 | 192 | 198 | 204 | 210 | 216 | 223 |
| 67 | 121 | 127 | 134 | 140 | 146 | 153 | 159 | 166 | 172 | 178 | 185 | 191 | 198 | 204 | 211 | 217 | 223 | 230 |
| 68 | 125 | 131 | 138 | 144 | 151 | 158 | 164 | 171 | 177 | 184 | 190 | 197 | 203 | 210 | 216 | 223 | 230 | 236 |
| 69 | 128 | 135 | 142 | 149 | 155 | 162 | 169 | 176 | 182 | 189 | 196 | 203 | 209 | 216 | 223 | 230 | 236 | 243 |
| 70 | 132 | 139 | 146 | 153 | 160 | 167 | 174 | 181 | 188 | 195 | 202 | 209 | 216 | 222 | 229 | 236 | 243 | 250 |
| 71 | 136 | 143 | 150 | 157 | 165 | 172 | 179 | 186 | 193 | 200 | 208 | 215 | 222 | 229 | 236 | 243 | 250 | 257 |
| 72 | 140 | 147 | 154 | 162 | 169 | 177 | 184 | 191 | 199 | 206 | 213 | 221 | 228 | 235 | 242 | 250 | 258 | 265 |
| 73 | 144 | 151 | 159 | 166 | 174 | 182 | 189 | 197 | 204 | 212 | 219 | 227 | 235 | 242 | 250 | 257 | 265 | 272 |
| 74 | 148 | 155 | 163 | 171 | 179 | 186 | 194 | 202 | 210 | 218 | 225 | 233 | 241 | 249 | 256 | 264 | 272 | 280 |
| 75 | 152 | 160 | 168 | 176 | 184 | 192 | 200 | 208 | 216 | 224 | 232 | 240 | 248 | 256 | 264 | 272 | 279 | 287 |
| 76 | 156 | 164 | 172 | 180 | 189 | 197 | 205 | 213 | 221 | 230 | 238 | 246 | 254 | 263 | 271 | 279 | 287 | 295 |

National Institutes of Health, National Heart, Lung, and Blood Institute, Obesity Education Initiative. (1998). *The practical guide: Identification, evaluation, and treatment of overweight and obesity in adults.* Bethesda, MD: U.S. Department of Health and Human Services.

open the nurse is when addressing this issue, the more likely clients will be to view their own patterns of alcohol use as an important aspect of health promotion.

Box 10–7 gives an assessment for alcohol abuse. Teaching the client about avoiding substance abuse issues is the next step after assessment (see Boxes 10–8 and 10–9).

Interventions targeted to groups and communities have demonstrated some efficacy in reducing substance abuse. School-based prevention programs directed toward altering perceived peer-group norms about alcohol use and helping develop skills in resisting peer pressure to drink are successful in reducing alcohol use among participants. Raising the minimum legal drinking age has reduced alcohol consumption, traffic accidents, and related fatalities among young persons less than 21 years of age. Higher cost for alcohol is also associated with lower alcohol consumption and lowered adverse outcomes. In college settings, one-to-one motivational counseling has been effective in reducing alcohol-related problems. It is important that the nurse direct efforts to reduce the proportion of adults using illicit drugs and engaging in binge drinking of alcoholic beverages.

## Responsible Sexual Behavior

In the United States, more than 65 million people are currently living with an incurable STD (CDC, 2001). Unprotected sex can result in unintended pregnancies and

| | 36 | 37 | 38 | 39 | 40 | 41 | 42 | 43 | 44 | 45 | 46 | 47 | 48 | 49 | 50 | 51 | 52 | 53 |
|---|---|---|---|---|---|---|---|---|---|---|---|---|---|---|---|---|---|---|
| **Very Obese** | | | | | | | | | | | | | | | | | | |
| Height (inches) | | | | | | | Body Weight (lbs.) | | | | | | | | | | | |
| 58 | 177 | 181 | 186 | 191 | 196 | 201 | 205 | 210 | 215 | 220 | 224 | 229 | 234 | 239 | 244 | 248 | 253 | 258 |
| 59 | 183 | 188 | 193 | 198 | 203 | 208 | 212 | 217 | 222 | 227 | 232 | 237 | 242 | 247 | 252 | 257 | 262 | 267 |
| 60 | 189 | 194 | 199 | 204 | 209 | 215 | 220 | 225 | 230 | 235 | 240 | 245 | 250 | 255 | 261 | 266 | 271 | 276 |
| 61 | 195 | 201 | 206 | 211 | 217 | 222 | 227 | 232 | 238 | 243 | 248 | 254 | 259 | 264 | 269 | 275 | 280 | 285 |
| 62 | 202 | 207 | 213 | 218 | 224 | 229 | 235 | 240 | 246 | 251 | 256 | 262 | 267 | 273 | 278 | 284 | 289 | 295 |
| 63 | 208 | 214 | 220 | 225 | 231 | 237 | 242 | 248 | 254 | 259 | 265 | 270 | 278 | 282 | 287 | 293 | 299 | 304 |
| 64 | 215 | 221 | 227 | 232 | 238 | 244 | 250 | 256 | 262 | 267 | 273 | 279 | 285 | 291 | 296 | 302 | 308 | 314 |
| 65 | 222 | 228 | 234 | 240 | 246 | 252 | 258 | 264 | 270 | 276 | 282 | 288 | 294 | 300 | 306 | 312 | 318 | 324 |
| 66 | 229 | 235 | 241 | 247 | 253 | 260 | 266 | 272 | 278 | 284 | 291 | 297 | 303 | 309 | 315 | 322 | 328 | 334 |
| 67 | 236 | 242 | 249 | 255 | 261 | 268 | 274 | 280 | 287 | 293 | 299 | 306 | 312 | 319 | 325 | 331 | 338 | 344 |
| 68 | 243 | 249 | 256 | 262 | 269 | 276 | 282 | 289 | 295 | 302 | 308 | 315 | 322 | 328 | 335 | 341 | 348 | 354 |
| 69 | 250 | 257 | 263 | 270 | 277 | 284 | 291 | 297 | 304 | 311 | 318 | 324 | 331 | 338 | 345 | 351 | 358 | 365 |
| 70 | 257 | 264 | 271 | 278 | 285 | 292 | 299 | 306 | 313 | 320 | 327 | 334 | 341 | 348 | 355 | 362 | 369 | 376 |
| 71 | 265 | 272 | 279 | 286 | 293 | 301 | 308 | 315 | 322 | 329 | 338 | 343 | 351 | 358 | 365 | 372 | 379 | 386 |
| 72 | 272 | 279 | 287 | 294 | 302 | 309 | 316 | 324 | 331 | 338 | 346 | 353 | 361 | 368 | 375 | 383 | 390 | 397 |
| 73 | 280 | 288 | 295 | 302 | 310 | 318 | 325 | 333 | 340 | 348 | 355 | 363 | 371 | 378 | 386 | 393 | 401 | 408 |
| 74 | 287 | 295 | 303 | 311 | 319 | 326 | 334 | 342 | 350 | 358 | 365 | 373 | 381 | 389 | 396 | 404 | 412 | 420 |
| 75 | 295 | 303 | 311 | 319 | 327 | 335 | 343 | 351 | 359 | 367 | 375 | 383 | 391 | 399 | 407 | 415 | 423 | 431 |
| 76 | 304 | 312 | 320 | 328 | 336 | 344 | 353 | 361 | 369 | 377 | 385 | 394 | 402 | 410 | 418 | 426 | 435 | 443 |

STDs, including HIV. About half of all new HIV infections in the United States are among individuals over 25 years of age, with the majority being infected through sexual behavior. Women bear the greatest burden of STDs, suffering more frequent and more serious complications than men. Recently, there has been an increase in abstinence among youth and an increase in condom use among sexually active adults. Condoms, used correctly and consistently, can prevent STDs, including HIV.

Nurses should never hesitate to assess sexual health. Here are some simple questions:

- Are you afraid you might have a sexually transmitted disease?
- Do you have questions about tests or treatment?
- If you need to find a doctor or clinic where you can get private, personal, and confidential care, you can call the National STD Hot Line at (800) 227-8922.

Health teaching is the most important disease prevention activity the nurse can use to address health issues related to sexual behavior. Again, sexuality must always be assessed, with teaching and interventions based on the client's knowledge base, concerns, and cultural sensitivities. As discussed in Chapter 9, young teens should be encouraged to delay age of first intercourse. Teaching about the effectiveness of various contraceptive methods and providing condoms are interventions that have been shown again and again to be essential to sexual health promotion.

## COMMUNITY-BASED NURSING CARE GUIDELINES

**Box 10–6** ▶ Quick Reference Guide for Clinicians Treating Tobacco Use and Dependence

| | |
|---|---|
| Ask | Systematically identify all tobacco users at every visit. |
| Advise | Strongly urge all tobacco users to quit. |
| Assess | Determine willingness to make a quit attempt. |
| Assist | Aid the client in quitting. |
| Follow up | Ask clients if they still smoke. Give ex-smokers a pat on the back. Send cards or call clients soon after their visit and just before their original quit day. |

Fiore, M., Bailey, W., Cohen, S., et al. (2000). *Quick reference guide for clinicians: Treating tobacco use and dependence.* Rockville MD: U.S. Department of Health and Human Services, Public Health Service. Retrieved February 5, 2003 from http://www.surgeongeneral.gov/tobacco/tobrg.htm.

## Mental Health

Twenty percent of the population is affected by mental illness during a given year, with depression as the most common disorder. Mental health is not just the absence of illness but a "state of successful mental functioning, resulting in productivity, fulfilling relationships, and ability to adapt to change and cope with adversity" (DHHS, 2000, p. 37).

Depression is a common condition that is often not recognized by health care providers. Home care nurses use the OASIS (outcome and assessment information set) method of assessment, which is discussed in Chapter 13. The recommended tool through OASIS for assessing depression is found in Box 10–10. Depression affects daily functioning and, in some cases, incapacitates the individual. Major depression is the leading cause of all disabilities and the cause of more than two thirds of suicides each year. Financial costs from lost work time are high. Unfortu-

### ▶ Box 10–7 Quick Assessment for Alcohol Abuse ◀

A "yes" answer to any of the following questions may be a warning sign that the client has a drinking problem and should talk to a health care provider.

- Have you ever felt that you should cut down on your drinking?
- Have people annoyed you by criticizing your drinking?
- Have you ever felt bad or guilty about drinking?
- Have you ever had a drink first thing in the morning to steady your nerves or to get rid of a hangover?

Agency for Health Care Research and Quality. (1998). *Personal health guide: Put prevention into practice.* (Publication No. APPIP 98–0027). Rockville, MD: Agency for Health Care Policy and Research. Retrieved May 30, 2003 from http://www.ahcpr.gov/ppip/adguide.

## COMMUNITY-BASED TEACHING

**Box 10–8** ▶ Tips to Reduce Substance Abuse Behaviors

- Don't use illegal (street) drugs of any kind, at any time.
- Use prescription drugs only as directed by a health care provider.
- Use nonprescription drugs only as instructed on the label.
- Tell your health care provider all of the medications you are currently taking.
- If you drink alcohol, do so only in moderation—no more than one drink daily for women and two drinks daily for men.
- Do not drink alcohol before or while driving a motor vehicle.
- If you have concerns about your alcohol or drug use, talk to your health care provider.

Agency for Health Care Research and Quality. (1998). *Personal health guide: Put prevention into practice.* (Publication No. APPIP 98–0027). Rockville, MD. Agency for Health Care Policy and Research. Retrieved May 15, 2003 from: http://www.ahcpr.gov/ppip/adguide.

nately, there is still widespread misunderstanding about mental illness and associated stigmatization, which often prevents individuals with depression from getting professional help.

Adults and older adults have the highest rates of depression, with major depression affecting twice as many women as men. Depression is also high among those with chronic conditions; 12% of clients hospitalized with heart disease or hip fracture are diagnosed with depression (DHHS, 2000).

Depression is a treatable condition—medications and psychologic treatment are effective in 80% of people suffering from depression. But to receive treatment, people with depression have to be identified and encouraged to seek help. An important role of the nurse in community-based care is to identify those experiencing depression and convince them to seek assistance early.

At least 90% of people who commit suicide have had or are experiencing mental illness, a substance abuse disorder, or a combination; therefore, it is essential that health care professionals be diligent about screening and intervention when mental illness is suspected. Again, nurses should not be afraid to ask questions regarding mental health concerns and to refer clients accordingly. It is important that the proportion of adults with recognized depression who receive treatment continues to rise.

## Injuries and Violence

The current yearly cost of injury and violence is estimated at more than $224 billion, which is an increase of 42% over the previous decade. Motor vehicle accidents are the most common cause of serious injury among adults. Nearly 40% of all traffic fatalities in 1997 were related to alcohol use, with drivers between 21 and 24 years old having the highest intoxication rate. About 3 in 10 Americans will be involved in an alcohol-related crash in their lifetimes (CDC National Center for Injury Prevention and Control [NCIPC], 2001).

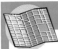

## COMMUNITY-BASED NURSING CARE GUIDELINES

**Box 10–9** ▶ Guidelines for Alcohol and
Substance Use Intervention

**Ask**

Ask clients if they use alcohol or other drugs, how much, and the frequency.
Ask about binge drinking (more than three drinks per occasion or seven
drinks per week). Congratulate recovering alcoholics and drug users.

Ask clients the assessment questions in Box 10–7. Also ask about any adverse consequences they have experienced from their drinking.

**Advise**

Ask what benefits the clients would enjoy if they reduced alcohol or
drug intake.

**Prepare**

Encourage client to set a date to quit drinking, attend Alcoholics
Anonymous, or get counseling for concerns related to his or her substance use.

**Follow up**

Follow up by asking about progress. Be straightforward, matter of fact,
and nonjudgmental. Praise and encourage any small steps taken.
Continue to validate any effort.

Certain types of injuries appear to affect some groups more frequently. Native
Americans and Alaskan Natives have disproportionately high death rates from
motor vehicle accidents, residential fires, and drowning. There are higher rates of
death from unintentional injury among African Americans. In every age group,
drowning rates are almost two to four times greater for males than females. Homicide is especially high among African-American and Hispanic youths. Nurses must
be involved in efforts to reduce death caused by motor vehicle accidents and
homicide. Box 10–11 provides recommendations for preventing injuries in general.

Injuries are among the leading causes of death for women in the United States.
Many injuries to women result from violent acts; others are caused by unintentional events such as falls, motor vehicle accidents, burns, drowning, and poison-
ings. Some injuries affect women more frequently than men, with hip fractures and
domestic violence being the most common.

Intentional injury, or physical assault, is a leading cause of injury to women,
with more women than men experiencing intimate partner violence. Research indicates that as many as 30% of women treated in emergency departments have injuries or symptoms related to physical abuse. Intimate partner violence is a major
cause of violence-related injuries. One in three women injured during a physical
assault or rape require medical care. Women are also more likely than men to be
murdered in the context of intimate partner violence (CDC NCIPC, 2001).

---

## ▶ Box 10–10   Criteria for Major Depressive Episode ◀

Five (or more) of the following symptoms have been present during the same 2-week period and represent a change from previous functioning: at least one of the symptoms is either 1) depressed mood or 2) loss of interest or pleasure.

1. Depressed mood throughout most of the day, nearly every day.
2. Markedly diminished interest or pleasure in all, or nearly all, activities most of the day, nearly every day.
3. Significant weight loss when not dieting or weight gain (eg, a change of more than 5% of body weight in 1 month), or a decrease or increase in appetite nearly every day.
4. Insomnia or hypersomnia nearly every day.
5. Psychomotor agitation or retardation nearly every day (observable by others; not merely a subjective feeling of restlessness or being slowed down).
6. Fatigue or loss of energy nearly every day.
7. Feelings of worthlessness or excessive or inappropriate guilt, nearly every day.
8. Diminished ability to think or concentrate, or indecisiveness, nearly every day.
9. Recurrent thoughts of death (not just fear of dying), recurrent suicidal ideation without a specific plan, or a suicide attempt or a specific plan for committing suicide.

Source: Raue, PA, Brown, E., & Bruce, M., (2002). Assessing behavioral health using OASIS: Depression and suicidality. *Home Healthcare Nurse, 20*(3), 154–161.

American Psychiatric Association. (1994). *Diagnostic and statistical manual of mental disorders.* (4th ed.). Washington, DC: Author.

---

The first and foremost responsibility of the nurse in cases where domestic abuse is suspected is to assess for domestic abuse. Nurses should never be afraid to ask the question, "Do you have any concerns about your personal safety?" In order to be comfortable with this type of assessment, the nurse should acquire basic information about domestic abuse as well as develop basic clinical skills for identifying and assessing domestic abuse. Next, the nurse must be familiar with resources within his or her own community for referral phone numbers and contact persons.

### Environmental Quality

An estimated 25% of preventable illnesses worldwide can be attributed to poor environmental quality. Poor air quality, including both ozone (outside air) and tobacco smoke (inside air), is one of the prime contributors. In the United States, air pollution alone is estimated to contribute to 50,000 premature deaths annually. Incidence of asthma has been on the rise for the past few decades among adults and children.

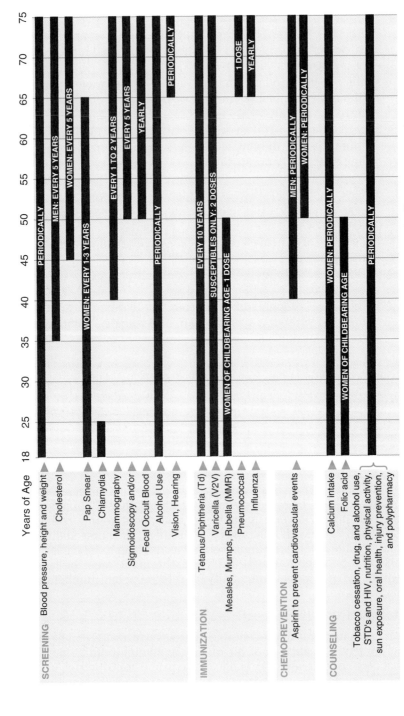

***Figure 10–3.*** ▲ Agency for Health Care Research and Quality. Personal health guide: Put prevention into practice. (Publication No. 98-027.) Rockville, MD. Agency for health care Policy and Research. Retrieved May 17, 2003 from http://www.ahcpr.gov/ppip/adguide.

## COMMUNITY-BASED TEACHING

**Box 10–11** ▶   Recommendations for Preventing Injuries

- Always wear a seat belt while in the car.
- Never drive after drinking alcohol.
- Always wear a safety helmet while riding a motorcycle or bicycle.
- Use smoke detectors in your home; check to make sure they work every month, and change the batteries every year.
- Keep the temperature of hot water less than 120°F, particularly if there are children or older adults living in your home.
- If you choose to keep a gun in your home, make sure that the gun and the ammunition are locked up separately and are out of the reach of children.
- Prevent falls by older adults by repairing slippery or uneven walking surfaces, improving poor lighting, and installing secure railings on all stairways.
- Be alert for hazards in your workplace and follow all safety rules.

Agency for Health Care Research and Quality. (1998). *Personal health guide: Put prevention into practice.* (Publication No. APPIP 98–0027). Rockville, MD. Agency for Health Care Policy and Research. Retrieved May 18, 2003 from: http://www.ahcpr.gov/ppip/adguide.

It is important that the proportion of individuals exposed to poor air quality is reduced, as well as the proportion of nonsmokers exposed to secondhand smoke. One intervention involves teaching clients about the importance of maintaining smoke-free indoor air and the hazards of secondhand smoke. Second, the nurse can teach clients the threat that poor outdoor air quality poses for health and the importance of supporting political candidates and legislation that protect air quality.

## Immunizations

Immunization is cited as one of the greatest achievements of public health in the 20th century. It is important to continue to increase the proportion of children who receive all vaccines, as well as the proportion of adults who are vaccinated annually against the flu. Figure 10–3 summarizes recommended screening, immunization, and health promotion activities.

## Access to Health Care

According to *Healthy People 2010,* access to quality care is important to eliminate health disparities and increase the quality and years of healthy lives for all Americans. One way to improve access is to improve the continuum of care. Until the 1980s, the proportion of people without health insurance gradually declined. Since the late 1980s, this proportion has remained the same, at 15%. The variation in access to health care by race and ethnicity is seen in Figure 10–4.

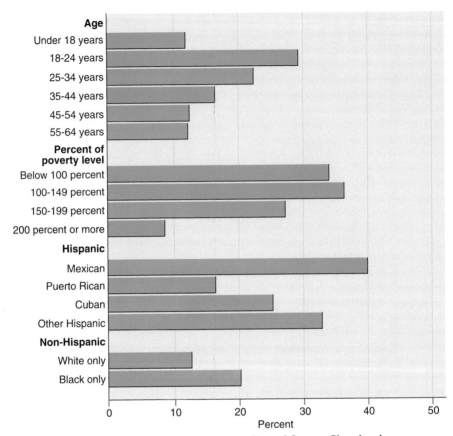

***Figure 10–4.*** ▶ Poverty rules by age and class: United States. Chartbook on health of the America's. (2002). Centers for Disease Control and Prevention, National Center for the Health Statistics, National Health Interview Survey.

## Conclusions

Current critical issues of health and health care have changed dramatically in the past 100 years. Today, most diseases and deaths result from preventable causes. The nurse plays an essential role in early identification of and intervention in these conditions. Nurses can be successful in this charge by screening, particularly in high-risk groups. By identifying conditions early in their course, nurses can provide interventions that will substantially minimize the effects of these conditions. By following the health indicators identified by *Healthy People 2010,* nurses can help adults live longer and healthier lives.

# What's on the Web

American Social Health Association
(ASHA)
P.O. Box 13827
Research Triangle Park, NC 27709
**Internet address:** *http://www.ashastd.org*
The ASHA has been providing health information to the American public since 1914.
They are recognized by the public, clients,
providers, and policy makers for developing and delivering accurate, medically reliable information about STDs.

*Personal Health Guide: Put Prevention into*
*Practice*
**Internet address:**
*http://www.ahrq.gov/ppip/adguide*
This on-line consumer guide from the
AHRQ explains preventive care for adults.
Print copies, available free of charge, can
be requested by calling (800) 358-9295.
The guide is also available in Spanish.

## COOKBOOKS

Heart-Healthy Home Cooking African
American Style
**Internet address:**
*http://www.nhlbi.nih.gov/health/public*
*heart/other/chdblack/cooking.htm*

Delicious Heart-Healthy Latino Recipes
(bilingual cookbook)
**Internet address:**
*http://www.nhlbi.nih.gov/health/public/*
*heart/other/sp_recip.htm*
Print copies can be ordered for a small fee
by phone at (301) 592-8573 or on the Web
at http://www.nhlbi.nih.gov/health/
infoctr/ic_ordr.htm

Obesity Education Initiative
**Internet address:**
*http://www.nhlbi.nih.gov/about/oei/*
*index.htm*
This excellent Web site offers abundant information for providers, clients, and public educators related to obesity, produced

by the National Heart, Lung, and Blood Institute.

## RESOURCES FOR ALCOHOLISM

Al-Anon Family Group Headquarters, Inc.
**Internet address**: *http://www.al-anon.*
*alateen. org/*
This Web site makes referrals to local Al-
Anon groups, which are support groups
for sponsors and other significant adults
in an alcoholic person's life.

Alcoholics Anonymous (AA) World Services, Inc.
**Internet address:** *http://www.aa.org*

National Council on Alcoholism and Drug
Dependence (NCADD)
**Internet address:** *http://www.ncadd.org*
This Web site lists telephone numbers of
local NCADD affiliates that can provide information on local treatment resources
and educational materials on alcoholism.

National Institute on Alcohol Abuse and
Alcoholism (NIAAA)
**Internet address:** *http://www.niaaa.nih.gov*
This site offers free publications on all aspects of alcohol abuse and alcoholism,
with some in Spanish.

## RESOURCES FOR
## CANCER SCREENING

American Cancer Society
**Internet address:** *http://www.cancer.org*

National Cancer Institute
**Internet address:** *http://www.nci.nih.gov*

National Cancer Institute Cervical Cancer
Information
**Internet address:**
*http://cancernet.nci.nih.gov*

National Cervical Cancer Coalition
**Internet address:**
*http://www.nccc-online.org*

## RESOURCES FOR CHRONIC DISEASE PREVENTION

Unrealized Prevention Opportunities: Reducing the Health and Economic Burden of Chronic Disease
**Internet address:**
*http://www.cdc.gov/nccdphp/upo/ factsheets.htm*
This Web site provides fact sheets, graphs and tables, and state-specific resource materials for all chronic conditions.

## RESOURCES FOR DOMESTIC VIOLENCE

National Domestic Violence Hot Line
**Hot line number:** 1-800-787-3224
**Internet address:**
*http://www.ndvh.org/*
The Web site and hot-line number provide information for individuals experiencing domestic abuse. The hot line is available 24 hours a day and 365 days a year. There is a database of 4,000 shelters and services across the United States, Puerto Rico, Alaska, Hawaii, and the U.S. Virgin Islands. With just one contact, those experiencing domestic violence can find out about the options available in their own community. Bilingual services are available.

## RESOURCES FOR SMOKING CESSATION

American Lung Association
Tobacco Control
**Internet address:**
*http://www.lungusa.org/tobacco*

National Center for Chronic Disease Prevention and Health Promotion
Chronic Disease Prevention: Risk Behaviors—Tobacco Use
**Internet address:** *http://www.cdc.gov/ tobacco/edumat.htm*

Nursing Center for Tobacco Intervention
**Internet address:** *http://www.con. ohio-state.edu/tobacco*
This Web site is designed to increase nurse provider participation in the delivery of tobacco cessation interventions with all tobacco users. This site has excellent information as well as links to other sites with outstanding teaching materials for health education.

Quick Reference Guide for Clinicians: Treating Tobacco Use and Dependence
**Internet address:** *http://www. surgeongeneral.gov/tobacco/clinpack.htm*
This guide summarizes the strategies for providing appropriate treatments for every client who could benefit from a smoking cessation program.

Virtual Office of the Surgeon General
Reducing Tobacco Use Report
**Internet address:** *http://www.surgeon general.gov/tobacco/smokesum.htm.*

## References and Bibliography

Agency for Healthcare Research and Quality. (1998). *Personal health guide: Put prevention into practice.* Rockville, MD. Retrieved from http://www.ahcpr. gov/ppip/adguide

Agency for Healthcare Research and Quality. (2000). *Addressing racial and ethnic disparities in health care* (AHRQ Publication No. 00–P041). Rockville, MD. Retrieved February 4, 2003, from http://www.ahrg.gov/research/disparit.htm.

Centers for Disease Control and Prevention. (2000). *Cancer prevention and control.* Retrieved June 1, 2003 from http:/www.cdc.gov/cancer

Centers for Disease Control and Prevention. (2001). *Tracking the hidden epidemics: Trends in STDs in the United States in 2000.* Retrieved March 18, 2003, from www.cdc.gov/nchstp/dstd

Centers for Disease Control and Prevention. (2002a). *2002 program fact sheet: Colorectal cancer.* Retrieved March 17, 2003, from http:///www.cdc.gov/cancer/ colerctl/colorect.htm

Centers for Disease Control and Prevention. (2002b). *2002 program fact sheet: The national breast and cervical cancer early detection program.* Retrieved March 17, 2003, from http:///www.cdc.gov/cancer/ nbccedp/about.htm

Centers for Disease Control and Prevention. (2002c). *Health topics: Overview.* Retrieved March 17, 2003, from http://www.cdc.gov/nccdphp/dash/ healthtopics/

Centers for Disease Control and Prevention. (2002d). *Minority cancer awareness.* Retrieved March 17, 2003, from http://www.cdc.gov/cancer/ minorityawareness.htm

Centers for Disease Control and Prevention. (2003). *Prostate cancer: The public health perspective.* Retrieved March 17, 2003, from http://www.cdc.gov/cancer/prostate/ prostate.htm

Centers for Disease Control and Prevention, National Center for Injury Prevention and Control. (2001). *Injury fact book: 2001–2002.* Atlanta, GA: Author.

Fiore, M., Bailey, W., Cohen, S., et al. (2000). *Quick reference guide for clinicians: Treating tobacco use and dependence.* Rockville, MD: U.S. Department of Health and Human Services, Public Health Service. Retrieved February 5, 2003, from http://www.surgeongeneral. gov/tobacco/tobrg.htm

Mukamal, K. et al. (2003). Roles of drinking pattern and type of alcohol consumed in coronary heart disease in men. *The New England Journal of Medicine, 348*(2), 109–118.

National Institutes of Health, National Heart, Lung, and Blood Institute, Obesity Education Initiative. (1998). *The practical guide: Identification, evaluation, and treatment of overweight and obesity in adults.* Bethesda, MD: U.S. Department of Health and Human Services.

Pastor, P., Makuc, D., Reuben, C., & Xia, H., (2002). *Health, United States, 2003, With chartbook on trends in the health of Americans.* Hyattsville, MD: National Center for Health Statistics. Retrieved January 10, 2003, from http://www.cdc.gov/nchs/hus.htm

Rice, V. H., & Stead, L. F. (1999). Nursing interventions for smoking cessation. *Cochrane Database System Review, 2,* CD001188.

*Treating tobacco use and dependence* [Fact sheet]. (2000, June). U.S. Public Health Service. Retrieved June 10, 2003 from http://www.surgeongeneral.gov/tobacco/ smokfact.htm

U.S. Department of Health and Human Services. (2000). *Healthy people 2010. National health promotion and disease prevention objectives.* Washington, DC: U.S. Government Printing Office.

# LEARNING ACTIVITIES

## JOURNALING: ACTIVITY 10–1

In your clinical journal, describe a situation where you have observed an adult client who was not receiving the health promotion or disease prevention care that he or she needed.

- How could or would you advocate for these issues when you begin to practice as an RN?
- What could you do now?
- Do you see evidence that the current health care system values and provides prevention and health promotion care? Why do you think that this type of care is or is not valued or provided? What arguments would you make that health care should provide such an emphasis in care?

## JOURNALING: ACTIVITY 10–2

1. In your clinical journal, describe a situation you have encountered when screening and doing health promotion and disease prevention teaching and planning with an adult client.
   *What did you learn from this experience?*
   *How will you practice differently based on this experience?*
2. In your clinical journal, describe a situation in which you have observed an adult client who was not receiving the health promotion or disease prevention care that he or she needed.
   *How could or would you advocate for these issues when you begin to practice as an RN?*
   *What could you do now?*

## CLIENT CARE: ACTIVITY 10–3

You are working as a home care nurse, caring for Richard, a 45-year-old client who has advanced chronic obstructive pulmonary disease (COPD) and is on oxygen constantly. Richard, a former smoker, has had several upper respiratory infections this winter, with one resulting in hospitalization for a week. Richard lives with his 25-year-old daughter and her husband, who are both teachers and heavy smokers.

   Which health indicators contribute to Richard's health status?
   What could you as the nurse for this family do to promote Richard's health?
   What steps will you take to address this issue?

## PRACTICAL APPLICATION: ACTIVITY 10–4

In a community-based setting, survey the people there to identify their health promotion and disease prevention needs. With some of the people from the agency, either staff members and clients or both participating in the discussion, determine the best way to provide health promotion and disease prevention teaching and care. Use the resources in the chapter to develop teaching sheets and classes. What's on the Web has several great sites listed in Chapters 10 and 11.

## CRITICAL THINKING: ACTIVITY 10–5

During a weekend visit to your parents' home, you are visiting with a friend of your parents who asks you about your studies in nursing classes. You explain that you are studying about disease prevention and health promotion. The friend, who is 45 years old, says, "I am not sick. What would someone my age need to do to prevent disease?"

   What would be your response to his question?

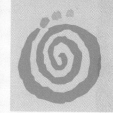

## CHAPTER 11

# Health Promotion and Disease Prevention for Elderly Adults

Roberta Hunt

## LEARNING OBJECTIVES

1. Identify the major causes of death for the elderly.
2. Discuss the major diseases and threats to health of elderly adults.
3. Summarize the major health issues for older adults.
4. Identify nursing roles for each level of prevention for major health issues affecting elderly adults.
5. Compose a list of nursing interventions for the major health issues of older adults.
6. Determine health needs of the elderly for which a nurse could be an advocate.

## KEY TERMS

life expectancy at birth
life expectancy at 65 or 85
medication safety
personal definition of health
polypharmacy

## CHAPTER TOPICS

- **Health Status of Elderly Adults**
- **Health Screening in Elderly Adults**
- **Interventions for Leading Health Indicators**
- **Conclusions**

## THE NURSE SPEAKS

Bea was unforgettable. She was a woman who had lived a hard life, which was reflected in her face and physical condition. She was short, thin, missing several teeth, and appeared older than her 73 years. Most remarkable was Bea's short vibrant red-orange hair, which spiked out in all directions. There were never any cards or flowers or visitors in Bea's room, but it was reported that her husband visited in the evening. Bea was not the kind of patient to inspire extra staff support, but Bea's continued presence on the unit and her weekly assignment to one of the students resulted in visits by almost all of the students each week. The students found her mysterious past, red hair, and one-of-a-kind smile hard to resist.

Spring break and on-campus activities had resulted in several weeks away from the unit. On our return, I was surprised to find Bea still on the unit. She had undergone additional major surgery and once again spent time in intensive care on mechanical ventilation. The staff noted that she was supposed to be up and walking, but when brought to a standing position, she would throw herself back on the bed, dead weight and hard to move despite her less than 100 pounds. The nursing staff felt I might be able to find a more interesting patient than Bea, so I assigned Bea to a student who had not yet cared for her. The next morning, I went in to check on the student and Bea. Bea still had that amazing red hair (which seemed a little more gray at the base), she was thinner (if that could be possible), she looked tired, and there was no smile. She was alone in a dark double room in the bed farthest from the door, a central line was infusing a variety of fluids, and she wore a nasal cannula for oxygen.

Two students were talking to Bea about their plans for the summer, beginning with a much-anticipated massage. I joined the conversation and agreed there was nothing more relaxing than a day at the spa. I asked Bea, if she would like to have a spa day and suggested that if she did, she and the student plan it for the next day. Bea was noncommittal. In postconference, Bea's spa day was discussed. The next morning, each of the students asked me if Bea's student was going ahead with the spa day.

About 9 o'clock, I finally made it to Bea's room. I had brought my lavender essential oil and planned to demonstrate how to use the oil to provide a hand massage. The student noted that Bea was presently resting, having received a complete bath and a long massage. Prior to the bath, the student had suggested that Bea get up for a short walk. According to the student, and to the amazement of the staff, Bea popped out of bed and circled the unit, leaving the student struggling to keep up. No wonder Bea was resting. Around 10 o'clock, we got Bea up in a chair, wrapped her in a warm bath blanket obtained from preop, and washed her hair using the hair-wash-in-a-hat. Bea's hair looked great—soft, shiny, clean, and, of course, very red. A foot soak was prepared using a few drops of lavender essential oil. The aroma of lavender began to fill the room. The student asked Bea is she would like a hand massage, and Bea agreed after some convincing. As the student began the steps of the hand massage, using Jane Buckle's 'M' Technique and a 5% lavender essential oil solution, Bea closed her eyes and snuggled into her blanket. When it came to massaging the second hand, Bea was ready. The aroma of lavender now filled the room and wafted into the hall. The students started stopping by. They reminded Bea who they were and asked her how her spa day was going. The students told Bea how relaxed and comfortable she looked and expressed some envy.

Eventually Bea was returned to a fresh bed with the curtains pulled back. Staff walking by the door started stopping in, wondering what was going on. They told Bea she smelled great and so did her room. The student told the staff about Bea's spa day as she reported off. Each of the nursing staff commented that this was what they had gone into nursing for and never had the time to do. Staff members also observed that they had never seen Bea look so great. During postconference, Bea's student shared how excited the staff was about Bea's spa day. The staff noted she looked much better and were definitely impressed by her walk around the unit, the first in a long time. The social worker decided she wanted to see for herself what this was all about, so she went in to see Bea and asked her how her morning had gone. Bea stated, "This is the first time I have felt like a real person in a long time."

Now whether this change in Bea was due to the massage, the hair wash, the warm blanket, the essential oil, an increase in positive social interaction, or Bea's own self-determination, it is hard to know. I like to think that it was a holistic intervention plan focused on Bea, helping her and those about her find Bea, a woman with strength, a great smile, a mysterious past, and amazing hair.

**Mary Kathryn Moberg, MS, RN**
**Associate Professor**
**The College of St. Catherine**

## Health Status of Elderly Adults

**Life expectancy at birth**, as well as **life expectancy at ages 65 and 85**, has increased over time as death rates for many causes of death have declined. Life expectancy at birth is the number of years that a person born in that year can expect to live. Life expectancy at 65 or 85 is the number of years that a person who is 65 or 85 years old can expect to live. The leading causes of death for elderly adults are listed in Table 11–1. The largest decrease in mortality has been in death rates for heart disease and stroke; death rates for pneumonia and influenza have increased in the past 2 decades (National Center for Health Statistics [NCHS], 1999).

The elderly population in the United States is growing. Life expectancies at ages 65 and 85 have increased over the past 50 years. People who live to age 65 can expect to live, on average, nearly 18 more years. Since 1900, the percentage of people 65 years and older has tripled (Fig. 11–1). This growth is expected to continue

**TABLE 11–1 •** Leading Causes of Death in Adults 65 Years and Older, United States, 2000

| Cause of Death | Number |
| --- | --- |
| Heart disease | 607,265 |
| Cancer | 390,122 |
| Stroke | 148,599 |

Centers for Disease Control and Prevention. (2002). National Center for Injury Prevention and Control. *Injury Fact Book: 2001-2002*. Washington, DC: U.S. Government Printing Office. Retrieved on February 4, 2003 from http://www.cdc.gov/ncipc/fact_book/04_Introduction.htm.

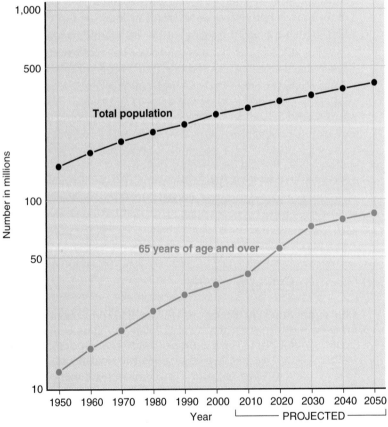

*Figure 11–1.* ▶ Total and elderly population: United States, 1950–2050. National Center for Health Statistics. (2002). *Chartbook on trends in the health of Americans*. U. S. Census Bureau, 1950–2000 decenial censuses and 2110–50 middle series population projections. (p. 18).

for some time, eventually accounting for more than 20% of all Americans by 2030. In addition, the elderly population will continue to be more and more diverse. This growing segment of the population has health care needs that are different from those of other segments of the population. Of people older than 70 years, 80% have one or more chronic conditions (U.S. Department of Health and Human Services [DHHS], 2001).

Living arrangements of persons over 65 years of age show that as people age, they are more likely to live alone. Further, they are more likely to have difficulty performing one or more physical activities, activities of daily living (ADL), or instrumental activities of daily living (IADL). Figure 11–2 shows selected chronic

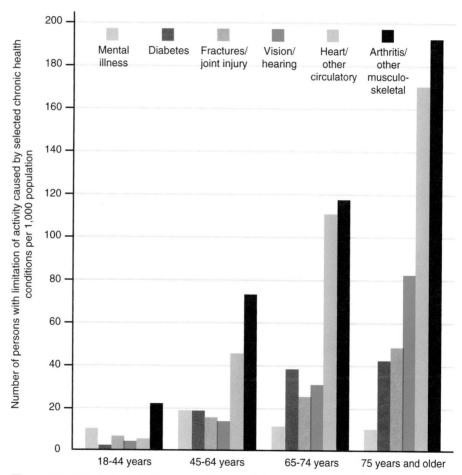

*Figure 11–2.* ▶ Selected chronic health conditions causing limitation of activity among adults by age: United States, 1998–2000. National Center for Health Statistics. *Chartbook on trends in the health of Americans.* (2002). Centers for Disease Control and Prevention, National Center for Health Satistics, National Health Interview Survey. (p. 411).

conditions limiting activity for people older than 70. All of these factors have implications for the ability of the elderly to perform self-care and live independently while managing a chronic illness, and the amount of nursing care this population may need as they age (DHHS, 2001).

##  Health Screening in Elderly Adults

As with clients at other ages, health screening for the elderly is intended for primary, secondary, or tertiary prevention. Primary prevention (to prevent the initial occurrence of a disease) with an elderly client could be immunization screening, recommendation of an annual flu shot, or a safety assessment of the home to identify areas where a fall could occur. Examples of secondary prevention are screening for hypertension and teaching breast self-examination to a group or an individual. Tertiary prevention could be initiating an exercise program for an elderly client who has heart disease. Screening is always performed so that people at risk for certain conditions can be identified, with interventions provided as appropriate.

One way to encourage the elderly client to put prevention into practice is to use the *Staying Healthy at 50+* guide developed by the Agency for Healthcare Research and Quality (AHRQ). This guide (AHRQ, 2000) is available on-line at http://http://www.ahcpr.gov/ppip/50plus/, or it can be ordered free by calling (800) 358-9295. It includes recommendations about lifestyle choices that prevent certain chronic diseases, primary prevention screening, and immunizations.

### General Screening

All screening discussed for adults also applies to elderly adults. This section discusses screening that is particularly important for elderly adults.

High blood pressure is more common in people over age 45, especially African Americans. Therefore, the elderly should have their blood pressure checked periodically with the frequency determined by their nurse practitioner or physician. Cholesterol levels start to increase in middle-aged men and women just before menopause and in anyone who has just gained weight; cholesterol should be measured in people meeting these descriptions.

Heart disease is the leading cause of death for people over 65 years of age. Heart disease is the number-one killer of women, yet only 8% of women realize that it is a greater threat than cancer. Box 11–1 provides more information about the disparity of care and knowledge of women with heart disease. Thirty-eight percent of women and 25% of men will die within 1 year of the first recognized heart attack, and 46% of female and 22% of male heart attack survivors will be disabled within 6 years. Women are almost twice as likely as men to die after bypass surgery (National Coalition of Women with Heart Disease, 2003).

As with other chronic conditions, the risk factors for developing heart disease should be identified and addressed in childhood (eg, poor diet, lack of exercise, smoking, and weight gain). It is essential that every adult be aware of his or her own risk factors for heart disease.

Type 2 diabetes is more common in people over age 45, with one in five individuals over 65 developing diabetes. Screening for diabetes is recommended for people who have a family member with diabetes, those who are overweight, and those who have had diabetes during pregnancy.

## RESEARCH IN COMMUNITY-BASED NURSING CARE

**Box 11–1** ▶ The Attitudes and Experiences of Women with Heart Disease

Despite the fact the cardiovascular disease is the leading cause of death in women, researchers have only recently examined women's knowledge of and attitudes about heart disease. This study assessed the knowledge, attitudes, and experiences of women with heart disease and the impact of the disease on their lives. A telephone survey contacted 204 women with heart disease who were asked about their diagnoses, symptoms, interactions with health care providers, knowledge of risks and symptoms, satisfaction with care and the effect of the disease on their lifestyle, psychosocial well-being, finances, interpersonal relationships, and spirituality. Most of the women surveyed had diagnoses of coronary artery disease (CAD) and took multiple medications. Almost half were unaware that they were at risk for coronary artery disease prior to diagnosis. After the condition was diagnosed, one fourth did not seek additional information about their condition or care because of physician-related knowledge and communication problems. Many reported they were unable or unwilling to make appropriate lifestyle changes, with less than 60% having received cardiac rehabilitation services. Significant changes in interpersonal relationships, mental, health, and financial and spiritual well-being were reported by the respondents. This study identified why women with heart disease have poorer medical outcomes than men with heart disease and recommends further investigation to improve outcomes for women with CAD.

Marcuccio, E., Loving, N., Bennett, S.D., & Hayes, S. (2003). A survey of attitudes and experiences of women with heart disease. *Women's Health Issues,13*(1),23-31.

Hearing impairment is common in older adults: More than 35% of people over 65 and 50% of people over 75 have some degree of hearing loss. Hearing loss can lead to miscommunication, social withdrawal, confusion, depression, and reduction in functional status (Demers, 2002).

Elderly individuals should also be screened for risk of osteoporosis, depression, alcohol abuse, and violence.

The adult immunization schedule applies to elderly adults as well. However, the current recommendation is that everyone older than 50 years receive an annual flu shot. Elderly people should be screened for tuberculosis (TB) if they have been in close contact with someone who has TB; have recently moved from Asia, Africa, Central or South America, or the Pacific Islands; have kidney failure, diabetes, or alcoholism; are positive for human immunodeficiency virus (HIV); or have injected or now inject illegal drugs. Making vaccinations more convenient is found to increase immunization rates among elderly and at-risk people (Grabenstein, Guess, & Hartzema, 2002). Nurses working in community-based settings are often the professionals who initiate this type of service.

### Cancer Screening

Most breast cancer occurs in women older than 50, so mammography is recommended every 1 to 2 years after a woman is 50 years of age. Women should have a Pap test every 3 years except in the presence of genital warts, multiple sex partners, or an abnormal Pap test, in which case, testing should be done annually. Women over age 65 with a history of normal Pap smears or with a hysterectomy may stop having Pap tests after consulting with a nurse practitioner or physician.

Colon cancer is more common in the elderly than in younger adults. Starting at age 50, fecal occult blood testing should be done every year and sigmoidoscopy every 5 to 10 years.

Prostate cancer is most common in men over age 50, African Americans, and men with a family history of prostate cancer. Screening includes digital rectal examination and prostate-specific antigen blood testing.

### Additional Screening

Environmental screening with a home safety check is an essential component of health promotion and disease prevention for the elderly client. As discussed in Chapter 5, other screening that is important for elderly clients is hearing and vision screening, functional assessment, and cognition status. With all clients, it is important to screen for all leading health indicators. Refer to Box 10–1 in Chapter 10 for a list of the leading health indicators from *Healthy People 2010* (DHHS, 2000). Interventions to address these indicators are covered in the next section.

##  Interventions for Leading Health Indicators

Once screening has been done, conditions that put the client at risk are addressed. Many factors have contributed to the decline in mortality from heart disease and stroke. Some of these include changes in health behaviors, a decrease in smoking, improvements in nutrition, increases in the overall educational level of the older population, and innovations in medical technology (Centers for Disease Control and Prevention [CDC], National Center for Chronic Disease Prevention and Health Promotion, 2002).

Because the average person is living longer, more attention is now focused on preserving quality of life than on extending length of life. Most elderly people have one or more chronic conditions, and as a result of increased longevity, they will be living longer with these conditions (Fig. 11–3). Nurses will be increasingly involved in efforts to decrease the adverse social and economic consequences of a high rate of activity limitation and disability of older persons. Thus, health promotion and disease prevention interventions for this segment of the population are important.

This shift in focus requires dispelling myths commonly held about the elderly, including seeing the elderly as sick and sedentary, sexless, and senile. Nurses can facilitate successful aging by considering the elderly client holistically, and they

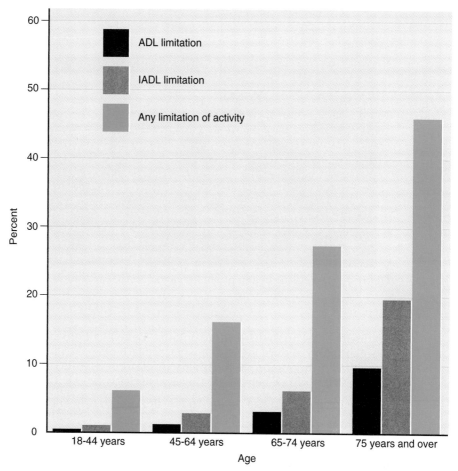

*Figure 11–3.* ▶ Limitations of activity caused by one or more chronic health conditions among adults by age: United States, 1998–2000. *Chartbook on trends in the health of Americans.* (2002). Centers for Disease Control and Prevention, National Center for Health Statistics, National Health Interview Survey. (p. 32).

can maximize functioning by addressing physical and psychologic well-being, as well as competence in adaptation (Fig. 11–4).

## Physical Activity

Older adults, both male and female, can obtain significant health benefits from a moderate amount of daily physical activity. Additional health benefits can be gained through even greater amounts of physical activity. Care should always be taken to avoid injury (AHRQ & CDC, 2002).

Previously sedentary older adults who begin physical activity programs should start with short intervals of moderate physical activity, from 5 to 10 minutes, and

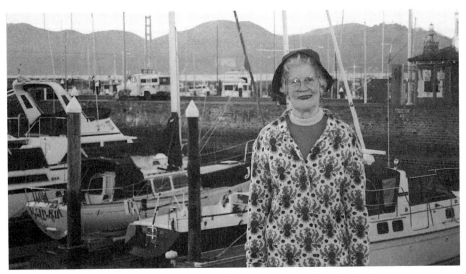

***Figure 11–4.*** ▶ Using health promotion and disease pervention strategies can create a longer and healthier life.

gradually build up to the desired amount. Benefits of physical activity include cardiorespiratory endurance and muscle strengthening. Stronger muscles reduce the risk of falling and improve the ability to perform routine tasks of daily life (AHRQ & CDC, 2002). Other benefits of physical activity include the following:

▶ Helps maintain the ability to live independently and reduces the risk of falling and fracturing bones
▶ Reduces the risk of dying from coronary heart disease and of developing high blood pressure, colon cancer, and diabetes
▶ Helps reduce blood pressure in some people with hypertension
▶ Helps people with chronic, disabling conditions improve their stamina and muscle strength
▶ Reduces symptoms of anxiety and depression and fosters improvements in mood and feelings of well-being
▶ Helps maintain healthy bones, muscles, and joints
▶ Helps control joint swelling and pain associated with arthritis (AHRQ & CDC, 2002).

Box 11–2 lists ways in which communities can promote physical activity for elderly adults.

## Overweight and Obesity

Because no consensus exists regarding optimal weight for older persons, it is difficult to make recommendations regarding weight loss in the elderly. In the past, it was believed that lean body weight throughout life is optimal, but stability in weight after age 50 is recommended. One study suggests that extra weight may be protective for the elderly. The researchers found that obese elderly people were less likely to die than those who were thin or normal weight, even after adjusting for differences in medical problems and income (Grabowski & Ellis, 2002).

---

▶ **Box 11–2.**  What Communities Can Do to Promote ◀
Physical Activity in Elderly Adults

- Provide community-based physical activity programs that offer aerobic, strengthening and flexibility components specifically designed for older adults.
- Encourage mall and other indoor or protected locations to provide safe places for walking in any weather.
- Ensure that facilities for physical activity accommodate and encourage participation by older adults.
- Provide transportation for older adults to parks or facilities that provide physical activity programs.
- Encourage health care providers to talk routinely to their older adult clients about incorporating physical activity into their lives.
- Plan community activities that include opportunities for older adults to be physically active.

Centers for Disease Control and Prevention. (1999). National Center for Chronic Disease Prevention and Health Promotion. *Physical activity and health: A report of the Surgeon General.* Available at: http://www.cdc.gov/nccdphp/sgr/olderad.htm.

---

## Tobacco Use

Smoking among adults has declined. However, because smoking remains the health indicator that is known to most negatively affect health, it is important to address the question of smoking with elderly clients and encourage them to quit. Box 11–3 can be used for teaching older clients about the advantages of quitting at any age.

## Substance Abuse

Not everyone who drinks regularly has a drinking problem. The questions in Box 10–7 in Chapter 10 can be used to help an elderly client recognize a drinking problem.

Older problem drinkers have a good chance for recovery because once they decide to seek help, they usually stay with treatment programs. A good resource is Alcoholics Anonymous (AA); local chapters can be found in the phone book. The National Institute on Alcohol Abuse and Alcoholism (NIAAA) at (301) 443-3860 is another resource.

## Responsible Sexual Behavior

Understanding normal changes in sexual response is the first step to sexual health promotion. With aging, women may notice changes in the shape and flexibility of the vagina and a decrease in vaginal lubrication. This can be addressed by using a vaginal lubricant. Men may find that it takes longer to get an erection or that the erection may not be as firm or large as in earlier years. As men get older, impo-

## COMMUNITY-BASED TEACHING

**Box 11–3** ▶ Check Your Smoking I.Q.

If you or someone you know is an older smoker, you may think that there is no point in quitting now. Think again. By quitting smoking now, you will feel more in control and have fewer coughs and colds. On the other hand, with every cigarette you smoke, you increase your chances of having a heart attack, a stroke, or cancer. Need to think about this more? Take this older smokers' I.Q. quiz. Just answer "true" or "false" to each statement below.

**True or False**

1. ○ True  ○ False   If you have smoked for most of your life, it's not worth stopping now.
2. ○ True  ○ False   Older smokers who try to quit are more likely to stay off cigarettes.
3. ○ True  ○ False   Smokers get tired and short of breath more easily than nonsmokers the same age.
4. ○ True  ○ False   Smoking is a major risk factor for heart attack and stroke among adults 60 years of age and older.
5. ○ True  ○ False   Quitting smoking can help those who have already had a heart attack.
6. ○ True  ○ False   Most older smokers don't want to stop smoking.
7. ○ True  ○ False   An older smoker is more likely to smoke more cigarettes than a younger smoker.
8. ○ True  ○ False   Someone who has smoked for 30 to 40 years probably won't be able to quit smoking.
9. ○ True  ○ False   Very few older adults smoke cigarettes.
10. ○ True  ○ False   Lifelong smokers are more likely to die of diseases like emphysema and bronchitis than nonsmokers.

**Answers**

1. False.   Nonsense! You have every reason to quit now and quit for good—even if you've been smoking for years. Stopping smoking will help you live longer and feel better. You will reduce your risk of heart attack, stroke, and cancer; improve blood flow and lung function; and help stop diseases like emphysema and bronchitis from getting worse.
2. True.   Once they quit, older smokers are far more likely than younger smokers to stay away from cigarettes. Older smokers know more about both the short- and long-term health benefits of quitting.

*(continued)*

## COMMUNITY-BASED TEACHING

**Box 11–3** ▶ Check Your Smoking I.Q. *(Continued)*

3. True.   Smokers, especially those over 50 years old, are much more likely to get tired, feel short of breath, and cough more often. These symptoms can signal the start of bronchitis or emphysema, both of which are suffered more often by older smokers. Stopping smoking will help reduce these symptoms.

4. True.   Smoking is a major risk factor for four of the five leading causes of death including heart disease, stroke, cancer, and lung diseases like emphysema and bronchitis. For adults 60 and over, smoking is a major risk factor for six of the top 14 causes of death. Older male smokers are nearly twice as likely to die from stroke as older men who do not smoke. The odds are nearly as high for older female smokers. Cigarette smokers of any age have a 70 percent greater heart disease death rate than do nonsmokers.

5. True.   The good news is that stopping smoking does help people who have suffered a heart attack. In fact, their chances of having another attack are smaller. In some cases, ex-smokers can cut their risk of another heart attack by half or more.

6. False.   Most smokers would prefer to quit. In fact, in a recent study, 65% of older smokers said that they would like to stop. What keeps them from quitting? They are afraid of being irritable, nervous, and tense. Others are concerned about cravings for cigarettes. Most don't want to gain weight. Many think it's too late to quit—that quitting after so many years of smoking will not help. But this is not true.

7. True.   Older smokers usually smoke more cigarettes than younger people. Plus, older smokers are more likely to smoke high-nicotine brands.

8. False.   You may be surprised to learn that older smokers are actually more likely to succeed at quitting smoking. This is more true if they're already experiencing long-term smoking-related symptoms like shortness of breath, coughing, or chest pain. Older smokers who stop want to avoid further health problems, take control of their life, get rid of the smell of cigarettes, and save money.

9. False.   One of five adults aged 50 or older smokes cigarettes. This is more than 11 million smokers, a fourth of the country's 43 million smokers! About 25% of the general U.S. population still smokes.

10. True.   Smoking greatly increases the risk of dying from diseases like emphysema and bronchitis. In fact, over 80% of all deaths from these two diseases are directly due to smoking. The risk of dying from lung cancer is also a lot higher for smokers than nonsmokers: 22 times higher for males, 12 times higher for females.

National Heart, Lung, and Blood Institute.

Available at: http://www.nhlbi.nih.gov/health/public/lung/other/smoking.html.

tence increases, with some chronic conditions contributing to this change (eg, heart disease, hypertension, and diabetes). For many men, impotence can be managed and reversed.

Having safe sex is imperative for people at all ages. In some areas of the country, the incidence of HIV among the elderly is on the rise. It is always essential that the nurse discuss the importance of safe sex, particularly regarding having sex with a new partner or multiple partners.

## Mental Health

Many issues related to mental health emerge as individuals age. The losses associated with aging, including loss of health, friends, and spouse, all contribute to the development of depression among the elderly (Fig. 11–5). The depression rate among older Americans who experience a physical health problem is 12% for persons hospitalized for problems such as hip fracture or heart disease. Depression rates for older persons in nursing homes range from 15% to 25%. Prevalence of dementia, such as Alzheimer's disease and other severe losses of mental abilities, is estimated at 12% at age 65 and more than 25% at age 85. The rate of completed suicide is highest among elderly men, who account for about 80% of suicides among persons age 65 and older. Elderly men have a suicide rate six times the national average (DHHS, 2000).

Box 10–10 in Chapter 10 provides criteria for identifying depression. Once depression is identified, it can be treated successfully. Support groups, other talk therapy, antidepressant drugs, and electroconvulsive therapy are some forms of treatment that may be used for clients with depression.

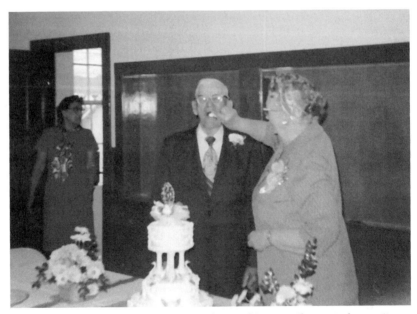

***Figure 11–5.*** ▶ A satisfying marital relationship contributes to longevity.

Preparing for major changes in life, keeping and maintaining friendships, developing interests or hobbies, and keeping the mind and body active may help prevent depression. Being physically fit, eating a balanced diet, and following the nurse practitioner or physician's recommendations regarding medication can also minimize depression. Other suggestions for the client facing depression include the following:

▶ Accept the fact that help is needed.
▶ Consult a health care provider who has special training in mental health issues of the elderly.
▶ Do not be afraid of getting help because of the cost.

If the depressed older person will not seek help, friends or relatives can help by explaining how treatment may help the person feel better. Sometimes the family can arrange for the health care provider to call the family member or make a home visit to start the process. Community mental health centers offer treatment and often have resources.

## Safety and Injury Prevention

Injuries are a leading cause of morbidity and mortality among the elderly. The primary causes of injury among this age group are motor vehicle accidents, falls, and mishaps related to polypharmacology.

Motor vehicle-related death rates for the elderly are the highest of any age group. Per miles driven, drivers older than 75 years have higher rates of vehicle-related death than all other age groups except teenagers. Measures that could benefit older people as well as other age groups are increased use of public transportation and restricted driving privileges when circumstances warrant. For example, in some states, the length of the license term for older drivers has been reduced from 4 years to 2 years. In some states, physicians are required to report to the state's licensing agency cases of certain medical conditions that could affect a person's ability to drive.

Falls are recognized as a leading cause of injury and death among the elderly. In the United States, one of every three people 65 years and older falls each year. Half of those older than 75 who fracture a hip as a result of a fall die within 1 year of the incident (CDC, National Center for Injury Prevention and Control [NCIPC], 2002). By 2020, the cost of fall injuries is expected to reach $32 billion (CDC, NCIPC, 2000b). The general risk factors for falling include gait and balance impairment, the use of sedative and hypnotic medications, incontinence, difficulties in performing ADL, inactivity, visual impairment, and reduced lower limb strength ("Predicting Falls," 2003). The elderly are at increased risk for injury from falls because of the high incidence of osteoporosis in this age group. Prevention of fractures is related to increasing bone density and preventing falls. See Box 11–4 for tips to prevent fractures in the elderly.

**Polypharmacy**, or the prescription of more than one medication, resulting in a complex medication regimen, is becoming more common. Elderly clients typically take more medications than other age groups. Medication errors are increasingly recognized as a potential for injury. Taking medication the wrong way or with other medications that cause harmful interactions can make the client worse rather than better. **Medication safety** should be practiced by all those taking a number of medications. *Prescription Medicines and You (Your Medication: Play It Safe.* National Council on Patient Information and Education, 2004) is an excellent guide designed to

## COMMUNITY-BASED TEACHING

### Box 11–4 ▶ Tips for Prevention of Fractures in the Elderly

Osteoporosis can be prevented by:
- Doing weight-bearing exercises, such as walking, stair climbing, jogging, yoga, and lifting weights
- Getting 1,000 to 1,300 mg of calcium per day
- Not smoking

For adults 65-years-old or older, 60% of all falls happen at home, 30% in public places, and 10% in health care institutions.

The risk of falling can be reduced by:
- Maintaining a regular exercise program
- Taking steps to make living areas safer:
  Remove tripping hazards
  Use nonskid mats in the bathtub
  Have handrails on both side of all stairs
- Reviewing all medication with the nurse practitioner or physician to reduce side effects and interactions
- Having a vision check every year

Adapted from Centers for Disease Control and Prevention. (2000). *Falls and hip fractures among older adults.* National Center for Injury Prevention and Control. Available on-line at: http://www.cdc.gov/ncipc/factsheets/falls.htm.

help avoid medication errors and get the most from the medication. See What's on the Web for information on how to obtain a copy.

### Environmental Quality

Because the elderly are more vulnerable to alterations in environmental conditions, poor air quality has a greater impact on this age group. The proportion of elderly individuals exposed to poor air quality, both secondhand smoke and other air pollution, must be reduced. With the elderly population increasing, maintaining air quality is even more essential to maintaining and improving the health of the nation.

### Immunizations

The most important intervention to improve the health of the elderly related to immunizations is to increase the number of elderly people vaccinated against influenza every year. Nurses play an important role in organizing, staffing, and evaluating immunization clinics. As nurses, we have some work to do in this area, particularly with diverse populations. The vaccination rate by rate is seen in Figure 11–6.

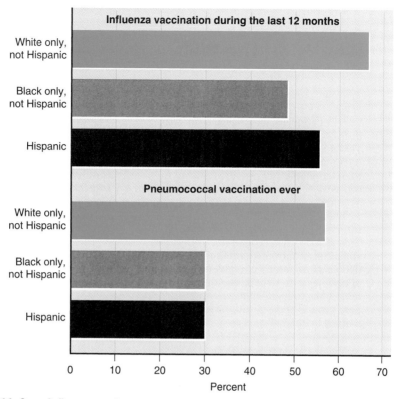

*Figure 11–6.* ▶ Influenza and pneumococcal vaccination among adults 65 years of age and over by race and Hispanic origin: United States, 2000. *Chartbook on trends in the health of Americans.* (2002). Centers for Disease Control and Prevention, National Center for Health Statistics, National Health Interview Survey. (p. 35).

## Access to Health Care

Access to care is important to increase the quality and years of healthy life for all Americans. Elderly individuals may perceive that they do not have access because they have unfounded concerns about cost for services. They also may have limited mobility as a result of either a chronic condition or lack of transportation. Perhaps the elderly person has a limited ability to speak English or is distrustful of health care providers. These are all issues of access that may affect the client's health. The nurse must always assess the client's perception of access and intervene accordingly.

 ## Conclusions

Life expectancy at birth, as well as at 65 and 85 years of age, has increased over the past decades. The elderly are growing in number and have special health needs. Because elderly people are living longer with more chronic conditions, attention is now focused on preserving quality of life. Nurses can use the leading health indicators to illuminate individual behaviors and physical, social, and environmental factors that require intervention to prevent disease and promote health in the older segment of the population.

# What's on the Web

*AgePage: Depression, a Serious but Treatable Illness*
**Internet address:** *http://www.niapublications.org/engagepages/depression.asp*
This document from the National Institute on Aging addresses depression as it relates to older people and provides a list of resources.

Alzheimer's Association
**Internet address:** *http://www.alz.org*
This site provides consumer and professional information, including a section dedicated to family caregivers and friends of people with Alzheimer's disease. Contains links to local chapters and other support groups and resources. Includes information in Spanish.

Centers for Disease Control and Prevention
**Internet address:** *www.cdc.gov/diabetes*
Information about diabetes statistics and state programs can be found at this CDC site.

*Health, United States, 1999 With Health and Aging Chartbook*
**Internet address:**
*http://www.cdc.gov/nchs/products/pubs/pubd/hus/2010/2010.htm*
This 1999 resource from the CDC National Center for Health Statistics includes a special report on the aging population in the United States.

Centers for Disease Control, National Center for Injury Prevention and Control. Internet address: *www.cde/gov/ncipc/pub-res/toolkit/toolkit.htm*

National Council on the Aging
**Internet address:** *http://www.ncoa.org*
This site provides information geared toward elderly people on topics including finances, housing, long-term care, rural aging, employment, health care, social security, senior centers, and end-of-life care.

National Institute of Diabetes and Digestive and Kidney Diseases

**Internet address:**
*www.niddk.nih.gov*
This National Institutes of Health (NIH) site provides information about research and recent advances related to diabetes.

National Diabetes Education Program
**Internet address:** *www.ndep.nih.gov/*
Consumer information about diabetes is available through this organization supported by NIH, DHHS, and CDC.

*Older Americans 2000: Key Indicators of Well-Being*
**Internet address:** *http://www.agingstats.gov*
This report of the Federal Interagency Forum on Aging-Related Statistics provides information on indicators that address the lives of the older population, including access to health care, home care, vaccinations, social activity, and dietary quality.

*Put Prevention Into Practice: Staying Healthy at 50+*
**Internet address:**
*http://www.ahcpr.gov/ppip/50plus/*
This on-line consumer guide from the AHRQ explains preventive care for older adults. Print copies, available free of charge, can be requested by calling (800) 358-9295. The guide is also available in Spanish.

Resource Directory for Older People
**Internet address:**
*http://www.nia.nih.gov/health/resource/rd2001.htm*
This site features a list of organizations compiled by the Administration on Aging and the National Institute on Aging.

*Your Medicine: Play It Safe*
**Internet address:** *http://www.talkaboutrx.org.resources.html*
This consumer guide from the National Council on Patient Information and Education and the AHRQ can be used as a teaching tool to facilitate medication safety. Print copies, available in six languages,

can be ordered for a small fee at *http://www.talkaboutrx.org/* or by calling (800) 358-9295.

## POTENTIAL PARTNERS FOR HEALTH PROMOTION ACTIVITIES FOR THE ELDERLY

American Association of Retired Persons
**Internet address:** *http://www.aarp.org*

American Council on Science and Health
**Internet address:** *http://www.acsh.org*

American Society on Aging
**Internet address:** *http://www.asaging.org*

Institute for Cancer Prevention
**Internet address:** *http://www.ifcp.us*

National Association for Home Care
**Internet address:** *http://www.nahc.org*

National Health Policy Forum
**Internet address:** *http://www.nhpf.org*

National Wellness Institute
**Internet address:** *http://www.nationalwellness.org*

People's Medical Society
**Internet address:** *http://www.peoplesmed.org*

## References and Bibliography

Agency for Healthcare Research and Quality. (2000). *Staying healthy at 50+* (AHRQ Publication No. 00–0002). Rockville, MD. Retrieved from http://www.ahrq.gov/clinic/ppipx/htm

Agency for Healthcare Research and Quality and Centers for Disease Control and Prevention. (2002). *Physical activity and older Americans: Benefits and strategies.* Retrieved December 10, 2002, from http://www.ahcpr.gov/ppip/activity.htm

Agency for Healthcare Research and Quality and National Council on Patient Information and Education. (1999). *Your medicine: Play it safe* (AHRQ Publication No. 03-0019). Rockville, MD, and Washington, DC. Retrieved from http://www.ahcpr.gov/consumer/safemeds/safemeds.htm

Centers for Disease Control and Prevention, National Center for Chronic Disease Prevention and Health Promotion. (2002). *Unrealized prevention opportunities: Reducing the health and economic burden of chronic disease.* Retrieved January 10, 2003, from http://www.cdc.gov/ndccdphp/upo/factsheets.htm

Centers for Disease Control and Prevention, National Center for Injury Prevention and Control. (2000a). *Falls and hip fractures among older adults.* Retrieved from http://www.cdc.gov/ ncipc/factsheets/falls.htm

Centers for Disease Control and Prevention, National Center for Injury Prevention and Control. (2000b). *The costs of fall injuries among older adults.* Retrieved from http://www.cdc.gov/ncipc/factsheets/fallcost.htm

Centers for Disease Control and Prevention, National Center for Injury Prevention and Control. (2002). *A tool kit to prevent senior falls* www.cdc.gov/ncipc/pub=res/toolkit/toolkit.htm. Retrieved January, 28, 2003.

Demers, K. (2002). Hearing screening. *Home Healthcare Nurse, 20*(2), 132–133.

Fowler, S. (1997). Health promotion in chronically ill older adults. *Journal of Neuroscience Nursing, 29*(1), 39–44.

Gillespie, L. D., Gillespie, W. J., Cumming, R., Lamb, S. E., & Rowe, B. H. (2000). Interventions for preventing falls in the elderly. *Cochrane Database System Review, 2,* CD000340.

Grabenstein, J., Guess, H., & Hartzema, A. (2002). Making pneumonia and influenza vaccinations more convenient may increase immunizations among elderly and at-risk people. *Journal of Clinical Epidemiology, 55,* 279–284.

Grabowski, J., & Ellis, D. (2001). High body mass index does not predict mortality in older people; Analysis of the longitudinal study of aging. *Journal of American Geriatric Society, 49,* 968–979.

Haber, D., Looney, C., Babola, K., Hinmand, M., & Utsey, C. (2000). Impact of a healthy promotion course on inactive, overweight or physically limited older adults. *Family and Community Health, 22*(4), 48.

Marcuccio, E., Loving, N., Bennett, S. D., & Hayes, S. (2003). A survey of attitudes and experiences of women with heart disease. *Womens Health Issues, 13*(1), 23–31.

National Center for Health Statistics. (1999). *Health, United States, 1999 with health and aging chartbook.* Hyattsville, MD: Author.

National Coalition of Women with Heart Disease. (2003). *Women and heart disease fact sheet.* Retrieved June 2, 2003, from http:// www.womenheart.org/

Predicting falls in the elderly. (2003). *American Journal of Nursing, 103*(5), 21.

National Council on Patient Information and Education (2004). *Your medication: Play it safe.* Retrieved March 24, 2004 from http://www.talkaboutrx.org

U.S. Department of Health and Human Services. (2000). *Healthy people 2010. National health promotion disease prevention objectives.* Washington, DC: U.S. Government Printing Office.

U.S. Department of Health and Human Services. (2001). *A profile of older Americans: 2001.* Washington, DC: U.S. Government Printing Office.

# LEARNING ACTIVITIES

## JOURNALING: ACTIVITY 11–1

In your clinical journal, describe a situation where you have observed an elderly client who was not receiving the health promotion or disease prevention care that he or she needed.

How would or could you advocate for these issues when you begin to practice as an RN?

What could you do now?

## JOURNALING: ACTIVITY 11–2

1. In your clinical journal, describe a situation you have encountered when screening and doing health promotion and disease prevention teaching and planning with an elderly adult.

What did you learn from this experience?

How will you practice differently based on this experience?

2 In your clinical journal, describe a situation in which you have observed an elderly client who was not receiving the health promotion or disease prevention care that was needed.

How could you advocate for these issues when you begin to practice as an RN?

What could you do now?

## CLIENT CARE: ACTIVITY 11–3

Roberta is a 62-year-old African-American woman employed as a housekeeper in a hotel. She does not have health insurance. As you are completing the Personal Health Guide, you learn that she has not had a pelvic or breast examination in 10 years.

What do you do?

Roberta says, "I used to be more active. I used to play basketball when I was a teenager, and now I can hardly walk up a flight of stairs. I would like to be more active and lose some weight. Would that help my high blood pressure?"

*What do you do?*

She tells you that she has smoked since she was 16 years old and has decided that she wants to quit.

*What do you do?*
*What resources do you use?*

## PRACTICAL APPLICATION: ACTIVITY 11–4

You are working in a community clinic that serves many senior citizens from the surrounding area. Last year, you noted that in November through March, most of the clinic visits were for colds, influenza, sore throats, bronchitis, and pneumonia, in order of frequency. As you are reviewing the clinic records, you learn that 80% of the clinic visits resulting in hospitalization resulted from bronchitis, pneumonia, and influenza.

1. What clinic activities related to health promotion and disease prevention would you plan for the next year in the late fall?

2. How would you go about assessing and planning the activities? (Consult Chapter 5 for some ideas.)

3. Develop a plan for the activities with a list of who would be involved in the planning, the goals and objectives of the plan, and a time line.

## PRACTICAL APPLICATION: ACTIVITY 11–5

A local senior citizens center has contacted your instructor and asks that a team of students provide a health fair for the center's fall festival held in late October or early November.

- What would you like to know about this group before beginning this project?
- When forming a group to work on this task, whom would you invite to participate in planning the project?
- How would you involve the various community partners in the planning?
- What screening activities would you suggest?
- What other activities would be important to offer based on the time of the year and the typical health needs of the elderly?

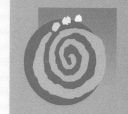

# SETTINGS FOR PRACTICE

The settings and roles of the nurse have changed over time. In the late 1800s, a nurse was a woman in a black dress and a long black cape with a black satchel, visiting homes to care for the sick. As health care shifted toward care of the ill in the hospital, the nurse was a woman with a severely starched white uniform, white stockings, and a starched white cap, bending over the bed of a sick person.

Today, male and female nurses work in a wide variety of settings, taking on many roles. These settings are discussed in Chapter 12. The nurse working in the community is no longer recognizable by sex, uniform, or setting, for nurses are now involved in all levels of health care delivery. Nurses practice in corporations, neighborhood schools, day surgery centers, churches, long-term care facilities, and a variety of ambulatory clinics. Their clients may be well children or they may be older people, abused women, homeless families, prisoners, or drug addicts.

Increasingly, the home is becoming the focus for many nurses practicing in the current health care system. Agencies providing home care, the significance of home care, and the transfer of acute care nursing to home care nursing skills are discussed in Chapter 13. Barriers to successful home care and skills and competencies are also addressed. The first visit is described, along with safety issues and lay caretaker involvement. Chapter 14 provides an overview of specialized home health care nursing, where hospice care, pain management, and wound care in the home setting will be discussed. In Chapter 15, the role of the mental health nurse in community-based settings will be outlined. This will include a discussion of the historical perspective, significance of community mental health, agencies and service available in community-based settings, and challenges to successful implementation of nursing care in these settings.

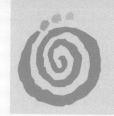

## CHAPTER 12

# Practice Settings and Specialties

Roberta Hunt

## OBJECTIVES

1. Describe different settings in which nursing care is provided.
2. Identify three settings in which children receive nursing care and the services that these settings offer.
3. Identify three settings in which elderly clients receive nursing care and the services that these settings offer.
4. Compare and contrast the role of the advanced practice nurse and the registered nurse.
5. Compare and contrast the roles of the nurse in a school setting and an industrial setting.

## KEY TERMS

adult day care
adult foster care homes
advanced practice nurses
ambulatory care centers
assisted living facilities
boarding care homes
case manager
certified nurse midwife
clinical nurse specialist
day surgery centers
detoxification facilities
employee assistance programs

employee wellness programs
extended care facilities
home health care
homeless shelter
nurse midwife
nurse practitioner
nursing centers
occupational health nurse
outpatient services
parish nurses
practice settings
rehabilitation center

residential center
retirement communities
school nurses
skilled nursing facilities
specialized care centers
subacute rehabilitation
   centers
transitional housing
wellness promotion
work-site health promotion

## CHAPTER TOPICS

- **Practice Settings and Practice Opportunities**
- **Nursing Specialties**
- **Conclusions**

For 5 years I have worked part time as a parish nurse at my church while also working 4 days a week at a clinic. In my job as a parish nurse, I conduct health screenings; provide programs and classes as requested by the members of the congregation; counsel people about health, family, and caregiving; make referrals; and do home, hospital, and nursing home visits. I really love the variety in terms of setting and working with people across the life span. One week, I may teach a class on sex education for teens and the next do an exercise class for the elderly members of our congregation. I write a monthly newsletter to insert in the church bulletin, which is very popular. Once a year, I am one of five parish nurses in our community who plan a community health fair. Last year, over 300 people attended. My favorite part of my job is just being there for people in times of crisis or illness. I have found that if I follow the family and person's lead, I either listen, read from a devotional book or the Bible, or we pray. Being a parish nurse is the most rewarding experience that I have had as a nurse.

**Marge Murlock, RN**
**Parish Nurse**

The settings for health care delivery have undergone rapid and dramatic changes in the past decade. This is due, in part, to escalating health care costs. It is also attributable to the self-care movement. Reduced infant mortality, control of communicable diseases, and the aging of "baby boomers" have increased the number of people living to older age. Life span has also increased for those with specific chronic diseases, such as cystic fibrosis, sickle cell anemia, diabetes, and acquired immunodeficiency syndrome (AIDS), and for those who have been paralyzed by stroke or trauma.

These recent changes have made it possible for nurses to choose fields or specialization from an infinite number of choices. Unlike the past, fewer than 60% of nurses currently work in hospital inpatient and outpatient departments, with more than 17% working in community or public health settings. Employment of registered nurses is expected to grow faster than the average for all occupations through 2008, with many new jobs being created. Although there will always be a need for traditional hospital nurses, a large number of nurses will be employed in home health, long-term care, and ambulatory care. Technologic advances in client care, which allow a greater number of health problems to be treated, will drive this growth. Further, as discussed in Chapter 11, the number of older people, who typically have more health care needs than other segments of the population, is increasing (U.S. Department of Labor, Bureau of Labor Statistics, 2000).

This chapter discusses the different settings for practice that a nurse may encounter. Schools of nursing are widening the experiences for clinical training of their students. However, no one school can cover all these settings within its curriculum. People entering nursing today must seek out ways of venturing into new and different settings by reading about, observing, and volunteering in some of these settings.

## Practice Settings and Practice Opportunities

With the increased emphasis on self-care, disease prevention, and health promotion, health care delivery is needed in settings other than traditional hospitals. Further, health care has had to extend to the areas where the population is (eg, to people who live in remote rural areas of the country).

As the need increases for local health care facilities that provide comprehensive services, the way the services are made available to consumers is changing. The growing number of nontraditional health care facilities reflects this trend. A glance at our social systems shows that almost every established institution provides some type of health care. Industrial plants, businesses, schools, prisons, churches, and civic groups provide varying degrees of care, usually with a focus on prevention. Although state laws govern the tasks nurses may perform, it is usually the work setting or the agency that determines day-to-day activities.

The number and type of **practice settings** for community-based nursing exceeds our capacity to count or examine in this book. However, an overview of a number of settings will be given. Further, it is difficult to place health care settings in precise categories; many of them overlap. For instance, a clinic may be located in a hospital, or some long-term care facilities may be specialized facilities. The categories in this section are arbitrary and were chosen for ease in identifying some of the settings and types of care that community-based nurses may provide (Box 12–1).

### Hospital Care

Hospitals remain the major site in which nurses practice. Technically, acute care nursing is community-based nursing because acute care nurses do take care of individuals and families in a specific community. They also perform much of the initial teaching of clients and caregivers for procedures to be done in the home. Most hospital nurses are staff nurses who provide bedside care and carry out the medical regimen prescribed by physicians. They may also supervise licensed practical nurses and aides. Hospital nurses usually are assigned to one specialty area.

### Care in the Home

**Home health care** is a growing area. Home health care nurses provide care mainly through home visits. Nursing agencies can contract directly with clients or with Medicare or private insurance plans to provide a selected number of visits to a particular client. Chapter 13 expands the discussion of home health care nursing.

Other community-based programs are designed to extend the period of time that seniors are able to remain in their homes. Most seniors prefer to stay in their own homes and communities rather then enter long-term care or assisted living facilities.

#### Block Nurse Program

This program was developed in Minnesota 20 years ago and is a community-based service that depends on professional and volunteer services of neighborhood residents to provide information, social and support services, skilled nursing care, and other assistance to the elderly to promote self-sufficiency and avoid nursing home placement. It is important to note that this program was started by a group

## COMMUNITY-BASED NURSING CARE GUIDELINES

**Box 12–1** ▶ Sampling of Variety of Nursing Functions in Health Care Settings

### Hospital: Acute Care
Serves as administrator or manager
Assesses and monitors client's health status
Provides direct care
Coordinates care of others
Teaches client and family
Provides support for family members
Makes referrals

### Home Care
Assesses client, family, and culture
Assesses home and community environment
Develops relationship based on mutual trust
Contacts physician regarding client's condition
Plans, implements, and evaluates plan of care
Provides direct care
Coordinates care given by others
Teaches client and family
Provides support for family members
Makes referrals

### Clinic (Ambulatory) Care
Makes health assessments
Assists primary care provider (may be primary care provider)
Provides direct care
Coordinates care given by others
Teaches client and family
Plans, implements, and evaluates the plan of care
Provides health promotion and disease prevention
Serves as a client advocate

### Nursing Home
Serves as administrator
Coordinates care of others
Assesses client's condition
Develops treatment plans
Provides direct care
Maintains contact with the client's physician

*(continued)*

## COMMUNITY-BASED NURSING CARE GUIDELINES

**Box 12-1** ▸ Sampling of Variety of Nursing Functions in Health Care Settings *(Continued)*

### Residential Centers
Provides direct care
Provides health assessments
Provides health promotion and prevention
Provides counseling and support
Makes referrals
Collaborates with other health team members
Coordinates services

### Schools and Industry
Conducts health screening
Completes health assessments
Provides first aid or initial emergency care
Provides health education
Provides health promotion and disease prevention
Provides counseling and support
Makes referrals

of nurses who wanted to provide better care for the elderly in their neighborhood. This concept depends on the grassroots community interest and active commitment of service groups, churches, businesses, schools, colleges, and universities. Evaluation of this program demonstrates that $3 is saved for every $1 spent keeping the elderly at home and out of long-term care facilities, which are primarily funded by Medicare. In the 37 sites in Minnesota, $10 million was saved during 1999–2000 by preventing premature nursing home placement. This model has been duplicated throughout the United States with great success. The program provides skilled nursing, case management, and supervision of home health aides and homemakers, often with nursing students as the care providers. The Web page for further information is http://www.elderberry.org/.

### Adult Day Care Centers
The **adult day care** center offers social, recreational, and therapeutic activities to seniors who are in need of supervision during the day. Nurses are frequently part of the professional staff and are responsible for health assessments and design and management of therapeutic regimens and medications. Often, physical care (eg, bathing) takes place at the day care center. These vital organizations offer more personal attention and have a quieter atmosphere than most senior centers. In addition, they provide care for the dependent individual who cannot manage alone but is not in need of nursing home placement. Adult day care is not reimbursable through Medicare.

### Adult Foster Care Homes

**Adult foster care homes** (AFCHs), also known as board and care homes or family care homes, are safe, small (usually fewer than six clients per home) residential sites that provide housing and protective oversight. Many AFCHs provide care to frail elderly adults and those with dementia. Nationwide, these facilities maybe referred to by many names, including residential, adult, foster, family, boarding, or assisted living. There is a lack of federal guidelines to standardize this type of care.

### Parish Nursing

**Parish nursing** is "a health promotion and disease prevention role based on the care of the whole person which encompasses seven functions" (Solari-Twadell & McDermott, 1999, p. 3). These functions are those of integrator of faith and health, health educator, health counselor, referral agent, trainer of volunteers, developer of support groups, and health advocate. Parish nursing has existed in the Midwest for more than 20 years. Before that, nurses sent by religious organizations practiced in many rural mountainous areas of the Southeast.

Parish nurses may offer screening, health education, resource and referral services, support groups, and holistic care to parishioners. According to one study, the most frequent nursing interventions of parish nurses are active listening followed by the NANDA diagnoses of Health-seeking behaviors, and Potential for spiritual well-being (Weis, Schank, Coenen, & Matheus 2002). Often, parish nurses reach out to vulnerable populations: older adults, single parents and their children, and grieving individuals. Many churches have nurses on their staffs, whereas others use volunteers. Clients view parish nursing as a useful, meaningful, and effective health intervention and setting. They describe parish nurses as effective and meaningful health providers (Wallace, Tuck, Boland, & Witucki, 2002).

## Residential Care for the Elderly

Some older adults, particularly those with chronic conditions, may be very isolated living at home. Living arrangements for these individuals in a **residential center** may be a better option. Successful placement, however, requires research, client and family involvement, planning, and a focus on the client's maintaining control of his or her own life. There are multiple levels of residential living from which to choose.

Extended care facility residents were queried in a study about factors that influence the quality of care they receive. They responded that the most important aspect was their ability to retain control of their lives. To provide effective care, the nurse must be familiar with the resident's health problems and needs. Aging is a normal, irreversible process. Many of the problems of aging can be prevented by considering that the older adult's physical, emotional, social, and spiritual needs are complex and interrelated. These factors are important to any older adult living in any kind of residential setting.

Residential facilities provide a unique setting for community-based nursing because the nurse has a captive audience. Here the nurse can take advantage of the close proximity of the residents to do health teaching, health promotion, and disease prevention. By building trust through good relationships with the residents, nurses expand their roles to become counselors and advocates, providing direct support.

### Retirement Communities

Designed for the functionally and socially independent, **retirement communities** provide a community living style for individuals who choose to live with other seniors. Accommodations include homes or apartments with supportive services provided by the retirement community.

### Assisted Living Facilities

Geared toward the individual who has need for some assistance in daily activities (medications, meals, dressing, bathing), but who is able to function fairly independently, **assisted living facilities** generally house residents in bedrooms located in a homelike environment.

### Extended Care Facilities and Skilled Nursing Facilities

More institutional in their design, with ongoing medical and nursing services and supervision, **extended care facilities** (known in some areas as nursing homes) provide care for individuals who need ongoing daily care, generally for the rest of their lives. **Skilled nursing facilities** provide nursing, medical, and therapy services for elderly people requiring ongoing medical or rehabilitative services but not hospitalization. Most individuals stay for a few weeks in a skilled facility and are then discharged home or transferred into an extended care facility because they can no longer manage at home after an acute illness or injury. For guidelines for consumers choosing a nursing home, see Box 12–2.

### Subacute Rehabilitation Centers

Focused on the rehabilitation of individuals who have suffered an illness or accident, **subacute rehabilitation centers** provide longer-term rehabilitative services, such as nursing and medical care and physical, occupational, and speech therapy. Residence in this category is for a limited time. Individuals are discharged when they have reached their rehabilitative goals or when they are no longer making progress. As one individual relates, these services assist in the development of independence:

---

## COMMUNITY-BASED NURSING CARE GUIDELINES

### Box 12–2 ▶ A Consumer Guide to Choosing a Nursing Home

- Consult long-term care ombudsmen (a person who investigates and resolves complaints) and citizen advocacy groups.
- Compare staffing information and quality measures from Nursing Home Compare at www.medicare.gov/NHCompare/home.asp.
- Consult state nursing home inspection reports.

National Citizens' Coalition for Nursing Home Reform (2002). A consumer guide to choosing a nursing home: Consumer information sheet. Retrieved on January 10, 2003 from www.nursinghomeaction.org.

Several years ago, I fractured my hip and had to have it nailed back together. Because of my age (77), the doctor and the physical therapist wanted to put me in a nursing home. When I insisted on a referral to a rehabilitation center, the social service department helped me find the best one in the area. Today, I can walk again, not as well as I used to, but I am walking and living at home. If I hadn't insisted on the rehab center, I'd be immobile in a nursing home today.

### Boarding Care Homes

Providing personal custodial care for residents who are not able to live independently, **boarding care homes** do not have nursing or medical supervision or care. Residents generally stay indefinitely.

## Residential Care Across the Life Span

Residential programs provide health care services across the life span in the areas of chemical dependency treatment facilities, group homes for the mentally ill or developmentally delayed, halfway houses for recovery from addiction, detoxification units for safe withdrawal from alcohol or drugs, shelters for battered women, and hospices for the terminally ill. Nursing functions and roles vary with the type of residential program or facility; they may consist of direct caregiver, case manager, health educator, discharge planner, counselor, and advocate.

### Shelters for Battered Women

Domestic violence crosses all social, economic, racial, and ethnic boundaries. Shelters have been built around the country to house battered women and their children. They provide a safe place where the women will have an advocate and easy access to counseling. The nurse functions primarily as advocate and collaborator and provides health assessment, referrals, and education for the women and their children. Individual and group meetings with residents are part of the nurse's regular routine. The nurse who works with battered women must have good communication skills and must be aware of the resources available to meet the needs of these women and children.

### Homeless Shelters and Transitional Housing

The percentage of people who are homeless has been increasing since 1970. The fastest-growing segment is women and children, making up more than 40% of the homeless population in many cities in the United States (U.S. Conference of Mayors, 2003). Most of these families are single-parent, female-headed families with up to three children who are primarily preschoolers (Helvie & Kuntsmann, 1999). The homeless population has three to six times higher rates of physical illnesses than the general population and is twice as likely to suffer from mental illness. Further, the homeless have greater difficulty gaining access to health care than do poor families with homes, with one study reporting that only 3% had any contact with mental health services in the previous year (Tischler, Vostaris, Bellerby, & Cumella, 2002). In addition, individuals without homes are exposed to nature's elements and to society's violence, placing them at increased risk for illness or injury. They also may be addicted to drugs and alcohol, have poor nutrition and poor hygiene, and live in overcrowded facilities.

In treating illnesses and injuries in the homeless population, the nurse practicing in a **homeless shelter** or **transitional housing** may offer a variety of services, such as immunizations, referral for further diagnosis of sexually transmitted dis-

eases, teaching for pregnant women, and instructions regarding health maintenance. Assessing and completing immunization status of children who are homeless is an important primary prevention intervention. Screenings for skin conditions and evidence of early signs of chronic conditions such as diabetes and
hypertension are secondary prevention interventions. Another example is screening for normal development in children by using the Denver Developmental
Screening Tool II to identify developmental delays. Assisting the client to follow up
with existing health issues and access to care, such as obtaining medication for
mental health conditions including depression, is tertiary prevention. Nurses play
an important role in the care of homeless individuals and families.

### Camps

Camp programs for children and adults employ nurses in private, church, YWCA,
YMCA, and Girl Scout and Boy Scout programs. Nurses may be employed as camp
nurses in camps for children with chronic illnesses, such as asthma, seizure disorders, and AIDS. Direct client care for acute situations, first aid, and health education are the primary roles. Camp nursing offers an opportunity to apply a variety
of skills in a unique setting.

### Rehabilitation Centers

A freestanding or hospital-associated **rehabilitation center** for drug dependency
treatment or for physical or emotional rehabilitation is another setting for care.
The goal of this type of facility is to help clients reach optimal health so they can
become part of the productive community again. Rehabilitation centers often
have a philosophy of improving quality of life and facilitating independent self-
care to the client's full ability. An interdisciplinary health care team collaborates
to plan and implement care. The role of the nurse includes direct care, teaching,
and counseling.

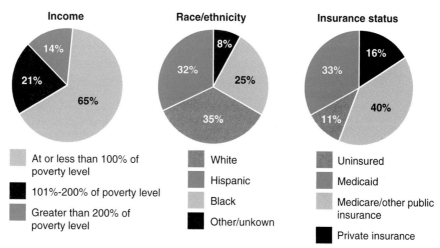

***Figure 12–1.*** ▶ Demographics of Health Center Patients U.S. General Accounting
Office (GOA). (2000). Source: The Alan Guttmacher Institute (AGI). Community
health centers and family planning, *Issues in Brief*, New York: AGI. Retrieved on
June 10, 2003 from http://www.guttmacher.org/pubs/ib_6-01html.

### Detoxification Facilities

Clients are admitted to **detoxification facilities** for the express purpose of detoxifying their bodies from chemicals. Nurses are responsible for health assessment, identification of immediate physical needs, and referral to community organizations at the time of discharge. Medication administration and ongoing monitoring of the client's physical well-being from the day of admission are critical to ensure the client's safety.

### Treatment Facilities for Addictions

Here again, the goal of the nurse is to return the client to optimal health. Clients in treatment facilities for addictions usually do not require close monitoring for physiologic changes after the first 48 to 72 hours of the detoxification period. The goal of treatment is for clients to begin their own recovery process to allow them to return to the community as better functioning and productive members of society. Recovery is a lifelong commitment that clients must make to address their addictions. The nurse is responsible for health assessment, planning, and management of identified problems. Direct care is provided through medication administration and management of acute problems. A multidisciplinary approach is used, and the focus for discharge planning is the successful reentry of the client into society.

## CLIENT SITUATIONS IN PRACTICE

### ▶ Role of the Nurse in a Residential Treatment Center for Teenagers

Jason is a nurse at a residential chemical dependency treatment program for male and female adolescents. Criteria for admission require that clients be between 11 and 17 years old and diagnosed as chemically dependent or have chronic substance abuse with legal consequences. The average length of the prescribed program is 30 to 45 days.

Jason has a small office close to the dormitory-style rooms where the clients stay. His responsibilities include medication supervision, oversight of self-administration of medications, health histories and assessments on each new admission, health education, disease prevention, health promotion, intervention in acute situations, collaboration during discharge planning, and teaching. He enjoys working with adolescents who have varied emotional and physical problems.

It is important that the teens trust Jason and develop a relationship with him that is different from the relationships established with the program's counselors. Establishing trust is always a challenge, but it is particularly so with teens who have addiction problems. Another challenge in this particular facility is that the population is coed. Sex education is imperative, as is problem solving about the many "attachments" the clients develop among each other. Jason states with a smile, "I just did not learn how to handle problems like this at nursing school. Some days, I really need to use every ounce of imagination I can muster." Jason has both independence and challenge in his practice.

## Ambulatory Care or Outpatient Services

### Clinics

Clients who do not require inpatient care (in an acute setting) can receive treatment, care, and education on an outpatient basis. **Outpatient services,** also called **ambulatory care centers,** are rapidly expanding and are now provided by hospitals, health maintenance organizations (HMOs), private and public hospitals, physicians' offices, community agencies, and public health departments (city, state, and federal). Services cover a broad range and include medical care, surgery, diagnostic tests, administration of medications (including intravenous therapy), physical therapy, kidney dialysis, counseling, birthing classes (Fig. 12–2), aerobics classes, well-child care, and health education. Ambulatory care centers are located around the community for ease of access. They may be found in hospitals, low-income neighborhoods, and shopping malls. They may be provided in conjunction with a physician's practice and a managed care facility. Some settings, such as urgent care centers, offer walk-in, emergency care during extended hours when physicians' offices may be closed.

Some ambulatory clinics offer services to select groups. For instance, community-based nurses practice in migrant camps (Fig. 12–3). Native American reservations, correctional facilities, and remote rural settings such as coal mining towns. Nurses can be an impetus for improved health and quality of life for such client populations.

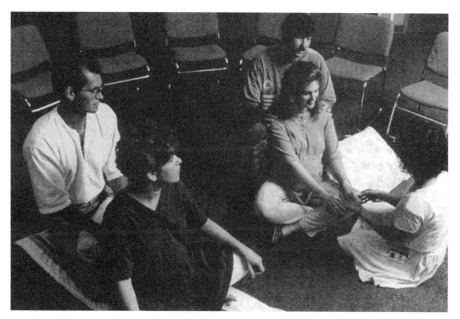

***Figure 12–2.*** ▶ Expectant parents learn techniques to promote relaxation and comfort during birth. Classes in breast-feeding, infant care, and child care are also provided by many maternity centers.

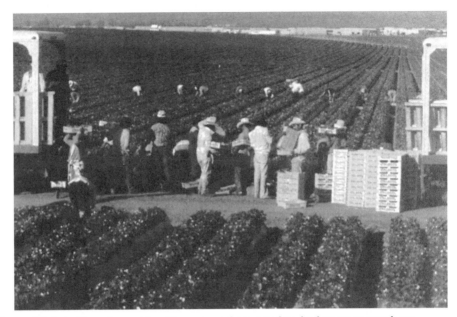

***Figure 12–3.*** ▶ Experienced health care workers need to find ways to reach underserved people, such as these migrant workers. Migrant workers are defined by their common occupation and lifestyle, but they may cross various ethnic or racial lines.

In some clinics, nurses have the primary role in conducting assessments and caring for clients who need health maintenance or health promotion. In some locations, nurse practitioners have established their own independent ambulatory services.

Clinic nurses take on a variety of roles, depending on the medical specialty of the physician in charge and the type of clients served. For example, a nurse working in an HMO wound care clinic may care only for clients with private insurance. Community clinics may have a more heterogeneous population, with some clients with and some without insurance. The clients' ability for self-care may vary between the two clinics, depending on the individual client, family and social support, and other resources. Further, continuity of care may vary depending on what the insurance coverage will pay for as well as the family and community support that is available for the client.

### Physicians' Offices

Physicians in private and group practices, in primary care or specialties, employ nurses. These nurses prepare clients, perform some assessments and routine laboratory work, assist with examinations, administer injections and medications, change wound dressings, assist with minor surgery, and maintain records.

### Day Surgery Centers

Advanced technologies have influenced changes in the care of the client and in the environment where care is provided. Minimally invasive procedures (eg, laparoscopy, use of flexible endoscopes and lasers, and microwave therapies) now allow surgical procedures to be done in an ambulatory setting. Nurses working in **day surgery centers** have a range of duties: case management and direct client care, admission and assessment, preoperative and postoperative monitoring, and discharge planning and teaching.

### Community Health Centers

For more than 3 decades, a network of federally subsidized community health centers has served as a major safety net provider for low-income Americans. Community health centers are private, nonprofit, community-based organizations. The number of community health centers doubled in the 1990s, from 1,400 to 3,200 in 2000. Last year, community health centers provided services to almost 10 million people, up from 5 million in 1990. Most of these people are poor or have low incomes. While 29% of people nationwide are minorities, at least 60% of community health center clients are minorities. Four in 10 community health center clients are uninsured, and one in three are covered through Medicaid (Fig. 12–1). Almost three in 10 community health center clients are women of childbearing age (Alan Guttmacher Institute [AGI], 2002).

These populations provide a challenge for experienced health care professionals to find ways to secure health care for the underserved (Fig. 12–4). Innovative nursing solutions to help develop appropriate services include working with community partners to develop programs and services. Nurses can also volunteer to staff a free clinic; participate in outreach, such as launching campaigns on health education; and speak to neighborhood gatherings, community forums, and church groups. Working in this setting is often reported as being exciting and rewarding.

**Specialized care centers** provide health care for a specific population or group. Some of these are walk-in clinics; others provide residential care. Specialized care differs depending on the population served. For instance, a walk-in clinic may serve only teens or homeless teens. Poor nutrition, poor hygiene, adolescent pregnancy, alcohol and drug abuse, and family violence may be prevalent in some urban and rural communities.

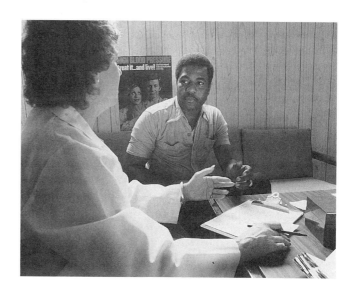

*Figure 12–4.* ▶ Nurses counsel men and women, children, and elderly clients in community health centers across the nation.

Specialized clinics for individuals with cancer or human immunodeficiency virus (HIV) and AIDS are available in most cities. Clients come from their homes for diagnosis, treatment, and care, including chemotherapy. These clinics are generally associated with a hospital or an HMO. Nurses provide direct client care, treatment, monitoring, and assistance with planning of interventions; they also attempt to minimize discomfort, manage pain, and maximize quality of life. The members of the multidisciplinary team collaborate closely. Nurses focus their time on care and support for the clients and significant others.

Day centers for older adults were discussed at the beginning of this chapter. Day care centers provide services for infants, children, or disabled adults. Care may be for children of working mothers after school before parents return from work. Some day care centers provide care for children with minor illnesses when the parents must work. Other centers provide day care for children with chronic illnesses who cannot attend public school or, because of physical, mental, or developmental disabilities, cannot find employment. Nurses usually serve on the staff, or a nurse may manage the day care center.

Mental health centers may be connected to a hospital or may be independent agencies. They may be part of a network of other coordinated social and health care services. Treatment provided may be short-term or long-term care or crisis intervention. The nurse may be involved in assessment, counseling, and administration of medications. Knowledge of the community for further referral is necessary. Nurses may be involved in 24-hour hot-line services. Clients may vary from mentally healthy people in a situational crisis to those with acute or chronic schizophrenia or Alzheimer's disease.

Maternal and well-child health care programs may be conducted at a specialized center. Prenatal and postnatal care may be provided in which assessment and education are the focus. Postnatal follow-ups are sometimes made by telephone or with home visits. The nurse may advise clients on exercise, nutrition, and family planning. These services are discussed in more detail in Chapter 9.

Nutrition centers may provide health counseling for mothers and children, older adults, and homeless or addicted clients. Government-sponsored Women, Infants, and Children (WIC) Programs help fortify the dietary intake of infants, children, and pregnant women. For every $1 spent on WIC, $3 is saved. Meals On Wheels and food pantries may be part of the program for older adults, homebound individuals, or clients and families living in poverty. Programs for adolescents with eating disorders, nutrition counseling for people with diabetes, and programs for the overweight client illustrate the variety of nutrition programs that can be offered in specialized clinics.

Senior citizen health clinics, designed to provide health care for seniors, are found in senior high-rises, neighborhood senior centers, and other locations where high concentrations of seniors live. These clinics provide blood pressure screening, medication review, hospital discharge follow-up, basic nursing screening and assessment, and disease prevention and health promotion interventions. Some clinics offer home visits.

In this setting, the clinic nurse may identify older adults who are in need of companionship or friendship. In some community-based senior citizen clinics, volunteers provide friendship on a one-to-one basis. These types of programs demonstrate success by providing older adults with the opportunity to have support and friendship, which has been shown to reduce depression and the number of clinic visits.

### Nursing Centers

Among the newer forms of community-based nursing are **nursing centers.** They may be located at various sites within a community. Managed by nurses, they deliver primary health care to specific populations. Physician backup is available, and consultation is used as needed. The National League for Nursing gives the following definition of a community nursing center (Murphy, 1995, p. 3):

▶ A nurse occupies the chief management position.
▶ Accountability and responsibility for client care and professional practice remain with the nursing staff.
▶ Nurses are the primary providers seen by clients visiting the center.

A nursing center is not only a setting for care; it is also a concept. A nursing center shapes broader services offered to the community. Nursing centers bring nursing care directly to communities to help maximize the health of diverse populations. One of the two broad goals for *Healthy People 2010* (U.S. Department of Health and Human Services [DHHS], 2000) is to eliminate health disparities. As a setting for community-based nursing, nursing centers are the perfect design to meet this charge.

Most academic nursing centers focus on community health, outreach, and **wellness promotion,** and many operate out of schools of nursing, with faculty and students providing the services. They often provide services to the underserved, uninsured, and disadvantaged populations, including women and children, the homeless, and minorities. However, there are nursing centers that serve insured populations as well. Many nursing centers exist in the midwestern United States.

Research on nursing centers is limited, but studies document changes in client and family knowledge, attitudes, behavior, and health status; client satisfaction; cost-effectiveness; and quality of care (Box 12–3). Surveillance of health issues and nutrition were found to be the most common types of nursing interventions in nursing centers (Schoenman, 2002). Several factors impede research on nursing centers, primarily lack of resources, time, staff, and money. However, the need for research is acute. Current accurate data on the number of nursing centers, diversity of missions, economic status, quality, and other issues are not available (Mackey & McNiel, 2002).

## Schools

In 1902, Lillian Wald placed a nurse, Lina Rogers, in a school setting in New York City as an experiment. The experiment, to determine if placing nurses in schools could reduce the spread of contagious diseases, proved to be successful. Today, schools of all kinds comprise a major sector of practice for community-based nursing: day cares, preschools, elementary schools, secondary schools, colleges, and universities. Children seen by **school nurses** reflect the changing society of the nation, with different racial and ethnic backgrounds, varying socioeconomic backgrounds, and complex disabilities. Often school nurses are the major source of health assessment, health education, and emergency care for the nation's children.

The school nurse focuses on the healthy, growing individual or specializes in educational settings for the mentally or physically disabled, a role that includes health education, collaboration, and client advocacy. A school health program may include identification of communicable, chronic, and disabling diseases; im-

## RESEARCH IN COMMUNITY-BASED NURSING CARE

**Box 12–3** ▸ Review of Studies of Whether Nurse Practitioners Working in Primary Care Provide Equivalent Care as Compared to Physicians

This was a systematic review of randomized controlled trials and prospective observational studies comparing nurse practitioners and physicians providing care at the first point of contact for clients with undifferentiated health problems in a primary care setting, which provided data on one or more of the following outcomes: patient satisfaction, health status, costs, and process of care. These studies were identified through Cochrane, MEDLINE, Embase, CINAHL, science citation index, database of abstracts of reviews of effectiveness, national research register, hand searches, and published bibliographies. Eleven trials and 23 observational studies were included in the review.

The review, which complied the data from the 34 studies, revealed the following:

- Clients were more satisfied with care by a nurse practitioner.
- No difference in health status was found.
- Nurse practitioners spent more time with clients and made more investigations than did physicians.
- No differences were found in prescriptions, return consultations, or referrals.
- Nurse practitioners seemed to provide a quality of care that is at least as good, and in some ways better, than doctors.

The researchers recommended that there should be an increased involvement of nurse practitioners in primary care. They also suggested that future research should explore the reasons that clients were more satisfied with nurse practitioner care than physician care. In addition, nurse practitioners and doctors did not necessarily work under similar circumstances or with similar pressures on their time, and this should be considered in future research. Further, research on nurse practitioners needs to be broadened to encompass a wider range of client groups with more complex psychosocial problems or chronic diseases.

Horrocks, S., Anderson. E., & Salisbury, C., (2002). *BMJ, 345*, 819-823.

munizations; safety; and health education. State laws determine if the school can provide emergency treatment for injuries, maintenance of health records, immunizations, referral for health and social services, physical assessments, and teaching (Fig. 12–5). One school nurse describes her position as follows:

I am responsible for about 1,200 high school students. Our office is open daily, and we serve 50 to 60 students each day with such complaints as headaches, sore

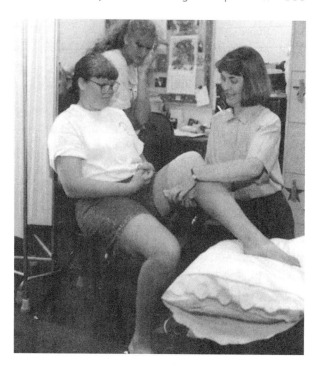

*Figure 12–5.* ▶ A school nurse assesses and treats an injured child. This is essential to a comprehensive school health program.

throats, and fever. The biggest change over the past few years has been the number of high-school-age single mothers we serve. I have developed a program of education for these young women. This includes safe sex, birth control options, child care, and child health. This takes up an enormous amount of my time—time we could not predict was in our future as school nurses. . . . I would say I am nurse, mother, confidante, baby-sitter, first-aid giver, record keeper, and friend as a school nurse.

Many school nurses have become "drop-in" counselors. Often the school nurse is the one to whom a child or adolescent goes with personal questions and problems. These nurses use an established network of referrals for students' personal needs. A school nurse may refer to speech and hearing services, individual and family counseling, gay and lesbian support and youth groups, the department of social services, crisis drop-in centers, drug and alcohol programs, foster care, drop-in health clinics, and parents-in-training groups.

School nursing requires competence in teaching, physical caregiving, and communication. Required educational preparation varies from that of a registered nurse to a nurse practitioner with a graduate degree.

Most families in a community are already associated with the schools. Expansion of school-based clinics into comprehensive neighborhood health and social service centers provides another opportunity for offering nursing care to people where they live.

## Industry

Business and industry provide another setting for nurses to care for people in a particular community. Occupational health nursing began in 1895 when Ida M.

Steward was hired by the Vermont Marble Company to visit mothers and infants, care for the ill at home, and curb communicable diseases.

Businesses began to recognize that having healthy employees was an important factor in good management. Currently, the toll of workplace injuries and illness remains significant. Every 5 seconds a worker is injured, and every 10 seconds, a worker is temporarily or permanently disabled in the United States. Every year, 137 people die from work-related diseases (DHHS, 2000). Employers acknowledge that the health and well-being of employees are vital to morale and enhance the productivity of the company. Consequently, most companies provide health insurance, and many have developed programs to enhance health through the promotion of healthy lifestyles. This has spawned new language and a new focus for health care with programs such as **work-site health promotion, employee wellness programs,** and **employee assistance programs,** all of which focus on the health of employees. Healthy snacks and meals, exercise programs and facilities, and educational classes are all used by companies to promote health.

The **occupational health nurse** works in a business or industry setting and fulfills a variety of roles, including health educator, advocate, collaborator, and coordinator. The focus is on keeping employees healthy, preventing illness and accidents, providing assistance to the employee who is returning to work after an illness or injury, and ensuring a safe business or industrial environment. Depending on the setting, any or all of the roles of teacher, manager, communicator, and caregiver are inherent in the occupational setting. The level of educational preparation varies.

Nurses can market their expertise to employers. They can provide programs aimed at job-related safety, weight reduction, and addiction-free lifestyles and promote nutrition, exercise, smoking cessation, and family planning. Box 12–4 shows the standards that guide nurses involved in occupational and environmental health practice.

## Disaster Nursing

Historically, most disaster nursing has been provided through the American Red Cross. Nurses have been central to the provision of services through the American Red Cross throughout the history of disaster nursing. Beginning with the 1880 Johnstown flood and the 1888 yellow fever epidemic, nurses have provided assistance during times of crisis. More than 40,000 nurses are involved in the American Red Cross in paid and volunteer positions. These activities consist of providing direct assistance in times of crisis, developing and teaching courses, and acting in management and supervisory roles. There are opportunities for both registered nurses and nursing students (American Red Cross, 2003).

There is renewed interest and appreciation for this type of nursing care following the attacks on the World Trade Center on September 11, 2001. Although we know more today about disaster nursing, terrorism, and bioterrorism preparedness than we did in September of 2001, some believe there is a need for additional education, training, and other preparation for all health care workers in anticipation of another terrorist event. Only 27% of family practice physicians surveyed through the American Academy of Family Physicians believe that the United States health care system could respond effectively to a bioterrorist attack. Only 18% of those physicians surveyed had received previous training in bioterrorism preparedness (Chen, Hickner, Fink, Galliher, & Burstin, 2002). Some believe that the health care community must take action to become better prepared for biolog-

## ▶ Box 12–4. Standards of Occupational ◀
## and Environmental Health Nursing

**STANDARD I. ASSESSMENT**
The occupational and environmental health nurse systematically assesses the health status of the individual client or population and the environment.

**STANDARD II. DIAGNOSIS**
The occupational and environmental health nurse analyzes assessment data to formulate diagnoses.

**STANDARD III. OUTCOME IDENTIFICATION**
The occupational and environmental health nurse identifies outcomes specific to the client.

**STANDARD IV. PLANNING**
The occupational and environmental health nurse develops a goal-directed plan that is comprehensive and formulates interventions to attain expected outcomes.

**STANDARD V. IMPLEMENTATION**
The occupational and environmental health nurse implements interventions to attain desired outcomes identified in the plan.

**STANDARD VI. EVALUATION**
The occupational and environmental health nurse systematically and continuously evaluates responses to interventions and progress toward the achievement of desired outcomes.

**STANDARD VII. RESOURCES MANAGEMENT**
The occupational and environmental health nurse secures and manages the resources that support an occupational health and safety program.

**STANDARD VIII. PROFESSIONAL DEVELOPMENT**
The occupational and environmental health nurse assumes accountability for professional development to enhance professional growth and maintain competency.

**STANDARD IX. COLLABORATION**
The occupational and environmental health nurse collaborates with employees, management, other health care providers, professionals, and community representatives.

**STANDARD X. RESEARCH**
The occupational and environmental health nurse uses research findings in practice and contributes to the scientific base in occupational and environmental health nursing to improve practice and advance the profession.

**STANDARD XI. ETHICS**
The occupational and environmental health nurse uses an ethical framework as a guide for decision making in practice.

Source: Standards of Occupational and Environmental Health Nursing. American Association of Occupational Health Nurses. Retrieved on July 12, 2003 from http://www.aaohn.org/practice/standards.cfm, with permission; revision possible.

ical terrorism (Jones, Terndrup, Franz, & Eitxen, 2002). This preparation requires a team approach.

To be prepared, nurses benefit from first developing their own individual family and home disaster plan. They must understand medical management of those exposed to biological agents as well as how to protect themselves when treating victims. According to the Centers for Disease Control and Prevention (CDC, 2002), protection varies according to the agent. The CDC provides education for the appropriate precautions on its Web site: http://www.bt.cdc.gov/Agent/agentlist.asp.

 ## Nursing Specialties

Although all nurses need to be communicators, teachers, managers, and care providers, nurses may specialize in certain areas. A nurse's title may reflect his or her setting, such as school nurse or occupational health nurse. Other titles may define the role the nurse plays in a setting, such as private duty nurse or a home visiting nurse.

The **home visiting nurse** has worked in community-based care since the middle of the 19th century. Currently, home visiting is most commonly seen with those recently hospitalized or those with chronic illnesses, primarily the elderly receiving home health care services. It is interesting to note that occupational health nursing and maternal and child care nursing originated in the home setting. In many industrialized nations, the home visiting nurse is central to promoting health and preventing disease in the maternal–child population. In fact, in the past few decades, various studies have demonstrated how home visits improve outcomes for high-risk pregnancies and at-risk infants (Cowley & Billings, 1999). As discussed in Chapter 9, one of the goals of *Healthy People 2010* (DHHS, 2000) is to reduce the rate of low-birth-weight infants. Pregnant teenagers receiving home visits from nurses deliver heavier babies than teenagers who are not visited by a nurse. Women who smoked before pregnancy who receive home visits are less likely to smoke during pregnancy than women without home visits, which decreases the risk of having a low-birth-weight infant. Numerous studies over the last 20 years have shown that postpartum home visits are associated with a decrease in recorded physical child abuse and neglect in the first 2 years of life, especially in unmarried teen mothers of low socioeconomic status (Olds, Henderson, Tatelbaum, & Chamberlin, 1986, 1988; Olds, Henderson, & Kitzman, 1995). Current research demonstrates enduring effects of nurse home visitation on maternal life course, evident in the rate of subsequent pregnancies, mean interval between the first and second birth, and mean number of months of welfare used (Kitzman et al., 2000).

Home visits with school children facilitate case finding as well as provide more intense assessment and intervention for children with chronic conditions. Home visiting allows the nurse to establish a trusting relationship with the family and the child so that additional interventions may follow. It enhances continuity of care for all populations with all conditions. Home visiting is proven to be an effective means to enhance health outcomes, yet it is used relatively infrequently in the United States, compared with many other countries.

A **case manager** coordinates an individual's care and manages services supplied by various health professionals. The case manager ensures that continuity of care is provided between the acute care setting and the home, among community referrals, and among the team of practitioners. Chapter 7 presents case management.

**Advanced practice nurses** include nurse practitioners and clinical nurse specialists. Over the last 15 years, epidemiologic studies have found that nurse practitioners provide client outcomes that are as good as or better than physicians' outcomes (Brown & Grimes, 1993; Dawson & Benson, 1997; OTA, 1988; Safriet, 1992; Horrocks, Anderson, & Salisbury, 2002).

The **nurse practitioner** is a registered nurse with advanced preparation, graduation from a nurse practitioner program, and successful completion of the licensing exam.

Nurse practitioners first began to appear in the United States and Canada in the late 1960s. Nurse practitioners may be generalists or may specialize in the care of particular types of clients. These include neonatal, pediatric, adult, geriatric, and family nurse practitioners and nurse midwives. They work in clinics, hospitals, and long-term care facilities, for public and private agencies, and in almost any setting providing health care.

Not only do nurse practitioners provide quality health care, but they also provide care at a fraction of the cost of physician care. It is estimated that nurse practitioner visits are 39% lower than the average cost for a comparable physician visit. The cost to society associated with not using nurse practitioners to their fullest potential is $6 billion to $9 billion a year, according to economist Nichols (1992).

A **clinical nurse specialist** (CNS) can practice in acute care or community settings. First formally recognized as a nursing specialty in 1965, such positions today generally focus on a particular expertise (eg, diabetes or oncology). The specialist may develop and oversee a specialty program, act as a resource and consultant for other staff, and establish educational programs for the general public. Nurses have different degrees of autonomy and responsibility, depending on the setting. Educational and professional role requirements differ as well. Most states require the nurse to have a master's degree to be a CNS. National certification by professional associations may be available. The role of the CNS is evolving as the health care delivery system continues to be transformed (Fulton, 2002; Beecroft, 2000).

A **certified nurse midwife** provides independent care for women during normal pregnancy, labor, and delivery since the inception of the certification and accreditation process in the early 1970s. The nurse midwife practices in connection with a health care agency in which medical services are available if the client develops complications. In the United States, a nurse midwife is required by law to have a baccalaureate degree in nursing and a graduate degree from an accredited nurse midwife program, and he or she must pass the certification examination from the American College of Nurse Midwives. The number of certified nurse midwives has more than doubled, from 3,000 to 7,000, in the last 10 years (Roberts, 2001).

## Conclusions

Rapid and dramatic changes have occurred in health care delivery in the community. Today opportunities exist for men and women to assume many roles in different settings in the community with a variety of clients. Because of the increasing elderly population, many nurses are entering the field of geriatric nursing, but many other opportunities exist for the practicing nurse. Such practice settings include, but are not limited to, the home, nursing centers, a variety of clinics and ambulatory care centers, specialized care centers, long-term care facilities, residential programs, schools, industry, and hospice care. The nurse may specialize in primary care, as a case manager, CNS, or nurse practitioner. Despite the variety in nursing practice, the principles of community-based care apply to all nursing roles in all settings. A creative, experienced nurse can find a variety of ways to use his or her expertise.

# What's on the Web

**Internet address:** *http://allnurses.com/*
To find an exhaustive array of information on different specialty roles in nursing, consult allnurses.com and click on the Nursing Specialties category. This site provides access to resources for more than 50 nursing specialties, including but not limited to many community-based nursing roles, such as school, ambulatory care, parish, and correctional health nursing; telephone triage; intravenous therapy; and advanced practice nursing or nurse practitioner duties.

American Academy of Ambulatory Care Nursing
East Holly Avenue, Box 56
Pitman, NJ 08071
Telephone: (856) 256-2350
Toll-free: (800) AMB-NURS
**Internet address:** *http://aaacn.inurse.com/*
This organization advances and influences the art and science of ambulatory care nursing practice and health care delivery systems to improve the health of individuals and communities.

American Academy of Nurse Practitioners (AANP)
Capital Station
P. O. Box 12846
Austin, TX 78711
Telephone: (512) 442-4262
**Internet address:** *http://www.aanp.org/*
This organization promotes high standards of health care as delivered by nurse practitioners and acts as a forum to enhance the identity and continuity of nurse practitioners.

American Association of Occupational Health Nurses (AAOHN)
2920 Brandywine Road, Suite 100
Atlanta, GA 30341
Telephone: (770) 455-7757
**Internet address:** *http://www.aaohn.org/*
This site provides information about occupational health nursing and the professional organization. AAOHN's mission is to advance the profession of occupational and environmental health nursing as the authority on health, safety, productivity, and disability management for worker populations.

American Holistic Nurses' Association (AHNA)
P.O. Box 2130
Flagstaff, AZ 86003-2130
Telephone: (800) 278-2462
**Internet address:** *http://www.ahna.org/*
The mission of AHNA is to unite nurses in healing. AHNA serves as a bridge between the traditional medical paradigm and universal complementary and alternative health practices. AHNA supports the concepts of holism: a state of harmony between body, mind and emotions, and spirit within an ever-changing environment.

American School Health Association (ASHA)
P.O. Box 708
Kent, OH 44240
Telephone: (330) 678-1601
**Internet address:**
*http://www.ashaweb.org/*
ASHA unites many school professionals

who are committed to safeguarding the health of school-age children. The goals of the organization are to advocate for children and youth, represent all school health professionals, and promote professional education, public education, research, and service to children and youth. The Web site offers information about publications and conferences related to school health.

*Healthy People 2010*
Educational and Community-Based Programs
**Internet address:** *http://www. healthypeople.gov/document/HTML/ Volume1/07Ed.htm*
This resource is one chapter in *Healthy People 2010,* which is full of information about various community-based settings (schools, work sites, and other commu-

nity settings) and the opportunities for community-based programs. It outlines issues and trends in each setting, identifies disparity considerations as well as opportunities for health promotion and disease prevention programming. Goals and objectives for each setting are articulated.

Visiting Nurse Associations of America (VNAA)
11 Beacon Street, Suite 910
Boston, MA 02108
Telephone: (617) 523-4042
**Internet address:** *http://www.vnaa.org/*
This Web site has information about visiting nurse agencies, conferences, and professional information, as well as caregiver information and home care resources.

## References and Bibliography

The Alan Guttmacher Institute. (2001). *Issues in brief: Community health centers and family planning.* New York: Author. Retrieved June 10, 2003, from http://www.guttmacher.org/pubs/ib_6-01.html

American Red Cross. (2003). *Nursing.* Retrieved June 5, 2003, from http://www.redcross.org/services/nursing

Beecroft, P. (2000). The new millennium: A change in perspective. *Clinical Nurse Specialist, 14*(1), 1–2.

Brown, S., & Grimes, D. S. (1993). *Nurse practitioners and certified midwives: A meta-analysis of studies on nurses in primary care roles.* Washington, DC: American Nurses Publishing.

Centers for Disease Control and Prevention. (2002). *Emergency preparedness and response.* Retrieved June 5, 2003, from http://www.bt.cdc.gov/

Chen, F., Hickner, J., Fink, K., Galliher, J., & Burstin, H. (2002). On the front lines; family physicians' preparedness for bioterrorism. *The Journal of Family Practice, 51*(9),745–750.

Cowley, S., & Billings, J. (1999). Identifying approaches to meet assessed needs in health visiting. *Journal of Clinical Nursing, 8*(5), 527–534.

Dawson, A., & Benson, S. (1997). Clinical nurse consultant: Defining the role. *Clinical Nurse Specialist, 11*(6), 250–254.

Fulton, J. (2002). Defining our practice. *Clinical Nurse Specialist, 16*(4), 167–168.

Helvie, C., & Kuntsmann, W. (1999). *Homelessness in the United States, Europe and Russia.* Westport, CT: Greenwood Publisher.

Horrocks, S., Anderson. E., & Salisbury, C., (2002). *BMJ, 345,* 819–823.

Jones, J., Terndrup, T., Franz, D., & Eitxen, E. (2002). Future challenges in preparing for and responding to bioterrorism events.

Kitzman, H., Olds, D., Sidora, K., Henderson, C., Hanks, C., Cole, R., Luckey, D., Bondy, J., Cole, K., & Glazner, J. (2000). Enduring effects of nurse home visitation on maternal life course. *JAMA, 283*(15), 1983–1989.

LeMon, B. (2000). The role of the nurse practitioner. *Nursing Standard, 14*(21), 49–51.

Mackey, T., & McNiel, N. (2002). Quality indicators for academic nursing primary care centers. *Nursing Economics, 20*(2), 62–65.

Meiner, S. (2000). Nursing documentation—Legal focus across practice settings. Thousand Oaks, CA: Sage Press.

Mundinger, M. (1993). Advance practice nursing—Good medicine for physicians? *New England Journal of Medicine, 330*(3), 211–214.

Murphy, B. (1995). *Nursing centers: The time is now* (NLN Publication #41-2629, pp. ix–xxiv, 1–279). New York: National League for Nursing.

National Coalition for the Homeless. (2001). *Homeless families with children.* Retrieved January 15, 2003, from http://nationalhomeless.org/families.html

Nichols, L. M. (1992). Estimating costs of underusing advanced practice nurses. *Nursing Economics, 10,* 343–351.

Office of Technology Assessment. (1986, December). *Nurse practitioners, physicians assistants and certified nurse-midwives.* (HCS 37) Washington DC: Congress of the United States.

Office of Technology Assessment. (1989). *The use of preventive services by the elderly: Preventive health services under Medicare. Paper 2.* Washington, DC: Congress of the United States.

Olds, D. L., Henderson, C. R., & Kitzman, H. (1995). Does prenatal and infancy home visitation have enduring effects on qualities of parental care giving and health at 25–50 months of life? *Pediatrics, 93,* 89–98.

Olds, D. L., Henderson, C. R., Tatelbaum, R., & Chamberlin, R. (1986). Improving the delivery of prenatal care and outcomes of pregnancy: A randomized trial of home visitations. *Pediatrics, 77,* 16–28.

Olds, D. L., Henderson, C. R., Tatelbaum, R., & Chamberlin, R. (1988). Improving the life course development of socially disadvantaged mothers: A randomized trial of home visitations. *American Journal of Public Health, 78*(11), 1436–1445.

Roberts, J. (2001). Challenges and opportunities for nurse-midwives. *Nursing Outlook, 49,* 213–216.

Safriet, B. (1992). Health care dollars and regulatory sense: The role of advanced practice nursing. *Yale Journal of Regulation, 9*(2), 417–487.

Salkever, D. (1992). Episode-based efficiency comparisons for physicians and nurse practitioners. *Medical Care, 20,* 143–153.

Schoneman, D. (2002). Surveillance as nursing intervention: Use in community nursing centers. *Journal of Community Health Nursing, 19*(1), 33–47.

Solari-Twadell, P. (1999). The emerging practice of parish nursing. In P. Solari-Twadell, & M. A. McDermott (Eds.), *Parish nursing: Promoting whole person health within faith communities* (pp. 3–24). Thousand Oaks: Sage Publishing.

Tischler, V., Vostanis, P., Bellerby, T., & Cumella, S. (2002). Evaluation of a mental health outreach service for homeless families. *Archives of Diseases in Childhood, 86,* 158–163.

U.S. Conference of Mayors (2003). Hunger and Homelessness Survey. Retrieved from www.USmayors.org/uscm/news/publications

U.S. Department of Health and Human Services. (2000). *Healthy people 2010. National health promotion and disease prevention objectives* (DHHS Publication No. 91–50212). Washington, DC: U.S. Government Printing Office.

U.S. Department of Labor, Bureau of Labor Statistics. (2000). *Occupational outlook handbook: Registered nurses.* Retrieved from http://stats.bls.gov/oco/ocos083.htm

U.S. General Accounting Office. (2000). *Community health centers: Adapting to changing health care environment; The key to continued success* (p. 11). Washington, DC: Author. Retrieved June 4, 2003, from http://www.agi-usa.org/pubs/ib-6-01.html

Wallace, D., Tuck, I., Boland, C., & Witucki, J. (2002). Client perceptions of parish nursing. *Public Health Nursing, 19*(2), 128–135.

Weis, D., Schank, M., Coenen, A., & Matheus, R. (2002). Parish nurse practice with client aggregates. *Journal of Community Health Nursing, 19*(2), 105–113.

Woodring, B. (2000). Home visits: Should they remain significant components of today's pediatric healthcare continuum? *Journal of Child and Family Nursing, 3*(3), 232–233.

# LEARNING ACTIVITIES

## JOURNALING: ACTIVITY 12–1

Contact a nurse in a specialty area that is of interest to you. Set up an appointment to interview him or her and spend some time observing the nurse perform in the clinical role.

- Develop questions prior to the interview (at least four to eight questions about aspects of the role that interest you). With permission from the nurse, audiotape the interview and transcribe it into written form. Complete a summary of the interview.
- As soon as you are home from the observation of the nurse, answer the following questions in your clinical journal.
  - o What did you see, hear, and feel today?
  - o How does it compare to what you expected?
  - o What would you enjoy doing regarding the role responsibilities?
  - o Which role responsibilities would you hate?
  - o Is this the type of practice that you would enjoy? Why or why not?

## JOURNALING: ACTIVITY 12–2

1. In your clinical journal, identify a practice setting that you would like to know more about. Identify three ways you can learn more about this setting and the roles that nurses have in it. Implement this plan.
2. Discuss the strategies you used to explore this setting and the roles of the nurse.
3. What did you learn from this experience?
4. How will you use this information?

## CLIENT CARE: ACTIVITY 12–3

Jose Martinez is an 85-year-old man who lives in a rural area of Texas. He was discharged 2 days ago from a hospital in Austin after breaking his hip herding his sheep into the corral behind his house. His wife died last year, and he has lived alone since then. He has eight children; all of them live in and around the small rural town where Jose has lived since he emigrated from Mexico 20 years ago.

Since fracturing his hip, Mr. Martinez has not been able to care for himself and is upset about his inability to tend to his sheep and be independent. His family has gathered to meet with the home health care nurse about plans for Mr. Martinez.

1. Discuss assessment questions related to culture that the nurse should ask when establishing a relationship with this family.
2. Identify some important questions the home health care nurse should ask during the client conference.
3. Determine what options exist for Mr. Martinez.
4. State ways the nurse can address Mr. Martinez's desire to be independent.
5. Determine Mr. Martinez's primary health care needs.
6. Given all the options, summarize the ideal place for Mr. Martinez to live.

## PRACTICAL APPLICATION: ACTIVITY 12–4

Interview a nurse in one of the settings described in this chapter. Use the following questions as a part of the interview.

1. How do you assist your clients to improve their self- care? Can you tell me a story about when you assisted or did not assist one of your clients to improve his or her self-care?
2. How do you alter care according to the context of the client's family, culture, and community? Can you tell me about a situation when you or someone else you work with did or did not alter care according to the context of the client's family, culture, or community?
3. How do you incorporate the concept of disease prevention and health promotion in the care you provide to your clients? Can you give me some examples?
4. How do you enhance continuity for your clients? Can you tell me about a time when you were or you weren't successful creating continuity?

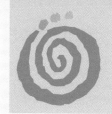

# CHAPTER **13**

# Home Health Care Nursing

Roberta Hunt

**THE NURSE SPEAKS**

"Please go out and see him. He's refusing hospitalizations and hospice, so there's not much more I can do." This was a fairly common request from AIDS-specialized physicians in the early to mid-1990s, so I was not surprised to find a very cachetic, disoriented patient when I arrived. Tom was lying in soiled sheets in an upstairs bedroom. He was too weak to be walked to the bathroom by his partner, and he had fallen twice in the past 3 days. He could answer some questions but frequently drifted off to sleep midsentence. Physical inspection revealed a severely wasted male in his middle years with a stage IV decubitus ulcer on his coccyx and 4+ pitting edema bilaterally to midthigh. When he was able to talk, he conveyed a strong will to live and gratitude for a supportive partner who was willing to assist in all of his care. Tom had tried the AIDS medications, but he had stopped them because he felt too weak to keep up with the regimen.

I immediately realized Tom still had a curative versus comfort focus. I also recognized it would take the effort of many people working together if we were to pull him back from the edge of death. Complex cases require thoughtful and effective case management, and Tom's case was no exception. I pulled in as many home health aide hours as his insurance would cover. I called and got orders for a dietitian consult, which led to NG tube feedings. From there, I involved a wound care specialist, who prescribed the best products to heal the decubitus ulcer. Tom was moved to the first floor of his home, providing more space for a hospital bed, commode, and wheelchair. This also allowed his partner to get more sleep so the family did not face the frequent problem of burnout. When the insurance company balked at the cost of all these services, I reminded them of the expense that would be incurred if Tom were staying in a hospital or long-term care facility for weeks on end.

Slowly, Tom's level of strength began to return and with it his ability to take his antiretroviral medications. Three months later, I was called to the front office by our receptionist. There stood Tom with a big smile on his face and a bouquet of flowers in his hand. He gave me a warm hug and asked me to wish him luck as he returned for his first day back at his job. The combined efforts of home care professionals guided by nursing case management had indeed helped Tom follow his desire to continue to focus on living.

**Teddie M. Potter RN, MS**
**Home Care Nurse**
**Instructor, Minneapolis Community and Technical College**

Home health care is the provision of health services to individuals and families in their places of residence for the purpose of promoting, maintaining, and restoring health. It is one of the most rapidly growing service industries in the United States. Nurses who work in this type of setting follow the nursing process in their provision of health care. They must have a competent knowledge of nursing care and communication, teaching, management, and physical caregiving skills. This chapter begins with a brief introduction to the history of home health care. **Home care agencies**, the purposes and goals of home health care, the advantages and disadvantages of home care, and barriers to successful home care are discussed. A large part of the chapter deals with nursing skills and competencies in this setting, including a summary of the first visit. Safety issues and lay caretaker involvement are included. The nurse's participation in care of the lay caregiver concludes the chapter.

## Historical Perspective

Although the current form of home care nursing is a relatively new phenomenon, the first home care agencies were established in the 1880s. It was almost 100 years later that changes in federal reimbursement for health care brought about vast growth in home health care. Figure 13–1 is a charming reminder of the long and rich history of the home care nursing profession.

Modern home care evolved from the Visiting Nurse Association (VNA), which originated at the beginning of the 20th century in New York City. The mission of home care has changed from that of the VNA in the early part of this century, when nurses were caring for mostly indigent tuberculosis clients in the tenements. Physicians were involved in home care before World War II. The war produced a shortage of physicians, however, so the use of nurses for home care services expanded. In the 1940s, **hospital-based home care agencies** were established. A piv-

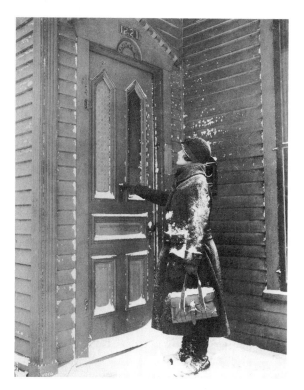

***Figure 13–1.*** ▶ A Minnesota home health nurse paying a visit to a client around the beginning of the 20th century. Copyright the Minnesota Historical Society. Used with permission.

otal change in home care came from the 1965 Medicare and Medicaid legislation that allowed payment for home care services for qualified recipients. With this legislation, home care became more narrowly defined as a medical model alternative to extended hospitalizations. The impact of this legislation is seen in the monumental growth in the home care industry. In 1963, there were 1,100 home health agencies; today, there are more than 8,000 (Table 13–1).

Governmental implementation of diagnosis-related groups (DRGs) during the late 1970s and early 1980s resulted from a need for cost containment. Most hospitals and health maintenance organizations (HMOs) began to recognize the importance of home care as a vital aspect of the health care system. Throughout the United States, insurance companies and HMOs have adopted home care as part of their standard health insurance package because the cost efficiency of care at home versus institutional care has been documented. With the trend toward shorter hospital stays, continuing care needs, and available reimbursement for home health care, the home care boom was born. Further, the increasing number of noninstitutionalized individuals over age 65, living longer and with multiple chronic conditions, has intensified the need for more home health care services. The acceleration in development of sophisticated technology that allows people to be kept alive and relatively comfortable in their own homes has also added to the need for nursing care in the home, as has consumer demand for improved end-of-life care at home.

## Significance of Home Health Care

The major role of home care is to educate, reinforce, and encourage clients, families, and caregivers about ongoing care needs. The goal of home health care nursing is to provide services to individuals and families and to promote, maintain, and restore health. In most cases, this is achieved through short-term, intermittent, direct nursing care made in home visits. Home care nurses provide direct services or supervise those services to assist with activities of daily living (ADL); teach clients, families, and caregivers how to provide self-care; and use communication skills to enhance continuity of care.

Governmental, private, and hospital-based programs employ home health care nurses. As most hospitals open their own home health care agencies, the fastest growing sector of home health care is the hospital-based sector. Home health care nurses come from all levels of educational preparation, but more than half are associate's degree or diploma nurses. Home health care includes not only skilled

| TABLE 13–1 • Number of Medicare-Certified Home Care Agencies | | | | |
|---|---|---|---|---|
| **Freestanding Agencies** | | | **Facility Based** | |
| YEAR | VNA | PUB | PROP | HOSP | TOTAL |
| 1967 | 549 | 939 | 0 | 133 | 1,753 |
| 1975 | 525 | 1,228 | 0 | 273 | 2,242 |
| 1985 | 514 | 1,205 | 832 | 1,277 | 5,983 |
| 1995 | 575 | 1,182 | 3.951 | 2,470 | 9,120 |
| 2000 | 436 | 909 | 2,863 | 2,151 | 7,152 |

Adapted from: National Association for Home Care (2000). *Basic statistics about home care.* Washington, DC: Author. Retrieved January 11, 2003, from http://www.nahc.org/consumer/hcstats.html

nursing care but also the services of physical, occupational, and speech therapists; social workers; and home health aides.

The National Association for Home Care and Hospice (NAHC) is the largest home care trade organization in the country. Its mission is to improve the quality of home care services. NAHC represents the interests of clients who need home care and caregivers who provide such services. Through a variety of activities and publications, NAHC attempts to be a unified voice for the home care and hospice community.

More than 68% of clients served in home care are older than 65 years. Recently hospitalized clients make up a large proportion of home care clients, with 16% of all Medicare hospitalized clients using home care within 30 days of discharge. Diseases of the circulatory system account for almost 30% of those receiving home care services with Medicare reimbursement (NAHC, 2000). There is also an increasing number of clients requiring high-technology medical interventions (eg, intravenous therapy, mechanical ventilation, parenteral nutrition).

## Agencies That Provide Home Care

Home health care has evolved into a major industry with three key components: home care agencies, **home care equipment vendors**, and home infusion therapy companies. Home infusion therapy will be discussed in Chapter 14. A change in the types of agencies that provide home care resulted from the federal legislation enacted in 1965 and 1983. Agency types today include official, hospital based, and proprietary.

**Official home care agencies** are often housed in city and county departments and only provide service certified by federal government mandates. Hospital-based agencies have no mandate and can offer services of their own choosing or Medicare and Medicaid service if they are certified by the federal government. They receive no tax support and operate as a unit or department of a hospital. Proprietary agencies are freestanding and for-profit home care agencies that provide services based on third-party reimbursement or self-pay.

All three types of agencies may choose to be certified by the federal government to provide services for clients with Medicare and Medicaid insurance. The services have to be skilled and provide home visits (30 minutes to 2 hours). Services include nursing; physical, occupational, and speech therapy; medical social work; and home health aide work. Most insurance companies now pay for home health care services, but few will pay for 24-hour nursing care. Few, if any, insurance carriers will pay for paraprofessional care without skilled care services. The growing managed care movement is following the Medicare guidelines for the development of home health care services, although the number of allowed visits may be fewer and may vary among insurance companies or managed care organizations.

Private duty agencies that primarily provide shift relief at health care institutions and for private clients are generally described as home care agencies. Private sources or private insurance pays for most of the care; time is scheduled in hourly blocks, and services are largely provided by paraprofessionals (aides and homemakers) and nurses. Home care is also a generic term used for the entire industry and can include all types of agencies. In this text, the term *home care* is used to include all at-home nursing services. Today, most hospitals own or contract with home care agencies to create a continuum of care or an alternative to hospitalization. HMOs frequently choose home care services over hospitalization

| TABLE 13–2 • Sources of Payment for Home Care | |
| --- | --- |
| **Source of Payment** | **Percent** |
| Medicare | 36.6 |
| Medicaid | 26.0 |
| State and local government | 12.3 |
| Private insurance | 18.9 |
| Out-of-pocket | 28.1 |
| Other | 5.2 |

From National Assocation for Home Care (2000). *Basic statistics about home care.* Washington, DC: Author. Reprinted with permission. Copyright 2001. National Association for Home Care.

for clients because of the cost-effectiveness of home care. Medicare is the largest single payer of home care services (Table 13–2). Only clients who are homebound and under the care of a physician are eligible for home care services under Medicare (Box 13–1). Many insurance companies follow the same criteria. For the most part, home care has become medical care in the home; clients are given care and treatment under the specific orders of a physician. The nursing focus, consequently, has changed from a broad public health model to a focus on specific needs that have to be addressed in a limited amount of time.

## Acute Care Nursing Versus Home Care Nursing

Because the setting for care has shifted to the home, the number of nurses employed outside the acute care setting has increased. As a result, many nurses with acute care experience are now branching out into community-based care, especially home care. There are critical differences between providing client care in the acute care and home care settings.

One obvious difference in the two settings is the environment. In the home setting, the nurse is a guest in the client's home, unlike the hospital or clinic setting, where the nurse is in control of the environment. The need for the nurse to be flexible and adaptable is essential in the home setting as the nurse visits many different clients living in a variety of home situations (Cullen, 1998).

---

▶ **Box 13–1.** Medicare Home Care Coverage Criteria ◀

To be eligible for Medicare reimbursement for home health care services, clients must meet the following criteria:
1. Homebound
2. Require a skilled intervention
3. Under the care of a physician

---

Zuber, R. (2002). Assessing Medicare eligibility. *Home Healthcare Nurse, 20*(7), 425.

Another difference between the two settings is the type and amount of family involvement. In the acute care setting, the staff makes decisions regarding the client's care; in the home, the client and family are encouraged to make the decisions regarding care. Client and family involvement requires the nurse to use different skills in decision making. Goals aim for long-term rather than short-term outcomes. Making decisions and setting priorities are shared activities.

A third difference is the nurse–client relationship. Often the home health care nurse cares for the same client and family over a long period of time. This allows for the development of a therapeutic relationship built on trust and caring that is much closer than in other settings.

Because home care requires assessing not only the client but also the family and environment, critical thinking, and organizational skills must be well developed. Further, because the nurse is only in the home for short periods of time, good communication, management, and documentation skills are essential (Cullen, 1998). Vital skills for a home care nurse are showcased in this text.

## CLIENT SITUATIONS IN PRACTICE

### Significance of Home Care

Rafael is a home care nurse who visits 91-year-old Norma Wilkinson three times a week. Ms. Wilkinson has several medical problems, the major ones being high blood pressure, a heart condition, and arthritis. Rafael takes Ms. Wilkinson's blood pressure, weighs her, and sometimes draws blood. He checks on Ms. Wilkinson's general well-being. Ms. Wilkinson never married and has no relatives nearby, but Ruth, a woman from her church, looks in on her now and then and takes her shopping. Ruth has a key to the apartment. Ms. Wilkinson does not always take her medications as prescribed because some of her friends tell her she is taking too many pills.

As usual, Rafael telephones before his Friday morning visit. There is no answer, but he decides to make the visit anyway. When he knocks on the door, there is no response and the door is locked. Should he leave? He knows Ms. Wilkinson has had some dizzy spells lately and has fallen several times in the apartment. Rafael decides to call Ruth to bring the key and check the apartment with him. They search the apartment, but Ms. Wilkinson is not there, and she has not slept in her bed. They realize Ms. Wilkinson did not take her pills the previous 2 days. They begin a search of the building and discover Ms. Wilkinson in a remote part of the basement where no one ever goes. She had fallen and is confused. If the home health nurse had not made his regular visit, Ms. Wilkinson might have been in the basement for several more days before anyone discovered she was missing.

## Advantages of Home Health Care

There are a number of advantages to providing care in the home as opposed to the acute care setting. The primary advantage is the lower cost. Table 13–3 shows the cost of inpatient care compared with home care for selected conditions. For clients, the advantage is the less-threatening, familiar comfort of

**TABLE 13–3** • Cost of Inpatient Care Compared with Home Care, Selected Conditions

| Condition | Hospital Costs per Patient, per Month | Home Care Costs per Patient, per Month | Savings per Patient, per Month |
|---|---|---|---|
| Low birth weight | $26,190 | $330 | $25,860 |
| Ventilator-dependent adults | $21,570 | $7,050 | $15,520 |
| Oxygen-dependent children | $12,090 | $5,250 | $6,840 |
| Chemotherapy for children with cancer | $68,870 | $55,950 | $13,920 |
| Congestive heart failure among the elderly | $1,758 | $1,605 | $153 |
| Intravenous antibiotic therapy for cellulitis, osteomyelitis, others | $12,510 | $4,650 | $7,860 |

National Association for Home Care (2001). *Basic statistics about home care.* Washington, DC: Author. Reprinted with permission. Copyright 2001. National Association for Home Care.

home, which enhances care and the quality of life. Home care allows for easier access to loved ones and their support, and clients are taught self-care and encouraged to be independent, which maximizes their quality of life. Being at home also removes the family burden of traveling to and from the hospital. Additionally, it contributes to the restoration of family control for the care being provided. These advantages are supported by the philosophy of community-based care, which focuses on enhancing self-care in the context of the family and the community.

## Disadvantages of Home Health Care

Home care also has disadvantages. The presence of the nurse or other professional is an intrusion on the family's privacy. This may affect family decision making and interaction among family members. For several decades, research has demonstrated that stress caused by multiple unfamiliar professionals coming into the home can also affect members of the family. In some instances, conflict may result if the nurse is not sensitive to the family's wishes and boundaries. Out-of-pocket expenses may accumulate as the result of home care not reimbursed by the third-party payer. These expenses may cause stress for the family. Financial pressure is often a precursor to the family assuming total responsibility for their loved one's care. In a classic study of 18 technology-dependent children, 72% of the parents indicated that financial problems were the most serious issues confronting them once the child was at home (Leonard, Brust, & Nelson, 1993). Caring for a loved one at home may also have a negative impact on siblings and may result in aggressive behavior.

The advantages of home care far outweigh the disadvantages. Disadvantages are more of an issue if the family member is ill for a long period of time. In home care, although the client and family experience a loss of privacy and interruption of the normal family decision-making process, they still can enjoy a life together that is not possible if the client is hospitalized.

## Barriers to Successful Home Care

Some of the disadvantages to home health care are also barriers to successful home care. For instance, family members express concerns about privacy, interruption of the family routine, loss of control, personality conflicts with the home care staff, and concerns about the competency of the nurses. Families express their difficulties with statements such as, "It changed our lives totally." Typically, loss of privacy interrupts the family structure, function, and communication patterns.

Families may understand the importance of regularity in the client's routine. Nurses can respect this concern by arriving on time for appointments and performing procedures consistent with the family's desire as long as they are within the parameters of safe care. Families tend to resent nurses who are too pushy or who try to control everything. They want the nurse to listen to them and respect the knowledge they have accumulated from being involved in care on a 24-hour-a-day, 7-day-a-week basis.

 ## Nursing Skills and Competencies in Home Health Care

The basic concepts of professionalism apply to nursing care in the home as they do in every setting. Promptness is imperative to good work habits. Nursing competency is critical. Families want procedures done carefully and in a manner similar to what was performed or taught in the hospital. Common needs of the home care client and family are psychosocial and learning needs: information about community resources, physical care, and management. Thus, as in other settings, communication, teaching, managing, and hands-on caregiving are important competencies and skills. Figure 13–2 shows "Don'ts for Young Nurses," an excerpt taken from a historic 1919 text for home care nurses. It is interesting that the tips provided are just as true today as they were so many years ago.

### Communication

A comfortable relationship between the nurse and the client is essential to successful home care. First and foremost, the successful nurse communicates effectively with the client and family. If the nurse can build a trusting relationship, all aspects of the care will be more effective.

The nurse must be able to deal with a myriad of psychosocial issues characteristic of the home care client. The nurse wears many hats when providing care in the home, including but not limited to, social worker, friend, spiritual comforter, psychologist, financial counselor, and translator of medical information. One home care nurse says this:

> I was not prepared for the numerous psychosocial demands of the job. I thought I was pretty good at dealing holistically with the clients I cared for in the hospital, but it was nothing like caring for someone in the home with the family present.

The psychosocial needs of the home care client primarily revolve around the client's adjustment to the illness, the anxiety it produces, and the possible social isolation that results. Nursing interventions that address the psychosocial needs of the client are primarily focused on building a trusting, therapeutic relationship.

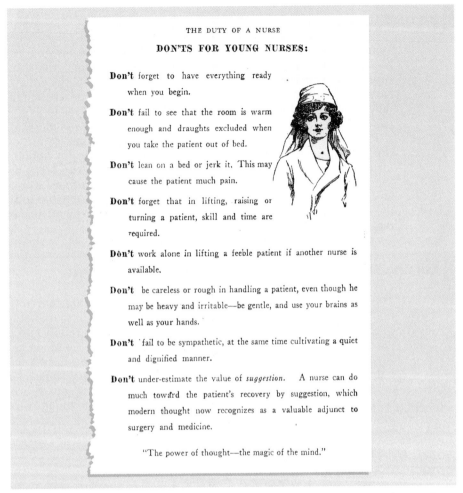

THE DUTY OF A NURSE

### DON'TS FOR YOUNG NURSES:

**Don't** forget to have everything ready when you begin.

**Don't** fail to see that the room is warm enough and draughts excluded when you take the patient out of bed.

**Don't** lean on a bed or jerk it. This may cause the patient much pain.

**Don't** forget that in lifting, raising or turning a patient, skill and time are required.

**Don't** work alone in lifting a feeble patient if another nurse is available.

**Don't** be careless or rough in handling a patient, even though he may be heavy and irritable—be gentle, and use your brains as well as your hands.

**Don't** fail to be sympathetic, at the same time cultivating a quiet and dignified manner.

**Don't** under-estimate the value of *suggestion.*   A nurse can do much toward the patient's recovery by suggestion, which modern thought now recognizes as a valuable adjunct to surgery and medicine.

"The power of thought—the magic of the mind."

*Figure 13–2.* ▶ Suggestions for visiting nurses from historic visiting nurse's text. Source: South, L. H. *Nurses in the home,* 11th ed. (1919). Buffalo, NY.

It is also helpful to elicit the client and family's thoughts and feelings about this situation, which has taken control away from them.

## Teaching

Teaching is a major role for the home care nurse (Fig. 13–3). Chapter 6 addresses teaching in detail. Teaching includes explaining care and treatment at a comprehensible level. The nurse remains open minded by listening and showing respect for the client and family's knowledge. Clients and families soon become experts and are generally accurate in their observations.

The nurse can follow the teaching principles outlined in Chapter 6 when assessing the client's learning needs, remembering that the learner may be the client, family member, or caregiver. The learner's readiness to learn, need to learn, and

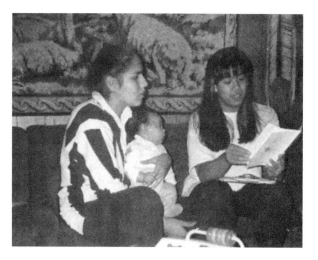

*Figure 13–3.* ▶ Teaching plays a major role in home care. Here a young woman is taught infant care by the community-based nurse involved in home care.

past experiences are assessed. Learning needs are then placed in the affective, psychomotor, or cognitive domain. Finally, the learning need is validated, and the teaching plan is mutually developed with the learner. After instruction, the teaching and learning are evaluated for their effectiveness. Several common areas of learning needs are the disease process, treatments, and medication.

### Disease Process

Most clients and families need assistance understanding the client's diagnosis and any related disease processes. Teaching about the disease process is similar to teaching about medications or treatments and varies depending on the client's specific condition and the complexity of the diagnosis.

The client who requires only two or three home visits after routine surgery would require less information than the client with multiple chronic diseases. The most effective way to teach complex information is to divide it into small, understandable parts and instruct the client over time. When a client's condition merits many home visits with care and treatment over an extended length of time, the nurse can use that time to teach and reinforce learning without having to give all of the information in the first visit.

### Treatments

Frequently, home care nurses are required to do treatments for clients and then assist the client or family to learn to complete the treatment. Treatment complexity varies. In some instances, the nurse may teach a dressing change by demonstration. In other cases, the family may have to learn to administer treatments with high-tech equipment. For example, a client may have brittle diabetes with a complicating large leg ulcer. The nurse changes the dressing, monitors the diabetes, and determines the learning and teaching needs of the client and family. If the client and family are capable, the nurse teaches them to change the dressing and monitor the diabetes. It is not unusual for a client with complex technical equipment to be home with either full-time or intermittent (visits of 30–90 minutes) nursing care. After instruction from the home care nurse, family members often provide daily intravenous line changes and irrigation, as well as infusions of intravenous fluids, medications, or hyperalimentation through peripheral or central venous lines.

They may also insert a Foley catheter or nasogastric tube and do tracheotomy care, including suctioning. Each year, more complex treatments and related equipment are available through home care. This trend requires home care nurses to provide teaching and rely on the client and family to perform procedures with a high degree of competence, identifying complicating issues and notifying the home care agency or physician appropriately.

### Medication

Low adherence to prescribed medication treatment is common, with typical adherence rates at about 50% (Haynes et al., 1999). Consequently, the client and family often require assistance with medication. A thorough assessment of their ability to set up medications is the essential first step to this important intervention. The assessment is initiated with a complete review of the medications the client is taking, compared with the most recent orders from the physician(s).

The need for assistance with medications will vary from client to client according to diagnosis, age, and competency in self-care. For example, clients recently diagnosed with diabetes may have complex learning needs for medication administration. Clients may need to learn about using a sliding scale for their insulin dosage based on taking a daily blood sugar level, drawing up the medication correctly, and injecting themselves. Some clients have a large number of medications with complicated doses that they must take several times a day. The more medications prescribed, the more likely the client is to not follow the prescribed regimen. Comprehensive teaching enhances compliance with the home care client.

## Management

As a manager of home care services, the nurse must apply leadership knowledge by performing the management functions of planning, organizing, coordinating, delegating, and evaluating care for a group of clients. The nurse must coordinate, through case management, an interdisciplinary team of practitioners, the client, family, physician, and various community providers (such as Meals On Wheels and equipment vendors). The nurse's role as case manager depends on the scope of services provided by the agency and the specific providers outside the agency who are involved in the care of the client. Continuity of care is a major function accomplished by effective communication among all members of the interdisciplinary team. To ensure comprehensive quality care, management also includes delegation and evaluation of care provided by paraprofessional caregivers, such as home health aides or homemakers and the family, as well as other professionals.

## Physical Caregiving

Although one of the primary functions of the home care nurse is physical caregiving, the nurse is required to be flexible in this role. This means allowing the family to participate in caregiving whenever possible. Before doing a procedure, the nurse must explain to the client and the family what is being done and why, adjusting the instruction to their particular developmental stage and cognitive abilities (Fig. 13–4). It is essential for the nurse to know his or her own strengths and weaknesses and to master new skills before attempting them. Confidence is not instilled in the client if the nurse is inept and unable to provide care proficiently.

The nurse should keep the work area neat and clean by carefully disposing of laundry, trash, and equipment. Medical researchers have known for several

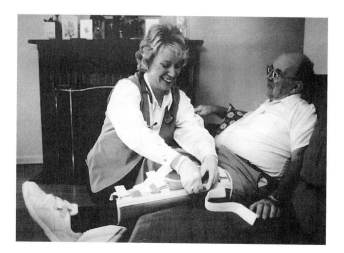

*Figure 13–4.* ▶ Home health nurses combine effective communication skills with their knowledge base of physical caregiving as they provide care for their clients.

decades that hand washing decreases transmission of pathogens between clients. People who receive nursing care in the home are at risk of acquiring infections, just as they are in the acute care setting. Thorough hand washing on entering the home, after procedures, and before leaving the home is an essential aspect of good care.

The Centers for Disease Control and Prevention (CDC) has issued new CDC Healthcare Infection Control Guidelines. Either antimicrobial or nonantimicrobial soap and water must be used when hands are visibly soiled or contaminated with blood or other body fluids. An alcohol-based hand rub may be used routinely for decontaminating hands that are not visibly soiled in the following clinical situations:

▶ Before and after direct contact with clients
▶ Before and after contact with a client's nonintact skin and wound dressings
▶ Before and after using gloves
▶ Before inserting an indwelling urinary catheter, peripheral vascular catheters, or other nonsurgical invasive devices (CDC, 2002)

## The Home Visit

The skill and competency central to home health care is the home visit. However, all nurses working in the community should be prepared to make home visits. Even nurses in schools or in occupational health care are sometimes required to make home visits. A home visit will often reveal information not obtained in other ways.

The main components of the home visit follow the nursing process. Observation of verbal and nonverbal patterns of family interaction helps the nurse make assessments. Nursing diagnoses (or problem statements) help the nurse make joint plans with the family and establish expected outcomes. Following through with these plans helps cement a therapeutic relationship.

### Preparation

Preparation for the initial visit involves reviewing the referral information to get basic information about the new client. Referrals come from a variety of sources, including hospitals, clinics, health care providers, physicians, nurses, individuals, and families. Home care referrals most often request intermittent or episodic care.

The client is contacted by telephone to inform him or her of the referral and to make an appointment for the first visit. The nurse identifies himself or herself, gives the name of the agency, and describes the purpose of the visit. A basic overview about the cost of services, eligibility, and alternative sources of support should also be discussed before the first visit. When applicable, the nurse must alert the client that he or she will need an insurance card or other evidence of coverage from a third-party payer, Medicare, or Medicaid on the first visit.

Unlike the acute care setting where a quick trip to the supply cart or utility room satisfies most equipment needs, the nurse must carry supplies in home health care. Before the first visit, the nurse should ask about supplies and determine what is needed. All home health care nurses use a bag to carry essential supplies to every home visit. This may consist of supplies and equipment the nurse uses daily for all clients, along with additional supplies. Each day, the nurse should review the needs of the clients to be visited that day and add specific items. Box 13–2 lists essential supplies and equipment often suggested for a home visit.

### Beginning the Visit

After introductions, the visit usually begins with casual, social conversation to put the client and family at ease. A friendly, warm manner helps when the nurse begins to ask the client questions about himself or herself and specific health care needs. It is important to begin building a trusting relationship from the first greeting.

During the initial interview, the nurse outlines a contract stating the purpose of the visit. The nurse uses a variety of communication tools to help the client and family understand the need for nursing care in the home.

### Assessment

Assessment on a home visit differs from that of the acute care setting (Fig. 13–5). The nurse incorporates the general elements of community-based care into the as-

---

▶ **Box 13–2.** **Essential Supplies and Equipment** ◀
for a Home Visit

- Handwashing equipment: disinfectant foam for hands, soap in container, paper towels, old newspapers (to set bag on in the home)
- Assessment equipment: thermometer, sphygmomanometer, stethoscope, tape measure, penlight, urine and blood testing equipment
- Treatment supplies: dressings, sterile and clean gloves, tape, alcohol swabs, scissors, lubricant jelly, forceps, syringes
- Occupational health and safety supplies: eye shields, mask, apron, gloves, plastic bag to double bag, sharps containers, disinfectant spray and clean-up supplies for spills, disposable scrubs, airway/mask
- Printed materials: map, agency forms, business cards
- Laboratory supplies: specimen containers, tubes, and equipment for venipuncture, culture, or urine specimen

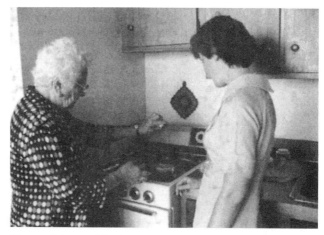

*Figure 13–5.* ▶ Home visits enable the nurse to assess whether the client can safely manage important self-care tasks such as cooking.

sessment process in the home and follows specific guidelines for documenting the status of each client receiving service. First and foremost, the nurse considers the issue of self-care by determining what the client's perceptions of his or her condition are and what the client identifies as personal problems and strengths. The client's ability to perform self-care and the family's acceptance of responsibility for care are explored. All assessments are made in the context of the family and community resources and support. Culture must also be considered. Continuity of care among various physicians and other professionals caring for the client is evaluated. A preventive focus, keeping in mind the principles of continuity of care, is used. The nurse assesses the client and family's knowledge of the client's condition, care, and treatment. Learning needs are assessed.

All individuals receiving Medicare-certified home care must be assessed following the Outcome and Assessment Information Set (OASIS) guidelines. OASIS is an assessment tool developed to measure outcomes of persons receiving home health care. The OASIS data provide a consistent format and standardized time points for documenting client care status. When OASIS information between two or more visits is compared, client outcomes can be identified (Richard, Crisler, & Stearns, 2000). All certified home healthcare agencies use OASIS as the assessment tool for home visits.

### Physical Assessment

Specifics of the physical assessment vary according to the client's needs. In most cases, the initial physical assessment will determine if the client is appropriate for home care services, what type of services are indicated, how long these services are likely to be needed, and who will pay for the care.

On the initial visit, and regularly throughout care, the nurse takes vital signs and conducts a full physical assessment of the client, including a review of all systems and a focused assessment of the client's presenting condition. During this assessment, the nurse collects information about the client's physical condition, functional status, ability to leave the home unassisted, ability to do self-care, and ability to perform ADL independently. Blood or urine specimens are often collected and sent to the laboratory.

### Family Assessment

Because community-based care is provided in the context of the client's family and community, assessment of the family is an essential ingredient to the success of home care. Family structure, stage of illness, developmental stage, and family functions may be assessed. The nurse must also determine if the client is isolated physically or socially from other members of the family or if the family is a close-knit, nurturing, and supportive family or kinship network.

### Financial Assessment

Information about the costs of home care services, insurance payment, and other financial concerns of the client and family should be discussed on the first visit. **Financial assessment** and options to reduce the cost of care while continuing the provision of safe, quality care should be explored. Some clients are insured 100% for home care services as long as the services are provided within the parameters of coverage. Others may have little or no insurance coverage. Clients and families may have little knowledge about their home care coverage and may be unaware that the number of visits may be limited or that they have a lifetime maximum as stipulated in the particular health insurance policy. All of these issues must be explored.

## Determination of Needs and Planning Care

After assessment, the nurse, client, and family discuss the nursing needs and develop a plan of care. They also determine who will be responsible for particular aspects of the care until the next nursing visit. The family support person may be responsible, or other professional health care or home care providers may be needed. An example of a home care interdisciplinary care plan is given in Box 13–3. Expected outcomes are developed and plans are made for a follow-up visit. Now and in the future, home health agencies have to demonstrate the client's progress toward achievement of desired outcomes. Medicare and insurance will not reimburse for a home visit if quality improvement and outcomes are not achieved.

## Implementation

Physical care, teaching, counseling, and referrals are completed according to the plan of care. Because home care replaces hospitalization in meeting acute medical needs, home care focuses on physical care of the client. Short visits of 30 minutes to 2 hours focus on hands-on care of the client, incorporating a large variety of nursing skills. These include giving injections, performing venipunctures for laboratory work, doing dressing changes, giving medications, teaching the client and family how to do the care on an ongoing basis, and being the eyes and ears for the physician in observing the client's progress toward recovery. While the nurse is performing skilled nursing care, he or she is also teaching, assessing, counseling, and advising the client and family.

## Termination of the Visit

The nurse reviews the purpose of the visit, outlines what was learned in the assessment phase, and reviews the mutually agreed on plan of care. The time and purpose of the next visit are discussed and agreed on by all involved. The nurse may end the visit with a small amount of casual conversation. Especially if the client lives alone, conversation will be anticipated and appreciated.

## Follow-up Visits and Evaluation

A thorough initial assessment allows for comprehensive planning for productive follow-up visits. Box 13–4 lists factors to consider when determining the need and

---

## COMMUNITY-BASED NURSING CARE GUIDELINES

### BOX 13–3 ▶ Home Care Interdisciplinary Care Plan

Client Name: _____ DOB: _____ Case Manager: _____

| Date | Client Issue | Intervention | Facilitator | Accomplished | | | Comments |
|------|-------------|-------------|-------------|-----|-----|-----------|----------|
| | | | | Yes | No | Partially | |
| | | | | | | | |
| | | | | | | | |
| | | | | | | | |
| | | | | | | | |
| | | | | | | | |
| | | | | | | | |

_____
Date Reviewed/Initials

_____
Date Reviewed/Initials

_____
Date Reviewed/Initials

_____
Date Reviewed/Initials

_____
Date Reviewed/Initials

_____
Date Reviewed/Initials

Disciplines on Case:
- ☐ RN      ☐ WNA
- ☐ PT      ☐ NMK
- ☐ OT      ☐ Volunteer
- ☐ ST      ☐ Chaplain
- ☐ MSW    ☐ Bereavement
- other _____

---

frequency of future visits. Each visit should have specific goals with plans implemented to meet those goals. Subsequent visits allow the nurse to build a trusting relationship with the client, which may lead to identification of additional nursing needs. In community-based nursing, the overall goal of every home visit is to maximize health functioning and self-care.

The nurse, client, and family or caregivers evaluate the visit and the care plan. Physical care, teaching, counseling, and referrals are discussed, and suggestions are made for ways to improve the care provided. The client may be asked to complete an evaluation survey (Box 13–5).

## Documentation

Generally, documentation for home visits follows specific regulations. To ensure that the agency will qualify for payment for the visit, the client's needs and the nursing care given are documented. This includes the client's homebound status and the need for skilled professional nursing care with Medicare, Medicaid, and

**ASSESSMENT TOOLS**

**BOX 13–4   Factors to Consider When Determining Need and Frequency of Follow-Up Visits**

- Client's current health status
- Home environment
- Level of self-care abilities
- Ability of family caregivers
- Level of nursing care needed
- Prognosis
- Teaching needs
- Mental status
- Level of adherence to treatment regimen

Adapted from Smeltzer, S. C., & Bare, B. G. (2000). *Brunner and Suddarth's textbook of medical-surgical nursing* (9th ed., p. 19). Philadelphia: Lippincott Williams & Wilkins.

most other third-party payers. If documentation is not done correctly, the agency may not be reimbursed for the visit.

At the beginning of this chapter, the Medicare coverage criteria that must be met for home care services to be reimbursed were discussed (Box 13–1). It is absolutely imperative that all of these criteria are met and documented. The nurse is responsible for documenting that the client is homebound. The primary dimensions of homebound status are that absences from the home are infrequent and, for the purpose of receiving medical treatment, that leaving home requires considerable and taxing effort. Homebound status must be documented in objective and measurable terms and include the following information about a client leaving home:

▶ How often
▶ For how long
▶ For what reason
▶ The effort and assistive devices required

Clients who leave the home to receive medical care not available in the home may still be considered for homebound status for the following reasons:

▶ Physician office visits
▶ Outpatient kidney dialysis services
▶ Attendance at adult day centers to receive medical care
▶ Outpatient chemotherapy or radiation (Zuber, 2002)

Documentation should always be focused on the client's illness, centering on the following:

▶ Statement of the problem(s)
▶ The skilled care provided to deal with the problem(s)
▶ Outcomes expected and achieved from the care provided ("Documentation tips," 1999)

## ASSESSMENT TOOLS

**Box 13–5  Client Satisfaction Survey**

To evaluate our services and continue our excellent standards of care, we need to hear from you. Please take a few minutes to complete this form and return it to us in the enclosed stamped envelope. Thank you!

1. Home health care services were provided in a timely manner when I needed them:

   _____ Very good          _____ Satisfactory          _____ Unsatisfactory

2. Home was the best setting for the care given to me for my comfort and recovery:

   _____ Very good          _____ Satisfactory          _____ Unsatisfactory

3. The number and frequency of visits provided were adequate to meet my needs:

   _____ Very good          _____ Satisfactory          _____ Unsatisfactory

4. The care I needed to improve my condition was received from home health care:

   _____ Very good          _____ Satisfactory          _____ Unsatisfactory

5. I am now able to care for myself with the procedures and instructions provided by the staff:

   _____ Very good          _____ Satisfactory          _____ Unsatisfactory

6. The home health care staff was courteous and respectful:

   _____ Very good          _____ Satisfactory          _____ Unsatisfactory

7. The names of community service agencies were given to me as needed and their services explained:

   _____ Very good          _____ Satisfactory          _____ Unsatisfactory

8. I felt my wishes about care were supported by the staff of the home health care agency:

   _____ Very good          _____ Satisfactory          _____ Unsatisfactory

9. I would use home health care services again:

   _____ Yes                _____ No

10. Home health care provided me with the following services:

    _____ Home health care  _____ Hospice          _____ Private duty

11. Comments (Please write on a separate sheet if more space is needed):

    _____

    _____

    _____

    _____

    _____

The plan of care also must be documented. Not only is a complete documentation of the care plan important for reimbursement and legal issues, but it is also critical to the evaluation of competent nursing practice used in quality assurance.

## Confidentiality

Confidentiality is essential to quality care in community-based settings. Sometimes nurses may care for someone they know or a friend or relative of someone they know outside of their professional role. Just as in the hospital setting, nurses must never discuss individual situations or the health status of clients and families with anyone except other professional staff within professional discussions.

## Safety Issues for the Nurse

The nurse should know the destination for the visit and have a route mapped out to get there. Depending on the neighborhood, asking directions can prove dangerous. When entering the client's neighborhood, the nurse begins an environmental assessment by doing a brief windshield survey (see Chapter 5). The purpose of the survey is to collect information about the community where the client lives and to determine if the neighborhood is safe. Occasionally, the nurse may not feel safe entering a client's home. In some areas, the nurse may need to be accompanied by a policeman or security officer. No nurse should ever disregard personal safety in an effort to visit a client. See Box 13–6 for a checklist of safety points to be followed by home care nurses.

## COMMUNITY-BASED NURSING CARE GUIDELINES

**Box 13–6** ▶ Personal Safety Checklist for the
Home Care Nurse

- Get to know the community, especially the differences between neighborhoods.
- Dress in sensible shoes and simple clothing, avoid long necklaces, expensive jewelry, or pins of political or religious nature.
- Get to know your client and family and determine if there is a history of violence.
- Know your agency policies and procedures and follow them.
- Keep your supervisor informed of any potential violent situations with your caseload.
- Have safety accessories in your car: a working cell phone, flashlight; and have a well-maintained car.
- Lock up equipment and your purse or valuables in the trunk of the car.
- Attend a course on safety, self-defense, or self-protection.

## CLIENT SITUATIONS IN PRACTICE

### Planning and Implementing a Home Care Visit

The discharge planning nurse calls your home care agency with the following information on a referral. Mrs. Gothie is an 85-year-old woman with severe congestive heart failure. She cared for her husband, who had dementia, for 7 years. He died 4 years ago. Mrs. Gothie has lived in the same third-floor apartment for 50 years. Although she has no children, she is close to her younger sister and brother and numerous nieces and nephews, who all live out of state. Her family is devoted to her, visiting her frequently, but most of her lifetime friends are no longer living. She has one friend who is able to help her on a limited basis, but most of her friends are aging.

When she came to the clinic 2 weeks ago, before being admitted to the hospital, her vital signs and laboratory values were as follows:

Temperature: 98.6°F
Blood pressure: 128/88 mm Hg
Respirations: 26 breaths/min
Lung sounds: rales in all lung fields
Lab values: prothrombin time 4 times normal
Digoxin level: 0.1 ng/mL

Mrs. Gothie stated the following at the clinic visit:

*I have had a terrible time getting my breath, especially at night. My ankles are three times as big as they used to be. I quit taking my water pill because it made me have to go to the bathroom all the time, and I couldn't sleep at night. I don't have any appetite, but I do eat fruit. Most days, I don't even bother to get dressed or take a shower because I'm so tired. What's the use—I never go any where—I'm always too tired. I have had a lot of bruises on my arms and legs.*

She was admitted to the hospital for acute congestive heart failure (CHF). After 3 days in the hospital, she was discharged to Happy Helpful Nurse HomeCare. After 1 week of physical therapy, she is scheduled to be discharged home. You are assigned to be the case manager for Mrs. Gothie's care. After reviewing the referral form in the figure plan your first visit with Mrs. Gothie.

- *List the points you will cover when you telephone Mrs. Gothie to set up an appointment for the first visit.*

You would call Mrs. Gothie to introduce yourself, give the name of the agency, and the purpose of the visits. If the visits are partially reimbursed by insurance, you may want to tell her that you will need to see her insurance card at the visit. You may also want to know if anyone will be home with her after she is discharged and if that person will be present at the visit. You may want to inquire if she has any concerns that she would like you to address during the visit so you can bring the appropriate supplies and educational materials.

- *Determine the primary purpose of the first visit and the focus of your physical assessment.*

The primary purpose of the first visit will be determined by the policies and procedures of the agency you are working for and the insurance coverage or Medicare requirements. In the latter case, the OASIS initial assessment would be initiated. The same goes for the focus of the physical assessment. You would be particularly concerned with the assessment of her cardiovascular status and any other assessment related to the symptoms of CHF. In her case, you would make sure that you assess her

| PATIENT REFERRAL FORM | AGENCY REFERRED TO: *Happy Helpful Nurse Home Care* |
|---|---|

| CONSENT FOR HOME VISIT GIVEN BY PATIENT OR FAMILY MEMBER?   YES   NO | | |
|---|---|---|
| ADMISSION DATE *1/8/07* | DISCHARGE DATE *1/15/07* | STATION *55* |

| STREET ADDRESS *Mrs Gothic Divisedere St.* | COUNTY *Marine* | HOME PHONE NO. *415-555-1212* |
|---|---|---|
| CITY, STATE, ZIP CODE *San Fransisco, Ca. 55157* | RELATIVE/FRIEND NAME *Ila Harris* | RELATIVE/FRIEND PHONE NO. *612-333-1212* |

| BIRTH DATE *4/15/23* | PRESENT AGE *84* | MALE / FEMALE *X* | MARITAL STATUS | | | |
|---|---|---|---|---|---|---|
| | | | SINGLE | SEPARATED | WIDOWED *X* | RELIGION (OPTIONAL) |
| | | | MARRIED | DIVORCED | | |

| MEDICAL INS. AND/OR | MEDICAL ABSTINANCE NO. *000-000-113* | MEDICARE NO. *000-000-113* | V.A. NUMBER *None* |
|---|---|---|---|

| PUBLIC ASSIST. COVERAGE | PRIVATE INSURANCE CO. AND POLICY NO. *Kaiser Group Health* |
|---|---|

### TO BE COMPLETED BY PHYSICIAN

MEDICAL HISTORY *Twenty year history of CHF with intermittant episodes of atral fib, ↑ symptom of CHF in the last year*

COMPLETE DIAGNOSIS/PROCEDURES THIS ADMISSION *CHF*

| PROGNOSIS *fair* | IS PATIENT AWARE? (YES) NO |
|---|---|
| | IS FAMILY AWARE? (YES) NO |

DOCTOR'S SPECIFIC ORDERS FOR HOME CARE *Nursing 2x wk x 3 week; 1x wk* ←

*O2 per nasal canola 3L/min. Monitor symptoms of CHF*

*PT drawn every other week*

*Monitor CHF; instruct in high-protein diet*

*Assess for PT*

*HHA 3x wk for personal care and meal prep.*

| DIET *high protein/high calorie* | ACTIVITY *ap ad lib* |
|---|---|

MEDICATIONS, TREATMENTS

| SUGGESTED FREQUENCY OF VISITS *2x a week x 3 then 1x week* | SUGGESTED DATE OF FIRST VISIT *Day after discharge from ECC* |
|---|---|
| PHYSICIAN'S SIGNATURE *Steven Hunt, M.D.* | DATE *Jan. 15, 2007* |
| PHYSICIAN'S IN CHARGE AFTER DISCHARGE *Dr. Kantor* | LOCAL PHYSICIAN'S NAME *Dr. Kantor* |

Medications

| Name | Amount | Time | Med Card | Comments/Instructions |
|------|--------|------|----------|----------------------|
| Coumidin | 10 mg | qd | yes | Watch for bruising on arms |
| Digaxir | 0.125 mg | qd | yes | Do not give if pulse ↓ 60 |
| Lasix | 60 mg | tid | yes | |
| K-LO4 | 60 mg | tid | yes | |
| | | | | |

DIET: (As desired unless indicate otherwise) _high protein diet needs help with meal prep_

ACTIVITIES: (As desired unless indicate otherwise) _encouraged to get up and dressed every day_

SPECIAL INSTRUCTIONS: (1) _Medication schedule received_
(2) _purchase slant pillow (40°) for nocturnal S.D.B._
(3) _call if ↑ S.D.B._

APPOINTMENTS:
a. Office appointment made: _Feb 1, 2007_
b. Call to make your appointment: _666-7666_

FOLLOW-UP:
a. If you have any questions after returning home, contact your doctor, _Dr. Kantor_

or you may call the hospital at _666-7666_

b. Referrals for follow-up care have been made to: _Happy Helpful Nurse Home Care_

SIGNATURES

Patient/Family Member _Ila Harris_
Signature indicates understanding of instructions above
Nurse (providing instruction) _Roberta Hunt, R.N._
Physician (Optional)

NURSING DISCHARGE INFORMATION

DISCHARGE TO:
Home ( √ )    Other ( )
Nursing Home ( )
METHOD OF DISCHARGE
Ambulatory/Carried/Wheelchair/Lifter
TRANSPORTATION:
Private ( √ )
Medibus/Ambulance ( )
ACCOMPANIED BY _sister_
DATE _Jan 16_    TIME _1:00 pm_

ALL VALUABLES RETURNED? _yes_
ALL MEDICATIONS RETURNED? _yes_
SUPPLIES/EQUIPMENT SENT:
_shower chair_
_O2 tank & tubing_

Discharge Nurse

PATIENT DISCHARGE INSTRUCTIONS    CHART COPY

appetite as she said at her last clinic visit that she doesn't have an appetite. She states that she is too tired to go anywhere, so you assess fatigue and what helps with that. Is she depressed? What about the bruises on her legs and arms? Was there a follow-up blood test done when she was in the hospital to explore this issue? Another concern will be what kind of support she needs to be safe at home. Then, you will assess the support she has and fill in the void with referrals. Obviously, you will be very concerned about the home environment and potential safety issues.

- *Identify your key areas of concern when you do your psychosocial and family assessment.*

You will do an assessment of the family structure, developmental stage, and functions. Another question you may have is whether Mrs. Gothie is physically or socially isolated from family or whether the family or her support network is close, nurturing, and supportive. Some of her statements at her last clinic visit indicated as much.

- *List the people who can provide support for Mrs. Gothie.*

According to the referral form, her sister accompanied her home when she was discharged. She also has one friend, but many of her friends are now deceased. You will want to assess the breadth and depth of any other support network. Does she need or want a home health aide for personal care and meal preparation?

- *Identify learning needs you will assess in the first visit.*

You note that she has had CHF for 20 years, with increased symptoms the last year. You will assess the learning need of both Mrs. Gothie and her sister. The first need that you will assess will be their understanding of the disease processes of CHF, her medications, and the use of oxygen. According to the notes from Mrs. Gothie's last clinic visit, it sounds like she is not taking the Lasix because she says that it makes her have to go to the bathroom too frequently to get adequate sleep at night. You assess when she takes the Lasix and recommend that she do so in the morning. You will also determine what her knowledge base is regarding the high-protein diet.

- *What referrals would you make?*

Your priority concerns are as follows:
1. Can she manage at home safely and make a reasonable recovery given her support system, her abilities, and other factors related to her living situation?
2. Does she need assistance managing her medications? Does she need someone either in her family or in the community to do this for her?
3. Does she understand the high-protein diet? Does she need to see a nutritionist?
4. How does she do grocery shopping? Are there services in the community to help her with this?
5. Is she open to home-delivered meals, such as Meals on Wheels?
6. Is congregate dining available in her community and transportation provided to the site?

- *What social opportunities would she consider?*

She states that she has no energy to go anywhere. Once she has more energy, what referrals could you make to address her social isolation (eg, church, community senior programs, other senior programs)?

## Support of the Lay Caregiver

Because so many clients are discharged from acute care settings earlier than in the past with conditions more serious or less stable, the home care environment has become the site of major caretaking activities. The use of families, relatives, and support systems such as caregivers is on the rise. In fact, **lay caregiving** is one of the world's fastest-growing unpaid professions. It is estimated that almost 75% of elderly persons with severe disabilities who receive home care services rely solely on family members or other unpaid assistance. Eight of 10 of these informal caregivers provide unpaid assistance for an average of 4 hours a day, 7 days a week. Three quarters of them are women, and one third are older than 65 years. A telephone survey estimated that more than 22 million households in the United States had at least one member who provided some level of unpaid assistance to a spouse, relative, or other person over age 50 (NAHC, 2000). Lost work caused by lay caregiving has cost businesses between $11.4 and $29 billion annually (Hunt, 2000).

Lay caregivers may have responsibilities for people at both ends of the age spectrum: children and older people with chronic health problems. "Parent caring" is the term used in the literature for sons and daughters caring for older parents. These caregivers are predominantly women. The "typical caregiver" is a middle-aged, married woman who is employed full time and is also spending about 18 hours a week caring for her mother who lives nearby (Weiland & Shellenbarger, 2002).

Sometimes the caregiver for an older person is an older person with his or her own functional disabilities. Recent research suggests that more men are becoming active in providing care in the home for an older spouse.

Caregiving includes providing emotional support, direct health services, and financial support; mediating with health and social service organizations; and sharing a household. It may include tasks such as bathing, toileting, shopping, preparing food, feeding, maintaining a household budget, and housekeeping. Family dynamics can be different from household to household. The nurse must be sensitive to this variety of family dynamics and work with the family and caregivers without being judgmental regarding their decisions.

## Stress on the Caregiver

Caring for a client who has acute needs that are treated with complicated technologic devices can be difficult. Such care may weigh heavily on the family. The nurse may need to provide not only client care and treatment but also a great deal of support for the family. For several decades, studies have documented the strain of caregiving on the caregiver's physical and psychologic health. One classic study found that more than half of the parents caring for children with high-technology equipment in the home had psychologic symptoms great enough to merit psychiatric intervention (Leonard et al., 1993). As family responsibility grows, parental distress increases. The nurse is in an ideal position to intervene.

The transition from visiting a family member in the hospital, where other people are responsible for care, to being a "paraprofessional" caregiver sometimes happens almost overnight. Suddenly the lay caregiver has 24-hour responsibility for tasks for which he or she has little or no knowledge and experience. The lay caregiver may have full- or part-time employment and other family members to care for. The strain on caregivers can be great, and risks for depression and illness are high. Other psychosocial problems raise the risk. The family may already have mounting bills with a mortgage and utilities. Safety in the community may be an issue. Transportation may be a problem, especially if the person requiring care was the family's means of transportation. Drug abuse on the part of a family member may add to the burdens. The lay caregiver may have no support person or outlets on which to rely.

The 24-hour responsibility for the client's care means more than supplying physical care for the client. It means that the lay caregiver always has the client and his or her care in mind. The role is unrelenting. The day is organized around the care activities and needs of the client, and sometimes the client must be under constant observation. Many times the client's personality, which may have changed with illness, places heavy demands on the caregiver's time and energy. The difficulty of the role has been associated with low levels of life satisfaction, high levels of depression, and symptoms of stress (Ruppert, 1996). If the care is to be provided temporarily, the stress may not be as great. If the length of time for care, however, is indefinite, as in chronic care, additional stress may be felt by the lay caregiver.

Because the stress on these lay caregivers is tremendous, community-based nurses need to consider this fact as they plan care. Although their clients are their main concern, a holistic nursing style means that nurses also provide care for family and other support persons.

## Assessment

The first home visit is an important time to discuss and clarify the relationship between the client and the caregiver. The OASIS provides items to assess caregiver presence, availability, and type of assistance needed. It is also essential to assess the caregiver's knowledge and physical and psychologic status. Caregiver needs must also be assessed because of the caregiver's increased risk for health problems.

## Interventions for Lay Caregivers

Nursing interventions may enhance quality of life for both the client and caregiver by ensuring that everyone has adequate preparation for ongoing care needs. Health care professionals need to be sensitive to caregivers, who handle many roles such as working outside the home or caring for other dependents in addition to being a caregiver. These individuals are often stressed, burdened, and depressed, as compared to those who have a single caregiver role (Chang, Brecht, & Carter, 2001). Nursing interventions may also assist in planning with the client and family to meet those needs. The nurse must do ongoing assessment of the family's financial status, coping ability, and emotional adjustment to the demands of giving care in the home, including assessment for signs of depression. If the situation indicates that a referral should be made for emotional or psychologic assistance, this must be done promptly.

The community-based nurse in any setting should be aware of the lay caregiver's circumstances and help the caregiver find solutions to problems. The nurse who initially establishes rapport with both the client and caregivers and builds on that trust is the most likely to successfully intervene. Sometimes working with the client to perform more self-care activities will take some of the responsibilities off the lay caregiver. Providing more teaching for the caregiver may help relieve the caregiver's feeling that the responsibilities are overwhelming. Other interventions include educational and support programs, burden-reducing programs, psychotherapeutic interventions, and self-help groups. Even a busy caregiver can find time in the schedule to attend a support group if it is deemed worthwhile. In these groups, people share their experiences and report on strategies that have or have not worked for them. Just knowing that other people are in

## RESEARCH IN COMMUNITY-BASED NURSING CARE

**Box 13–7** ▶ Predictors of Social Support and
Caregiver Outcomes

This study identified the predictors for caregiver's burden, satisfaction, depression and social support. The purpose of the study was to both examine the ability of social support to predict caregiver's levels of burden, satisfaction and depression, and to examine the caregiver/care-recipient characteristics that may predict social support. Caregivers who participated in the study all spoke English, the care recipients all had some some level of dementia and had difficulty with dressing or eating. Eighty-one dyads, caregiver/care recipients, were interviewed for the study which used appraisal tools to measured caregiver burden, satisfaction, depression, anxiety and hostility. The study found that difficulty arranging support from close friends significantly correlated with caregiver burden and depression and negatively correlated with satisfaction. Intensity of contact with social support was found to correlate with caregiver satisfaction. Caregiver participants who were married had more social support while those participants who were handling several roles (employment and caring for other dependents) had less social support. This research has several implications for health care providers. Nurses must be sensitive to caregivers who handle many roles such as working outside the home and caring for other dependent persons. They may need special assistance in identifying and utilizing a support network. The ability to obtain assistance from a close friend is the most important factor to add to a social support assessment.

Chang, B., Brecht, M., & Carter, P. (2001). Predictors of social support and caregiver outcomes. *Women and Health, (33)*1/2, 39-61.

the same situation or have the same feelings is helpful. Box 13–7 provides current research and nursing interventions for caregiver stress.

The nurse helps caregivers cope by sharing realistic prognostic information, discussing alternative levels of care, and providing information regarding **respite care**. A community day care program may be available for the client to relieve the lay caregiver of constant responsibility. Some communities help with housekeeping provisions or meal programs. Churches may have volunteers who can provide respite care. Additional resources for caregivers are found at the end of the chapter in What's on the Web.

Respite care provides a temporary break for the caregiver. The care may include someone coming into the house for an hour or two so the caregiver can shop, do errands, or keep his or her own doctor's appointments. Respite care is an important aspect of hospice care. Another form of respite care is the client's temporary visit to a nursing home or other facility. While the client is cared for in other surroundings, the caregiver and family are free to vacation, perform household maintenance duties, or simply relax.

## The Future of Home Care

There are several trends in home care that have been reported by Humphrey (2002). First, there is more focus on practice, including client care, pharmacology, best practices, and cost-saving clinical approaches to client care. Agencies are accomplishing this through the educational strategies of practice rounds, journal clubs, increased library holdings, expansion of orientation, and teleconferences. Changes in the emphasis of client care is another trend. Accentuating empowerment with families and clients is one example. Further, individualizing the care plan so that the home visits follow what the client and family needs rather than what is typically expected for the diagnosis is gaining more legitimacy.

It is anticipated that home care will assume an increasingly important role in community-based care in the future. The client advocate role will continue to be a central element of both as complexity of health care delivery and concern for cost containment continue. Flexibility and accountability will remain fundamental as the pressure to meet professional practice standards intersects with the pressure to contain costs. Challenges facing home care nurses will require that the nurse keep up with ever-changing regulations regarding coverage, as well as the documentation requirements that will follow. In addition, nurses will be called on to counsel clients and families as they have increasing responsibility for acutely ill family members at home. As in all nursing specialties, it will be vital for home care nurses to welcome the increased use of technology (Harris, 2000).

## Conclusions

The setting for the provision of health care has shifted several times from the late 1800s to the present. Care of the ill in the home was at one point primarily physician care. The setting for care moved from the home to the hospital or acute care setting in the mid-1900s, but it has now relocated back to the home and community. The major roles of home care are to educate, reinforce learning, and encourage clients and families to provide ongoing self-care. In home care, the family and client experience a loss of privacy and an interruption in normal decision making, but the advantages for the client and family outweigh the disadvantages when compared with inpatient care. Regardless of the client's diagnosis, the nurse in home care encourages self-care with a preventive focus, which is provided in the context of the client's family and community and follows the principles of continuity of care.

# What's on the Web

Administration on Aging (AOA)
Telephone: (202) 619-0724
**Internet address:** *www.aoa.dhhs.gov*
This Web site presents information on AOA and its programs. Resources for practitioners, statistics, and consumer information on obtaining services and age-related issues are included.

Canadian Home Care Association
17 York Street, Suite 401
Ottawa, Ontario, Canada K1N 9J6
Telephone: (613) 569-1585
**Internet address:** *http://www. cdnhomecare.on.ca/*
The Canadian Home Care Association is dedicated to the accessibility, quality, and development of home care and community support services that permit people to stay in their homes and communities with safety and dignity. The Web site contains information on publications, related sites, employment opportunities, and education programs, as well as information related to the organization.

Centers for Disease Control and Prevention
Hand Hygiene in Healthcare Settings
**Internet address:**
*http://www.cdc.gov/handhygiene*
This site provides access to the guidelines and materials to promote hand hygiene in health care facilities.

Family Caregiver Alliance
Telephone: (800) 445-8106
**Internet address:**
*www.caregiver.org/caregiver/jsp/home.jsp*
This site focuses on information and services to families and professionals caring for adults with cognitive disorders, as well as fact sheets on topics applicable to a variety of caregivers.

National Association for Home Care and Hospice
228 Seventh St. SE
Washington, DC 20003
Telephone: (202) 547-7424
**Internet address:** *http://www.nahc.org*
The National Association for Home Care and Hospice (NAHC) is a professional organization that represents a variety of agencies providing home care services, including home health agencies, hospice programs, and homemaker or home health aide agencies. The Web site contains news and information about home care and hospice, including publications, statistics about home care and hospice, a job search vehicle, and a locator for hospice and home care agencies and their affiliates. It also has information about NAHC membership, meetings and conferences, grassroots activities, and state associations.

National Family Caregivers Association
Telephone: (800) 896-3650
**Internet address:**
*http://www.nfcacares.org/*
Free membership is available to any family caregiver. Both the newsletter and Web site provide good resources for "caring for the caregiver" information.

Visiting Nurse Associations of America
99 Summer Street, Suite 1700
Boston, MA 02110
Telephone: (617) 737-3200
**Internet address:** *www.vnaa.org*
The Visiting Nurse Associations of America is the official national association for non-profit visiting nurse associations. It supports community-based VNAs in their mission to provide home and hospice care through skilled nursing, therapy services (physical therapy, occupational therapy), and home health aide care to elderly, children, homebound, disabled, and other types of clients.

## References and Bibliography

Centers for Disease Control and Prevention. (2000). *Infections associated with home health care: Focus of health experts.* Retrieved January 2, 2003, from http://www.cdc.gov/od/oc/media

Centers for Disease Control and Prevention. (2002). *Guideline for hand hygiene in health-care settings.* Retrieved June 4, 2003, from http://www.cdc.gov/mmwr/preview /mmwrhtml/rr5116a1.htm

Chang, B., Brecht, M., & Carter, P. (2001). Predictors of social support and caregiver outcomes. *Women and Health, (33)*1/2, 39-61.

Clark, D. (2000). Old wine in new bottles: Delivering nursing in the 21st century. *Image: Journal of Nursing Scholarship, 32*(1), 11–15.

Cullen, J. (1998). How student nurses see home healthcare nurses today. *Home Healthcare Nurse, 16*(2), 75–79.

Documentation tips. (1999). *Home Healthcare Nurse, 17*(3), 193–194.

Frequently asked questions about OASIS. (2000). *Home Healthcare Nurse, 18*(4), 229–230.

Harris, M. (2000). Challenges for home healthcare nurses in the 21st century. *Home Healthcare Nurse, 18*(1), 39–44.

Haynes, R., Montague, P., Oliver, T., McKibbon, D., Brouwers, M., & Kanani, R. (1999). Interventions for helping patients to follow prescriptions for medications. Cochrane Database of Systematic Reviews, (2) CD000011; PMID; ID796686.

Humphrey, C. (2002). The current status of home care nursing practice. *Home Healthcare Nurse, 20*(10), 677–684.

Hunt, G. (2000). Caregiving in the workplace. In C. Levine (Ed.), *Always on call: When illness turns families into caregivers,* (pp. 101–112). New York: United Hospital Fund.

Layton, S. (1999). A patient's prayer. *Home Healthcare Nurse, 17*(5), 293.

Leonard, B., Brust, J., & Nelson, R. (1993). Parental distress: Caring for medically fragile children at home. *Journal of Pediatric Nursing: Nursing Care of Children & Families, 8*(1), 22–30.

National Association for Home Care. (2000). *Basic statistics about home care.* Washington, DC. Retrieved June 4, 2004 from http://www.nahc.org/Consumer/hcstats. html

Pfaadt, M. (2000). A review of the basics—Understanding the categories of skilled nursing services. *Home Healthcare Nurse, 18*(5), 297–300.

Richard, A., Crisler, K., & Stearn, P. (2000). Using OASIS for outcome-based quality improvement. *Home Healthcare Nurse, 18*(4), 232–237.

Ruppert, R. A. (1996). Caring for the lay caregiver. *American Journal of Nursing, 96*(4), 40–45.

Schwarz, K., & Roberts, B. (2000). Social support and strain of family caregivers of older adults. *Holistic Nursing Practice, 14*(2), 77–90.

Shyu, Y. (2000). Patterns of caregiving face competing needs. *Journal of Advanced Nursing, 31*(1), 35–43.

Smith, B., Appleton, S., Adams, R., Southcott, A., & Ruffin, R. (2000). Home care by outreach nursing for chronic obstructive pulmonary disease. *Cochrane Database System Review, 2,* CD000994.

Smith-Stoner, M. (2000). Palliative care . . . 2000. *Home Healthcare Nurse, 18*(1), 32.

Turkoski, B. (2000). Home care and hospice ethics: Using the code for nurses as a guide. *Home Healthcare Nurse, 18*(5), 309–317.

Weiland, S., & Shellenbarger, T. (2002). Family caregiving at home. *Home Healthcare Nurse, 20*(2), 113–119.

Zuber, R. (2002). Assessing Medicare eligibility. *Home Healthcare Nurse, 20*(7), 425.

# L E A R N I N G   A C T I V I T I E S

## Journaling: Activity 13–1

The Home Visit

1. In your clinical journal, reflect on a home visit you have made in clinical. Identify the nursing skills and competencies you used as you provided care.
2. What did you expect the visit to be like and how did the actual visit compare?
3. How was caring for the client in the home different from an acute care setting? How was it similar? What did you do differently in the home setting?
4. What did you learn from this experience?
5. How will you use this information in your future practice?

Lay Caregiver

1. In your clinical journal, reflect on an experience you have observed or a client you have cared for in clinical who has been cared for by a lay caregiver for an extended period of time. Outline the case.
2. Discuss what you observed with this situation and how it applies to the theory in the text.
3. How did or would you support the caregiver based on what you learned reading the text?
4. How will you use what you learned from this experience in your future practice?

## Critical Thinking: Activity 13–2

Consider the psychosocial needs of home care clients in the following situations. Comment about the likelihood of their condition to produce anxiety or social isolation. Give a reason for your answer.

1. A 50-year-old retired government employee who is caring for his 50-year-old wife who has severe dementia
2. A 20-year-old woman caring for her 5-month-old baby, who has frequent episodes of apnea. The apnea has required frequent immediate action and, on one occasion, necessitated cardiopulmonary resuscitation to revive the baby.
3. A 70-year-old woman caring for her husband, who has terminal lung cancer.
4. An 80-year-old woman with severe chronic obstructive pulmonary disease who lives alone and is homebound.
5. A 60-year-old man with congestive heart failure who has frequent episodes of shortness of breath at night.

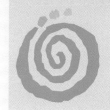

## CHAPTER 14

# Specialized Home Health Care Nursing

Roberta Hunt

## THE NURSE SPEAKS

One day when I came in to pick up my assignments, I was asked to visit Mrs. Black, who I had just seen for the first time the day before. She had called in to triage that morning to request another visit because of increased pain from pancreatic cancer. I was relatively new to **hospice care**, so I reviewed the procedure to increase the dose of morphine on the CADD pump. As I drove to her home, I was thinking about the home visit I had made to Mrs. Black the day before for pain management and anxiety issues. I remembered that at that time, she did not want the dosage of morphine or lorazepam increased. During that visit, I noticed the sadness in her eyes and had taken time to sit down next to her and hold her hand to ask her to tell me about her life. She reached under her bed and pulled out her wedding album and talked about the joy she felt on that particular day. I could tell there was sadness and worry behind the words she spoke that she was not willing to share.

When I arrived at her home, I expected that this second visit in as many days would be very short and would be focused on increasing the morphine on the CADD pump. After a pain assessment, I decided to increase the morphine to 2 mg/hour more than she had been receiving. As we sat side by side on the sofa, I concentrated fully on the unfamiliar procedure and tuned out the words she was speaking. In fact, I remember wishing that she would be quiet so I could finish the task at hand. But there was something in the sound of her voice that jolted me into hearing her words. I realized that she was sharing deep regrets about choices she had made in her life that could not be easily rectified in the time she had left. A sudden overwhelming feeling washed over me. What could I do about this information? I stopped fumbling with the pump and listened for a long time, acknowledging her pain and her suffering but offering no solutions or answers. She seemed to gain in personal strength as she shared. This experience reminded me to never lose sight of the compassionate and caring role of the nurse in the alleviation of suffering.

**Kathleen Dudley, MSN, RN**
**Hospice Nurse**
**Assistant Professor**
**College of St. Catherine**

In the last 20 years, home health care has become more specialized and complex as nursing care is increasingly provided in community-based settings. As in basic home health care, nurses must be competent in communication, teaching, management, and physical and emotional caregiving. In addition, they must develop expertise in a specialized area. Specialized home health care nursing, which will be discussed in this chapter, includes home telemedicine, infusion therapy, **wound care**, maternal–child home care, pain management, and hospice care.

## Infusion Therapy

**Home infusion therapy** is a broad area incorporating chemotherapy, pain management, fluid replacement therapy, immunosuppressive drug therapy, thalassemia treatment with deferoxamine mesylate, inotropic therapy, and blood and platelet transfusion. These medications are infused by a variety of methods. The actual administration of the therapy is performed by home infusion nurses or self-administered by clients or their caregivers. Because the therapy and technology of infusion therapy has become increasingly advanced, reimbursement criteria are stricter. Preauthorization is essential before any home infusion therapy is initiated, or the result could be nonpayment for the services provided (Sinkinson, Cammon, Curry, & Foley, 2001).

### Role of the Nurse

It is imperative that nurses who seek employment in infusion therapy have sharp problem-solving and interpersonal skills, detailed knowledge of the therapies and their effects, and technical skill in working with equipment. Although all nursing roles are important in the specialized area of infusion therapy, the primary one is that of direct caregiving (Figure 14–1). Before the visit, the nurse must be sure that the visit has been preauthorized and that the medication dosage, rate, route, and site-change frequency are all indicated in the physician order. In addition, all necessary equipment and supplies must be in the home or brought to the home by the nurse. Box 14–1 details the numerous safety requirements of this type of therapy.

Another important nursing function involves completing a full assessment, including intake and output, weight, and signs of reactions to therapy. This assess-

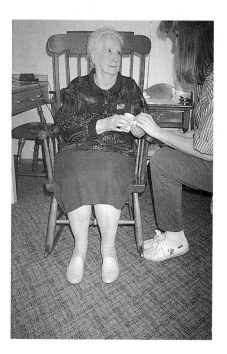

*Figure 14–1.* ▶ It is imperative never to lose sight of the importance of compassion and caring in the alleviation of suffering in our role as nurses.

---

> ▶ **Box 14–1.** Safety Requirements for Infusion Therapy ◀

- Emergency plan and access to functional phone and list of emergency phone numbers
- 3-prong grounded outlet to maintain proper grounding of the machine
- Adequate refrigeration capacity to store medication requiring cool storage and chemical spill kit in the home
- Notification to the fire and police departments and telephone and electric companies of person on life support equipment or medically necessary oxygen or infusion
- Systems established to ensure adherence to a complex medication regimen
- Information on medications, including dosage, adverse effects, interactions, and safe storage
- Identification and correction of environmental hazards and patient-specific concerns
- Fire evacuation plan, functional smoke detectors, and access to functional fire extinguisher

Adapted from Sinkinson, G., Cammon, S., Curry, J., & Foley, M. (2001). *Pocket guide to home care standards.* Springhouse, PA Springhouse (p. 273).

---

ment should also include the infusion site, operation of the infusion pump, care for the access site, signs of infection, allergic response, fluid overload, and dehydration or other signs of complications. Response to the therapy must always be assessed and documented. Reimbursement for home care infusion therapy is often limited because it is expected that all clients and their families will assume some or all aspects of the care. It is more common for the infusion therapy nurse rather than the discharge planning nurse to teach the family caregiver or client how to do the infusion. It is important that the nurse teach the client and family regarding the safe infusion of the medication. In the rare case when the teaching is done before discharge from the hospital, the client and family members are often so overwhelmed and anxious that they may have difficulty learning the procedure. What may happen is that the client or family is unable to complete the skill independently once they are home. The content of this teaching incorporates using proper technique for infusions and solving common problems related to intravenous (IV) therapy, site care, and use of the infusion pump, as well as the purpose, route, and dosage of the medications. The family must also know how to document the rate and time of all infusions, symptoms of IV infiltration and infection, and times to call or contact the nurse or physician (Gorski, 2002).

## Trends in Infusion Therapy

As previously mentioned, nurses who seek employment in infusion therapy must have sharp problem-solving and interpersonal skills, detailed knowledge of the therapies and their effects, and technical skill in working with equipment. Although not required at this time, there is some interest in requiring certification for employment as an infusion therapy nurse. At this time, the Joint Commission on Accreditation of Healthcare Organizations states that nurses must be appropriately qualified and competent in the infusion field to be employed as an infusion nurse. Some research indicates that certified nurses experience fewer adverse events and errors in care than their noncertified counterparts. There is a trend to require agencies to hire nurses who are certified through the Infusion Nurses Certification Corporation and maintain this certification to be reimbursed for services. However, there is a downside to requiring home infusion therapy nurses to become certified in that it may create a shortage of certified nurses and consequently limit access to home infusion care (Sexton & Seldomridge, 2002).

 ## Wound Care

Wound care is a common specialized home care function. A variety of problems can occur in wound healing, stemming from a combination of factors and situations. These include the client's general health, nutritional status, skin texture and turgor, body weight, and mobility, all of which impact healing (Sinkinson et al., 2001). Wound care is not simply a technique of dressing application; there is a discipline of specialized practice for wound care that includes advanced training, education, and certification. There is a lack of wound care specialists, caused by area-specific shortages and the expense of contracting for such services (Biala, 2002).

### Role of the Nurse

In wound care, the nurse acting as the physical caregiver must focus on ongoing evaluation of the wound and any particular risk factors for healing. Before the first visit, the nurse must be familiar with the type of wound, wound care orders, cleaning method, and frequency of dressing change, as well as any pressure-relieving or support devices, dietary restrictions and caloric allowance, medications, and activity orders and restrictions. Mobility enhancement and pain assessment should be initiated at the first visit and done periodically as needed. Scrupulous documentation following the Outcome and Assessment Information Set (OASIS) assessment or the agency policy is an essential aspect of wound care. For additional information on the OASIS documentation, see Chapter 13. Box 14–2 outlines other safety considerations.

---

▶ **Box 14–2.** Safety Considerations for Wound Care ◀

- Universal precautions for infection control and disposal of sharps and used dressings
- List available to the client and all caregivers of signs and symptoms to report to the nurse or physician
- Documentation of medications and allergies
- Identification and correction of environmental hazards and patient-specific concerns (Sinkinson, 2001)

It is important that the nurse be comfortable educating the client and caregivers in wound care skills. Lay caregivers must become competent in several aspects of wound care, as they often are the main care providers. They need to be able to describe and demonstrate wound care and signs and symptoms of infection. Knowledge of the importance of medicating 30 minutes before a painful dressing change is essential. Nutritional practices profoundly impact wound healing, and one way to monitor this is through a dietary log. The client should be encouraged to participate in activity as appropriate for the condition. For those with limited mobility, caregivers must understand range-of-motion exercises and initiate them at least three times a day. Techniques for turning and positioning the client every 2 hours to alleviate pressure are also essential caregiver skills (Sinkinson et al., 2001).

## Trends in Wound Care

Care conferencing for wound care is one trend. A care conference is a meeting to discuss specific cases and need for revisions to the plan of care. Most agencies have identified criteria for cases that must be examined by a care conference. It is important that these criteria explore the causes or factors contributing to the wound and how the plan of care addresses these. The past and current status of the wound and the current orders for the dressing and treatment must also be clearly documented and must be compatible. The client or caregiver's role in the wound plan of care must be examined, as should the frequency of physical therapy visits. The barriers to wound healing should be identified and addressed. Discharge goals and time frame should be realistic (Biala, 2002).

Through technology, new tools are being developed, along with different, targeted approaches to provide more effective care to those with wounds that require advanced care and supervision. The first trend is the use of telemedicine. Telemedicine is an integrated, innovative system of care "that provides a variety of health and education services to clients unhindered by space and time" (Dimmick, Mustaleski, Burgiss, & Welsh, 2000). Home-based telemedicine can involve teleconsulting, conferencing, reporting, and transmitting.

One trend for wound care is the use of cameras and Internet consultation for wound care. Telewound care, or the use of ordinary digital cameras to document the status of a wound for better care tracking and planning, is becoming commonplace. An ongoing photographic history of the wound provides excellent continuity between the home, clinic, and hospital. Cost savings of 50% have been documented as a benefit of using telewound care (Kinselia, 2002).

Another trend is specialty wound services delivered directly to the home via a computer screen. The photographs of the wound are transmitted to a specialty wound care service that provides consultation for management of difficult wounds. These virtual specialists work together with the home care nurse to assess and plan care. Both of these trends are offering hope for healing difficult wounds in a more cost-effective manner.

##  Maternal–Child Home Care

Women who are identified as having high-risk pregnancies may require home care for several pregnancy complications, including preterm labor, **pregnancy-induced hypertension**, and **hyperemesis** gravidarum. The main advantage of home care for high-risk pregnancy is that it reduces costs by preventing hospitalization and decreases the percentage of low-birth-weight infants. Increasingly, woman experiencing these complications require high-technology care, such as infusion therapy or telemedicine in the form of home monitoring.

## Role of the Nurse

Nursing roles depend on the client's condition. Hyperemesis, or protracted vomiting with weight loss and fluid and electrolyte imbalance, sometimes requires IV replacement therapy at home to maintain hydration. In women at risk for preterm labor, home care prevents premature birth. Nursing roles include assessment of the mother's weight, fetal heart tones, fundal height, nutrition, psychosocial status, compliance with the plan of care, and knowledge of signs and symptoms of preterm labor.

Pregnancy-induced hypertension (PIH) is the second leading cause of maternal mortality in the United States. Seven to 10 percent of all pregnancies are complicated by PIH (Yerge-Cole, 2001). PIH is a hypertensive disorder of pregnancy that includes preeclampsia, eclampsia, and transient hypertension. Home monitoring of those individuals experiencing PIH has been shown to reduce mortality and health care costs. Skilled nursing care includes assessment of the mother's weight, presence of edema and hyperreflexia, signs and symptoms of a worsening condition, fetal heart tones, compliance with the plan of care, nutrition, psychosocial status, and knowledge of symptoms.

## Postpartum/Well-Baby Home Care

Postpartum home care is a growing area of perinatal services. It is common for insurers to reimburse at least one visit for families after early discharge in the presence of high-risk factors. These may include conditions with the infant such as hyperbilirubinemia, low birth weight, and failure to feed well or gain weight appropriately. Any woman who manifests signs of postpartum depression merits a referral for follow-up with a home care nurse after discharge. Again, the role of the nurse involves assessing and monitoring postpartum status and referring for follow-up as appropriate. There is an impressive body of research that documents the long-term value of nurse home visiting for perinatal care (Box 14–3).

## Pediatric Home Care

The need for home care services for the pediatric client has grown substantially in recent years. Most of these services are for postsurgical clients released from the hospital so early that they need skilled nursing care at home through the rehabilitation phase of care. A second common group, children with chronic conditions such as bronchial pulmonary dysphasia, cystic fibrosis, and cancer, are now being cared for at home rather than in the hospital setting. Children may need some of the same nursing care that has already been discussed: infusion therapy, wound care, or other high-technology care. All of the general principles and guidelines discussed in Chapter 13 that apply to the home care of adults also apply to children. It is particularly important when caring for children that all nursing functions are formulated, implemented, and evaluated in collaboration with the parents or caregiver.

**RESEARCH IN COMMUNITY-BASED NURSING CARE**

**Box 14–3** ▶ Enduring Effects of Nurse Home Visitation on Maternal Life Course

For decades there has been evidence that nurse home visiting creates benefits for the families who receive the service. This research was designed to determine the effectiveness of prenatal or infancy home visits on the maternal life course of women in an urban setting over a 3-year period of time. Pregnant women were randomly assigned to either the control group with no visits or to weekly visits by a nurse. The 743 participants received an average of 7 visits during their pregnancy and 26 visits from birth to their child's 2nd birthday. The women who received home visits had fewer subsequent pregnancies, longer intervals between the birth of the first and second child, and fewer months of using AFDC (welfare) and food stamps. This study concluded that there are enduring effects of home visiting program on the lives of the women who participate in these programs.

Kitzman, H., Olds., D., Sidora, K., Henderson, C., & Hanks, C., et al. (2000). Enduring effects of nurse home visitation on maternal life course: A 3-year follow-up of a randomized trial. *Journal of the American Medical Association, 283*(15),1983-1989.

### Trends in Maternal–Child Home Care

Some of the trends in home care of high-risk pregnancy include use of telemedicine for the management of preterm labor. In one program, clients who were diagnosed with preterm labor or had a history of preterm labor were provided with daily assessment of uterine activity through home uterine activity monitoring by telephone along with standard care. The other group did not receive home uterine activity monitoring or telemedicine. The mean cost for the telemedicine group was $7,225, whereas the mean cost for the group who did not receive daily home uterine monitoring was $21,684. This represented an average savings of $14,459 per pregnancy using telemedicine services (Morrison, Bergauer, Jacques, Coleman, & Stanziano, 2001).

Although pediatric home health care represents a small portion of all the home health care services, increasing technologic advances and the continued movement of health care from the acute care to the community setting is expected to lead to higher use.

## Pain Management

For many conditions, pain management is central to effective nursing care. It is common for clients and their caregivers to fear uncontrolled pain. They may need frequent reassurance that pain control can be achieved. Many factors contribute to successful assessment and management of pain, but the relationship and trust

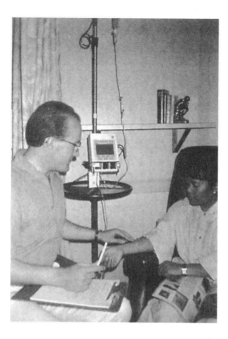

***Figure 14–2.*** ▶ Intravenous therapy and other technologic treatments are performed in the home.

between the nurse and client is central to this process. Caring and compassion are essential to this relationship (Fig. 14–2).

### Role of the Nurse

Effective pain management is based on a comprehensive pain assessment. In the home environment, where the nurse may see the client for limited periods of time, it is imperative that the nurse develops skills in assessment and management of pain. Because pain is subjective and an individual experience, the client's report of pain must be considered accurate and valid. Generally, acute pain is defined as pain that lasts less than 6 months, whereas chronic pain lasts more than 6 months. As in all community- based nursing care, prevention and early intervention is always the first consideration in the assessment and management of pain (Johnson & Smith-Temple, 1998). Box 14–4 contains a method for assessing pain.

The pharmacologic interventions for the management of pain are too numerous to address in this chapter. Most fundamentals or medical–surgical textbooks comprehensively address this issue. Sometimes physical pain relief techniques can be used with success. Positioning and good hygiene often relieve pain for those individuals who spend long hours in bed. Cutaneous stimulation, such as massage, vibration, heat, and cold are often effective for temporary relief from pain. Anticipatory guidance, distraction, guided imagery, and hypnosis also contribute to pain management. There are also behavioral pain relief techniques including relaxation and meditation.

### Trends in Pain Management

One trend in pain management is the increasing use of alternative and complementary therapies. A great deal of research documents the benefits of relaxation and

## ASSSESSMENT TOOLS

### Box 14–4  Pain Assessment

Describe any pain you have now.
What makes it worse?
What makes it better?
When does it occur? How often? How long does it last?
What else do you feel when you have this pain?
Show me on this drawing (or figure) where you have pain.
Rate your pain on a scale of 1 to 10, with 10 being the most severe pain.
   (Have a child use the Oucher scale, with faces ranging from frowning to crying.)
Has pain impacted your daily activities? How has your pain affected your activities of daily living?

Adapted from Weber, J. (2001). *Nurse's handbook of health assessment* (4th ed.). Philadelphia: Lippincott Williams & Wilkins (p. 27).

meditation for conditions such as pain management. National Institutes of Health (NIH) authorities recommend that practitioners use relaxation and meditation for pain management given their low cost and demonstrated health benefits and judge them as among the best alternative therapies for widespread use (McCann, 2003).

As in other areas of medical research, there is a great deal of research focusing on the role of medication in pain management. Notable among these are researchers working to develop a morphine-like drug that will have the same pain-deadening qualities without the drug's negative side effects. Another group is working to develop pain medications that take advantage of the body's natural ability to block or interrupt pain signals (NIH, 2003).

##  Hospice Care

Hospice care provides an essential alternative for the terminally ill client. Agencies that provide hospice care are committed to maintaining supportive social, emotional, and spiritual services to the terminally ill, as well as support for the client's family. Caring for the terminally ill includes caring for the family and caregivers. Care varies according to the client and family's needs; however, the focus is always on the client and family as the unit of care. Hospice care is often interdisciplinary care that reaffirms the right of every individual and family to participate fully in the final stage of life.

Dr. Cecily Saunders founded the hospice movement in London in the late 1960s. Dr. Sylvia Lack established the first hospice in the United States based on the model developed in Great Britain. Since 1982, when the Medicare hospice program was established, the number of hospices has grown dramatically. According to the Hospice Association of America (HAA, 2002), there were 31 Medicare-certified hospices in 1984. In 1985, there were 151. In 1991, there were 1,011, and by 2000, the number had increased to 2,273. In addition to all the other benefits to clients and family provided by hospice care, the daily cost is substantially less than the cost of stays in the hospital and in skilled nursing facilities.

When a client is diagnosed with a terminal illness and has 6 months or less to live, the client qualifies for hospice care through Medicare. Payment for hospice services under Medicare is based on four levels of care:

1. Routine care
2. Continuous home care (24 hours in a crisis situation)
3. Inpatient respite care not to exceed 5 days at a time
4. General inpatient care (AHA, 2002)

Hospice care is offered in a variety of settings. These include the freestanding hospice house where inpatient hospice services are provided at the end of life, hospital- and home-based services provided by freestanding hospice agencies, and home care-affiliated hospice agencies. Most of the programs in the United States are provided through autonomous, community-based, in-home hospice programs. Nurses develop and supervise many hospice agencies.

Intermittent hospice care is provided in the home by nurses; medical social workers; physical, occupational, and speech therapists; home health aides; and homemakers. Hospice programs provide short periods of continuous care in which a client is provided with shift nursing and aides for an acute episode and respite care for the family by placing the client in a nursing home for a few days. Hospice-trained volunteers provide emotional and physical support for clients and families by assisting with transportation, household care, child care, errands, and companionship. Volunteers also provide a vital link between the client and health care providers.

## The Role of the Nurse

In hospice, the focus of care shifts from aggressive, curative treatment to palliative care and strengthening of the client and family's quality of life as the client faces death. The goal of hospice in the home is to maintain the client's quality of life, keep him or her as comfortable as possible, and provide support and instruction to caregivers. The purpose of the care is to make the dying process as dignified as possible while keeping the client comfortable physically and providing emotional and spiritual support. Nursing care in this context also assists the client and family to define their needs at the end stages of life and to have the resources necessary to carry out their wishes. With hospice care, terminal illness no longer means dying alone in a hospital. People can remain in the comfort of their own home, surrounded by family and loved ones, and die peacefully without fear of major medical intervention and resuscitative measures. Death with dignity is the motto of hospice.

The specific role of the nurse varies according to the client's diagnosis and treatment plan. The nurse should be competent in all the roles important for any community-based setting, but it is particularly important in communication, teaching, and direct physical caregiving.

Good communication is essential in hospice care. It is self-evident that the client is vulnerable at this time, and family members are vulnerable as their loved one is dying. It is very important in this specialization that the nurse is skilled in therapeutic communication. Managing psychologic conditions in palliative care is central to this role. It is common for the client to experience anxiety, depression, and delirium at the end of life. Each of these conditions can occur as a result of the primary disease, concurrent physical conditions, inadequate pain management, medication side effects, or a combination of all of these (Paice, 2002). It is imperative that all hospice nurses are knowledgeable about various types of pain management techniques.

As in any situation providing direct physical care, the nurse must carefully assess the particular needs of the client, family members, and caregivers. This assessment should follow the main premises of this book. In other words, the nurse should consider the needs of the client within the context of his or her family, culture, and community. The focus should be on maximizing the potential of the individual and family through health promotion and disease prevention, even at the end of life. For example, the simple intervention of good hand washing can prevent an infection that could cause pain and suffering during the client's last days. Encouraging activity that the client finds pleasurable promotes health, even when death is near. Anticipating medication needs is one important role for the hospice nurse.

Planning for medication needs even if they occur after regular pharmacy hours is another role in comfort care with end-of-life care. These situations should be anticipated before such a need arises by careful advance planning and assessment. Hospice nurses should have excellent pain management skills. Adequate pain relief is assured by the following measures:

▶ Obtaining and maintaining a standing order for analgesia that incorporates consideration of increasing pain levels
▶ Assessing for all causes of pain, including anxiety, positioning, and environment
▶ Documenting every medication dose and any changes in dose, response to medication, and nonpharmacologic interventions that are effective for pain relief for this individual

Following the death of the client, bereavement counseling and support for the family continue for a year. Spiritual counseling is a common aspect of care. Spirituality expressed through the religious beliefs of the client and family can be a useful tool in the care of people who are dying.

## Trends in Hospice Care

Public and political consciousness, research allocation related to end-of-life issues, emphasis on personal choice, and increased public awareness of the limits of medical technology have all increased interest in hospice care. Recognition of the importance of pain management, along with the joining of forces between palliative care and hospice, have also contributed to increased availability and quality of pain management in hospice care (Head, 2000). It is anticipated that hospice care will assume an increasingly important role in community-based care in the future (Harris, 2000).

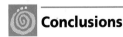

## Conclusions

Both specialized home care and hospice care will be important for the future of community-based care. The client advocate role will continue to be a central element of both as complexity of health care delivery and concern for cost containment continue. Flexibility and accountability will remain fundamental as the pressure to meet professional practice standards intersects with pressure to contain costs. Challenges facing home care nurses will require that the nurse keep up with ever-changing regulations regarding coverage, the documentation requirements that will follow, and the evolving certification requirements for nurses in these specialties. In addition, nurses will be called on to teach and support clients and families because of increasing responsibility for acutely ill family members at home. As in all nursing specialties, it will be vital for specialized home care and hospice nurses to welcome the increased use of technology (Harris, 2000). High tech and high touch will continue to be the practice imperative.

# What's on the Web

American Society of Pain Management Nursing (ASPMN)
**Internet address:** *http://www.aspmn.org/*
This organization of nurses is dedicated to promoting and providing optimal care for individuals with pain, including the management of its sequelae. All of this is accomplished through education, standards, advocacy, and research.

Home Care Guide: Caring for Young Persons With Cancer at Home
**Internet address:**
*http://www.hmc.psu.edu/pedsonco/Homeguide.html*
This wonderful site outlines practical suggestions for typical issues that arise with pediatric home care for children with cancer. It takes the nurse step by step through nursing interventions for common symptoms that arise with cancer care.

Infusion Nurses Society
220 Norwood Park South
Norwood, MA 02062
(781) 440-9408
**Internet address:** *http:/www.ins1.org/*
The Infusion Nurses Society (INS) promotes excellence in infusion nursing through standards, education, advocacy, and outcome research. They are committed to supporting access to the highest quality, cost-effective infusion care for all individuals. INS achieves this mission by providing opportunities for advanced knowledge and expertise through professional development and resource networking.

Nursing: Specialties: Wound Care
**Internet address:** *http://www.nursewebsearch.com/Specialties/Wound_Care/*
This Web site lists numerous links related to the nursing specialty of wound care.

Pediatric Home Care Association of America (PedHCAA)
**Internet address:**
*http://www.nahc.org/PedHCAA/home.html*
This site provides valuable information about this affiliate of the National Association for Home Care and Hospice (NAHC). One of the goals of this organization is to strengthen communication between pediatric hospices and home care providers. It also represents the interests of pediatric hospice and home care providers to the U.S. Congress and regulatory bodies. Another goal is to develop pediatric resources and educational opportunities at national, regional, and local organization meetings.

Palliative Care: One Vision, One Voice
**Internet address:** *http:/www.palliativecarenursing.net/*
This site is the leading source of on-line information about initiatives related to improving care at the end of life. If offers information on conferences, educational opportunities, initiatives, publications, and resources and research on end-of-life issues. This is an outstanding source of information for the beginning practitioner.

## References and Bibliography

Biala, K. (2002). Case conferencing for wound care patients. *Home Healthcare Nurse, 20*(2), 120–125.

Dimmick, S., Mustaleski, C., Burgiss, S., & Welsh, T. (2000). A case study of benefits and potential savings in rural home telemedicine. *Home Healthcare Nurse, 18*(2), 124–135.

Gorski, L. (2002). Effective teaching of home IV therapy. *Home Healthcare Nurse, 20*(10), 666–674.

Harris, N. (2000). Challenges for home health care nurses in the 21st century. *Home Health Care Nurse, 18*(1)39–44.

Head, B. Corporate compliance and the hospice nurse. *Hospice Today, 18*(5), 290–291.

Hospice Association of America. (2002). *Hospice facts and statistics.* Retrieved June 11, 2003, from http://www.nahc.org/consumer/hpcstats.html

Johnson, J. & Smith Temple, J. (1998). *Nurse's guide to home health procedures.* Philadelphia: Lippincott-Raven.

Kinselia, A. (2002). Advanced telecare for wound care delivery. *Home Health Nurse, 20*(7), 457–461.

Kitzman, H., Olds, D., Sidora, K., Henderson, C., Hanks, C., et al. (2000). Enduring effects of nurse home visitation on maternal life course: A 3-year follow-up to a randomized trial. *Journal of the American Medical Association, 283*(15), 1983–1989.

McCann, J. (2003). *Nurses's handbook of alternative and complementary therapies* (2nd ed.). Philadelphia: Lippincott Williams & Wilkins.

Morrison, J., Bergauer, N., Jacques, D., Coleman, S., & Stanziano, G. (2001). Telemedicine: Cost-effective management of high-risk pregnancy. *Managed Care.* Retrieved February 7, 2003, from http://www.managedcaremag.com/

National Institutes of Health, National Institute of Neurological Disorders and Stroke. (2003). Pain—hope through research. Retrieved June 16, 2003, from http://www.ninds.nih.gov/health_and_medical/pubs/pain.htm

Paice, J. (2002). Managing psychological conditions in palliative care. *American Journal of Nursing, 102*(11),36–42.

Sexton, J., & Seldomridge, L. (2002). The characteristics and clinical practices of nurses who perform home infusion therapies. *Journal of Infusion Nursing, 25*(3),176–181.

Sinkinson, G., Cammon, S., Curry, J., & Foley, M. (2001). *Pocket guide to home care standards.* Springhouse, PA: Springhouse.

Yerge-Cole, G. (2002). On the alert for pregnancy-induced hypertension. *Home Healthcare Nurse, 19*(11), 727–728.

# L E A R N I N G   A C T I V I T Y   1 4

## JOURNALING: ACTIVITY 14–1

In your clinical journal:

- Discuss your own attitudes and beliefs regarding pain control. How do you think they could impact the way that you provide pain control for your clients? What do you think that you can do to prevent your own attitudes about pain from interfering with the needs of your clients?
- Describe what you learned from reading this chapter (or saw when you observed a nurse in one of the specialized roles outlined in this chapter).
  - Discuss what you thought was important and how it fits into what you have learned so far about the role of the nurse in the community.
  - How has your view of the nursing role in the community changed after reading this chapter (and observing the role of the nurse in the community)?

## CLIENT CARE: ACTIVITY 14–2

Maureen is a 57-year-old widow who was referred to hospice home care. She was diagnosed with stage IV breast cancer 1 year ago. After extensive surgery, chemotherapy, and radiation, she has been diagnosed with metastasis to her liver and bones. Her referral states that she has almost constant pain. Her daughter lives in another state and has three preschool children. Her son is living temporarily in Africa for 6 months. You are the home care nurse doing the admission intake by following the agency forms. However, you will have some particular concerns given what you read on Maureen's referral form, including the following:

1. On what do you concentrate your assessment?
2. What questions do you use to assess?
3. What combination of interventions do you use to help keep Maureen comfortable (both pharmacologic and other methods)?
4. What safety considerations do you have and how do you assess them?

## PRACTICAL APPLICATION: ACTIVITY 14–3

Contact an agency that employs nurses to work in one of the roles described in this chapter. Arrange to observe a nurse working in the setting. After the observation, arrange for a short interview with the nurse. Develop several questions before the observation and interview. You may decide to use some of the following questions as a part of the interview.

1. What do you enjoy about this type of work?
2. What is difficult about the work?
3. How has the role changed over the last 5 years? Ten years?
4. How do you use the concept of self-care in your practice?
5. What place does health promotion and disease prevention have in your daily work?
6. What do you need to know about families, culture, and community to do this type of work?
7. What type of special training is now required or would you recommend in preparation to do this type of work?

8. Do you have any recommendations for a new graduate who may be interested in entering this type of work in the future?
   - Send a thank you note to the nurse and agency after the visit. (Not only is this a great strategy for getting a job in the future, building goodwill with some people you may work with in the community, but it is also just plain good manners.)
   - Summarize your observation and interview in a 2- to 3-page paper.

## PRACTICAL APPLICATION: ACTIVITY 14–4

Find an article or book on the Internet on CINAHL or MEDLINE about one of the specialized settings and roles from the chapter that interests you. Get the article or book (pick a chapter) and respond to the following.

1. What was the main point of the article or chapter from the book?
2. What did you think was the most important aspect of the article or chapter for your learning?
3. How do you think that you can use this new information in the future?

## CRITICAL THINKING: ACTIVITY 14–5

Identify a topic related to one of the specialized home care settings or roles discussed in this chapter. If you have discovered a specialized home care role not included in the chapter, it can also be used as the topic for this activity. Some examples could be the following:

- Why should nurses have to be certified to practice in the specialty (eg, pain management, infusion nursing, pediatric home care, high-risk obstetrics home care, hospice home care)?
- What are the current issues in one of the settings or roles? (For example, in high-risk home care, one issue is whether home uterine monitoring prevents preterm birth. In pediatric home care, one issue is how to work with the parents to plan and implement care.)
- How has the nursing shortage impacted these specialized roles?
- What issues related to funding impact the availability of specialized care?

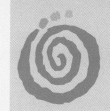

## CHAPTER 15

# Mental Health Nursing in Community-Based Settings

Marva Thurston

## LEARNING OBJECTIVES

1. Describe the historical evolution of mental health care.
2. Identify the behaviors of the major mental illnesses.
3. Discuss the significance of mental illness.
4. Describe the risk factors affecting those with mental illness.
5. Outline the elements of a therapeutic relationship.
6. Identify agencies that serve the mentally ill.

## KEY TERMS

culture of poverty
deinstitutionalization of the mentally ill
professional relatedness
psychotropic medications

seriously mentally ill (SMI)
seriously and persistently mentally ill (SPMI)
staff splitting
stigma of mental illness

## CHAPTER TOPICS

- **Historical Perspective**
- **Significance of Community Mental Health**
- **Nursing Skills and Competencies**
- **Mental Health Assessment**
- **Community Mental Health Agencies and Related Services**
- **Challenges to Successful Implementation**
- **Conclusions**

## Historical Perspective

The earliest ancient civilizations attributed mental illness to possession by evil spirits or having divine or inspirational power. Later (BC) views of mental illness explained the condition as magical, caused by guilt, or created by excessive heat, cold, or moisture. Hippocratic physicians were the first to label symptoms of depression as melancholia caused by the accumulation of black bile.

Further views of mental illness in the Middle Ages included the idea of madness and demonic possession. Witches and midwives were seen as evil members of a dangerous class of sinful women. The overriding view of treatment was that of moral judgment, persecution, and degradation, with the mentally ill seen as social outcasts, living on the fringes of society in jails or poor houses. During the mid-1500s, St Mary's of Bethlehem (Bedlam) was opened to house the insane. People were chained in rat-infested cells, where the public paid 1 penny to see the "loonies." Individuals suffering from mental illness were seen as incompetent and dangerous. They possessed no rights in society.

By the end of the 18th century, there was greater understanding of mental illness, and those who suffered from mental illness were being treated more humanely. Asylums were constructed where actual treatment protocols, however primitive, were in place. Far from anything like today, there remained great stigma, coercion, and degradation of people with mental illness. The first half of the 20th century saw the evolution of modern psychiatry but with continued inhumane institutionalized care.

Two women in nursing known for their progressive awareness of mental illness are Linda Richards and Jane Taylor. Richards, who graduated in 1873, is designated as American's first trained nurse and is also honored as the first psychiatric nurse in the United States. Taylor was the first professor of psychiatric nursing at the Yale School of Nursing in 1926.

Not until the mid-1950s did the first **deinstitutionalization** of the mentally ill occur and a move to community-based mental health services. Unfortunately, many of the clients released from institutions were unprepared to live outside their institutions and were ill served in the community. The deinstitutionalization caused increased stigma for mentally ill persons, but it also forced society to look at the needs of the mentally ill, who were no longer locked away, out of sight.

The 1950s and 1960s brought about other significant changes related to treatment of mental illness. Hildegard Peplau, RN, promoted the "therapeutic use of self" for nurses and brought forth the concept of "Milieu Therapy."

Medication development dramatically changed psychiatric care for the seriously mentally ill (SMI); in 1952, chlorpromazine (Thorazine), the first antipsychotic medication, was introduced. In 1960, haloperidol (Haldol) brought calm and order to the noisy and chaotic psychiatric wards. In 1962, the revolution of treatment of bipolar disorder occurred with the use of lithium. Currently, we are in the midst of yet another era of evolution of psychopharmacologic treatment. The neurotransmission theory has brought about major changes in the medication management of persons with depression and schizophrenia.

The 1970s brought third-party reimbursement for RNs who could bill for counseling services. Following this came prescriptive authority for mental health clinical nurse specialists.

Today, we continue to struggle with placement of our mentally ill, as well as with the stigma of mental illness. We still have hard questions to answer, such as these:

Why are 90% percent of adults with SMI unemployed?

What are the barriers that keep adults with mental illness from productive work and children with serious emotional disturbances from success in school?

Although there have been ad campaigns promoting the awareness of depression and schizophrenia, there remains much to do in terms of progress. The 1999 surgeon general's report addresses these issues, and *Healthy People 2010* further emphasizes mental illness as a major health focus (U.S. Department of Health and Human Services [DHHS], 2000). As nurses in the community at the beginning of the 21st century, we have the unique opportunity to address the mental health needs of our clients through promotion, advocacy, and education.

 ## Significance of Community Mental Health

Historically in Western medicine, the mind and body have been treated as separate entities. It is over time that the mind–body connection has been made and mental and physical functioning are seen as parts of a whole. In the 1990s, much emphasis was placed on research related to mental illness and what constitutes mental wellness. Congress declared the 1990s the "Decade of the Brain," and DHHS published *Healthy People 2010,* declaring mental health among the top 10 leading indicators of health (2000). According to *Healthy People 2010*, in established market economies such as the United States, mental illness is equal to heart disease and cancer as a cause for disability.

Another report by the surgeon general, *Mental Health: Culture, Race and Ethnicity* (DHHS, 2001), ranks mental disorders second only to cardiovascular disease as far as the impact of disability in the United States. The report goes on to state that one third of disabled adults ages 18 to 55 living in the community report having a mental disability.

Suicide, another major public health concern, is most often a consequence of a mental disorder. Approximately 40 million Americans age 18 to 64 years, or 22% of the population, had a diagnosis of a mental disorder or of a co-occurring mental and addictive disorder in the past year. At least one in five children and adolescents between ages 9 and 17 have a diagnosable mental disorder in a given year. An estimated 25% of older people (8.6 million) experience mental disorders. The World Health Organization (WHO) reports that four of the 10 leading causes of disability for people 5 years and older are mental disorders (WHO, 1999). The multitude of risk factors that contribute to mental illness, shown in Box 15–1, speaks to the tremendous challenge in treatment and prevention that must be addressed.

The cost of inpatient mental health treatment has also come to the forefront in the 1990s with a move away from high-cost, hospital-based treatment to community health management and treatment for mental illness. Health insurance and the economic challenges of payment for mental health services, while still lagging behind medical care coverage, is moving toward greater reimbursement of community mental health services. Today, in order to be hospitalized for mental health reasons, one has to be dangerous to themselves or others. All other mental health issues are now dealt with in the community.

The need for community mental health nurses continues to grow. A broad knowledge base and understanding of mental illness becomes the springboard for effective community-based mental health nursing.

 ## Nursing Skills and Competencies

Because of the pervasiveness of mental health issues, nurses working in all settings are called on to have skills and knowledge to work with individuals who have mental health issues. Clients with mental illness are seen in clinics, on every unit in hospitals, often in crisis at hospital emergency rooms, and everywhere in the community.

Knowledge of the major mental illnesses is important in understanding behavior and planning for intervention. A guideline for diagnosis and treatment of mental illness, published by the American Psychiatric Association, is the *Diagnostic and Statistical Manual of Mental Disorders (DSM-IV-TR)*. The manual classifies mental illnesses and provides diagnostic criteria for approximately 300 mental disorders. The diagnostic criteria for several of the major mental illness are listed along with general information relevant to quality nursing care.

A summary of several of the major diagnostic criteria with integration of nursing process information follows.

### Mood Disorders

The mood disorders range from major depressive disorder to acute mania. The definitions used in relation to the mood disorders are as follows:

Major Depressive Disorder: A major mood disorder with one or more episodes of major depression, with or without full recovery

Dysthymic Disorder: Depressed mood with loss of interest or pleasure in activities of daily life

Cyclothymic Disorder: A mood disorder of at least 2 years with numerous periods of mild depressive symptoms mixed with periods of hypomania

Hypomania: Behaviors that are less than manic; a lesser degree of mania

▶ **Box 15–1.**   Risk Factors That Contribute ◀
to Mental Illness

## Emotional Factors

*Self-esteem—many factors can affect one's self-esteem and impact mental health.*
- Developmental factors such as the changes that are experienced in adolescence, and middle and old age
- Relationships that are neglectful and/or abusive
- Body image, how one sees one's physical self (eg, as in anorexia and bulimia)

*General mood*
- Fluctuations in mood such as mania and depression—these are not willful, but are phenomena of mental illness
- Psychological stress
- Multiple unresolved losses

*Attachment/bonding issues*
- Research proves that lack of maternal or paternal attachment in infancy and childhood predisposes children to issues of abandonment.
- Child abuse and neglect

## Biologic Factors

*Neurobiologic and genetic factors*
- Family history of mental illness
- Birth defects
- Low birth weight
- Language disabilities
- Below average intelligence

*Physical health problems with associated mental illness*
- Diabetes/depression
- Heart disease/depression
- Chronic physical illness of any kind/depression

*General physical conditions that predispose to mental illness*
- Traumatic injuries
- Prenatal damage due to diet, chemical abuse, or smoking
- Alcohol and drug abuse

## Relationship/Role Model Factors

- Abuse/neglect
- Assault
- Manipulation
- Abandonment
- Severe family discord
- Overcrowding or large family size
- Paternal criminality
- Maternal mental illness
- Admission to foster care

*(continued)*

▶ **Box 15–1.   Risk Factors That Contribute** ◀
to Mental Illness *(Continued)*

**Support System Factors**

- **Negative**—support systems that are a detriment to functioning
- **Lack of**—inability to develop relationships that are supportive in nature
- **Burn out**—due to the chronic nature of mental illness, families and friends may become exhausted in their ability to provide support. Lack of understanding of why the client can't just "get over it" leads to major frustration and ineffective treatment.

**Environmental Factors**

- **Climate and seasonal changes**—Seasonal Affective Disorder (SAD) is an example of a mental disorder that exists as a phenomenon of seasonal change.
- **Crime**—often mentally ill clients who are chemically dependent will resort to criminal activity such as stealing and prostitution as a means of gaining resources for survival. By virtue of their vulnerability, the mentally ill can also be easy victims of crime.
- **Stigma**—is an unjustifiable mark of shame as a result of misunderstandings and myths about mental illness. Stigma also arises from lack of knowledge about how mental illness occurs and how it can be treated.

**Economic/Financial Factors**

**Economic stress**
**Poverty**
**Homelessness**—The vast majority of our homeless are mentally ill, chemically dependent, or both. For some, the downhill slide into homelessness can in itself lead to symptoms of mental illness. There are numerous clients with bipolar illness and schizophrenia who find themselves homeless because of their mental illness as well as their drug/alcohol addiction used to self-medicate.

**Social Factors**

Racial and ethnic minorities are over-represented among the most vulnerable to be homeless, incarcerated, and have higher rates of mental disorders. Clinicians' inability to speak the language of the minority client and a lack of awareness of cultural issues of mental health in minority populations contribute to the social stigma of mental illness and fear and mistrust of treatment.

Major Depresson → Dysthymia → Cyclothymia → Hypomania → Bipolar I → Bipolar II → Mania

*Figure 15–1.* ▶ The continuum of mood disorders.

Bipolar I Disorder: A major mood disorder characterized by episodes of major depression and mania (requires one or more episodes of mania or hypomania)

Bipolar II Disorder: A major mood disorder with the occurrence of one or more major depressive episodes with at least one episode of hypomania

The continuum of mood disorders (see Fig. 15–1) further defines the dynamic nature of depression and mania.

### Depression

Depression affects approximately 15 million Americans each year. The direct costs for mental health care for those suffering from depression are in the billions of dollars. Other factors to consider are the loss of productivity and the value of lost workdays. As nurses working with clients in a variety of settings, we need to look more closely for signs of depression in clients who present with physical symptoms, particularly chronic symptoms of all kinds, and those who have recently suffered major loss. We need to look at those clients who are chemically dependent and anyone with whom we come in contact who is feeling the effects of oppression or abuse. It is essential that the risk factors for depression (Box 15–2) are considered with each individual cared for, considering the pervasiveness of depression.

The word *depression* has a variety of definitions that can range from feelings of sadness and loss to the symptoms of major depression. The clinical definition of depression goes beyond sadness and seriously affects an individual's functioning and feelings about life and self. In addition, depression has a high rate of co-occurrence with other psychiatric disorders (anxiety disorder, substance-related disorders, eating disorders, and obsessive-compulsive disorder [OCD]), as well as with other general medical conditions such as stroke, diabetes, coronary artery disease, chronic fatigue syndrome, and a history of traumatic brain syndrome.

---

▶ **Box 15–2.  Risk Factors for Depression** ◀

Female gender (twice as likely as men to become depressed)
Weight gain or loss
Chronic illness
Substance use and abuse
Chronic stress (ie, relationship, financial)
Family history of depression
Lack of support systems
A prior episode of depression
Postpartum status
Current or history of physical, sexual, or emotional abuse
Family history of mood disorders and schizophrenia
Recent major losses (spouse, child, job, etc.)

The major indicators of depression are summarized here and are also outlined in Box 15–3. Behaviors include withdrawal, negativism, and unhappiness with self-deprecating, guilty, or self-blaming comments and expressions of hopelessness. The sense of hopelessness that one presents is a defining factor in clinical depression. There is decreased attentiveness to oneself, with decreased energy, an inability to concentrate, and excessive indecisiveness. Additional physical signs are changes in weight or eating patterns, changes in sleep patterns, and changes in sexual interest and activity.

Nursing interventions in depression include an ongoing assessment of behavioral symptoms related to self-care, medication compliance, general well-being, and suicidal thoughts or actions. The nurse should take into consideration a client's limited concentration and reaction time by waiting patiently for answers to questions. The nurse wants to provide positive feedback about a client's seeking help for depression or any improvements in the client's behavior. Try not to be overzealous, but rather calm and supportive. It may be appropriate to offer hope, particularly if you have an ongoing care-giving relationship with the individual, and to acknowledge that you understand the tremendous energy it takes when depressed to just get up in the morning or to get dressed.

Ongoing assessment of suicide is an important aspect of working with the depressed client. To be comfortable with suicide assessment, the nurse must address any misconceptions or fears he or she has about it. Suicidal thoughts or actions can occur at anytime in the course of depression. One important time in the course of treatment that is risky for suicidal clients is when they start on medications and begin to feel some energy. This energy can make them more vulnerable to the risk of acting on a suicidal plan. Awareness of the risk of suicide allows you to set up a safety net for the client during his or her most vulnerable time. The next section addresses further aspects of suicide.

### Suicide

Suicide is a major public health issue. The National Institute of Mental Health (NIMH) identified suicide (in 1999) as the 11th leading cause of death in the United States, and the 3rd leading cause of death among young people ages 15 to 24 years of age. Refer to Box 15–4 for further information on statistics of at-

## ASSESSMENT TOOLS

### Box 15-3   Assessing Behaviors in Major Depression

Individuals with depression may exhibit any or all of the following behaviors:

- A sense of hopelessness
- Depressed mood most of the time
- Loss of interest or pleasure in usual activities
- Changes in weight, either loss or gain
- Inability to concentrate, difficulty focusing or processing information
- Changes in sleep habits, either an increase or decrease in sleep
- Frequent thoughts of death and suicide, with our without a plan or attempt

## ▶ Box 15–4. Suicide Facts ◀

**Completed Suicides, U.S. 1999***

- Suicide was the 11th leading cause of death in the United States.
- It was the 8th leading cause of death for males, and 19th leading cause of death for females.
- The total number of suicide deaths was 30,622.
- The 2001 age-adjusted rate** was 10.7/100,000 or 0.01%.
  - 1.3% of total deaths were from suicide. By contrast, 29% were from diseases of the heart, 23% were from malignant neoplasms (cancer), and 6.8% were from cerebrovascular disease (stroke)—the three leading causes.
  - Suicides outnumbered homicides (20,308) by 3 to 2.
  - There were twice as many deaths due to suicide than deaths due to HIV/AIDS (14,175).
- Suicide by firearms was the most common method for both men and women, accounting for 55% of all suicides.
- More men than women die by suicide. The gender ratio is 4:1.
- Among the highest rates (when categorized by gender and race) are suicide deaths for white men over 85, who had a rate of 54/100,000.
- Suicide was the 3rd leading cause of death among young people 15 to 24 years of age, following unintentional injuries and homicide.
- The suicide rate among children ages 10-14 was 1.3/100,000 or 272 deaths among 20,910,440 children in this age group.

**Attempted Suicides**

- No annual national data on all attempted suicides are available.
Other research indicates that:
  - There are an estimated 8-25 attempted suicides for each suicide death; the ratio is higher in women and youth and lower in men and the elderly.
  - More women than men report a history of attempted suicide, with a gender ratio of 3:1.

---

*1999 U.S. mortality data are based on the International Classification of Disease, 10th revision (ICD-10), whereas ICD-9 has been used for the last several years of mortality data. For this reason, comparisons between 1999 and earlier mortality data should be made carefully. For a full explanation of the implications of this change, see http://www.cdc.gov/ncipc/wisqars/fatal/help/datasources.htm#6.3.

** Age-adjusted rates refer to weighting rates by a population standard to allow for comparisons across time and among risk groups. The 1999 mortality data are calculated using figures from the 2000 census, whereas previous years have been calculated using 1940 census data. For this reason, comparisons between data from years 2000 to 2001 and earlier mortality data should be made carefully. For a full explanation of the implications of this change, see http://www.cdc.gov/ncipc/wisqars/fatal/help/datasources.htm#6.2.

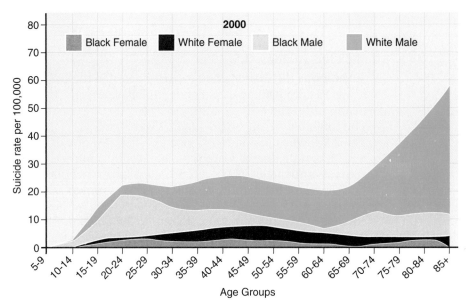

***Figure 15–2.*** ▶ U.S. suicide rates by age, gender, and racial group (retrieved February 7, 2003, from http://www.nimh.nih.gov/research/suichart.cfm.

tempted and completed suicides and Figure 15–2 for U.S. suicide rates by age, gender, and racial group. It is important to consider this information in terms of the risk factors for suicide. In addition, those who are at risk for suicide can suffer from any number of conditions. Persons who suffer from depression, schizophrenia, panic disorder, substance abuse, and chronic medical conditions all are at risk for suicide.

Signs to look for when assessing for suicide risk are recurrent thoughts of or preoccupation with death; ongoing suicidal ideation with or without a plan; a bleak, hopeless attitude toward life; or a sudden change from being depressed to being upbeat or "at peace," which may include preparations for "putting one's house in order." Other major factors are possession of means to commit suicide and a history of or recent suicide attempt.

Suicide is the most difficult and devastating type of death faced by family, friends, health care professionals, and society as a whole. For family and friends, there is overwhelming guilt for not having prevented it. For health care professionals, there is sadness and frustration for not seeing the signs.

As a nurse, the first aspect of assessment for suicide risk that must be understood is that asking someone if he is suicidal does not give him the idea, and it does not make him any more likely to act on suicidal thoughts. In fact, the opposite is true. By asking, "Have you had or are you having thoughts of hurting yourself?" you are giving the client the opportunity to talk about it and ask for help if needed. You may also provide a great sense of relief that someone is willing to talk about the guilt and sadness surrounding thoughts of suicide. If the client states that he or she has suicidal thoughts, the next question to ask is does he or she have a plan. If the client says he or she has a plan, you should ask about the plan, availability of the method, and lethality of the method. For example, a client who plans to shoot himself and owns a gun is at a high immediate risk compared to the client who tells you she wants to overdose but doesn't have the pills to do it. If the client presents with a lethal method and a means, immediate hospitalization may be necessary.

Less lethal means may require a contract for safety in which the client signs a document stating that he will not hurt himself, and if he feels like he will, he will have an alternative plan, such as someone to call or a place to go for help. Box 15–5 lists guidelines for suicide assessment and includes questions to ask. Don't ever feel like you are alone in deciding what steps to take for suicidal behavior. The team approach in community mental health nursing means that you have other professionals whom you can call for consultation and support.

### Mania

The primary symptoms you will observe in manic behavior are any degree of the following: a decreased need for sleep with increased motor activity or agi-

## ASSESSMENT TOOLS

### Box 15–5   Suicide Assessment

**General Questions**
- Are you feeling like you want to hurt yourself?
- Are you feeling like ending it all?
- Do you have thoughts of wanting to end it all?
- Do you ever feel like it would be easier to not go on?
- Does this feel so overwhelming that you do not feel like living?

**Specific Questions**
If there is an answer of yes to any of the above, you want to assess frequency of thoughts and methods:
- How often do you feel this way?
- Have you had any thoughts about how you would end your life?
- What thoughts have you had about ending it all?
- When you feel this way, what do you feel like doing?

**Assess Lethality**
Assess how lethal the methods are and the availability of those methods. Lethality has to do with how easy it is to rescue someone as well as what access he or she has to the means.

| *Highly Lethal Methods* | *Less Lethal Methods* |
| --- | --- |
| Gunshot | Driving into a tree |
| Jumping from a bridge | Taking pills |
| Hanging | Walking out into traffic |

tation, pressured speech, decreased appetite, grandiosity, and impulsivity and focus on pleasurable activities, such as spending large amounts of money or promiscuous sexual behavior. The individual will exhibit a flight of ideas by jumping from one topic to another and will be easily irritated. The client may exhibit an inflated opinion of himself and a loss of normal inhibition. Because of the flight of ideas and impulsiveness, there is a lack of follow-through on meaningful activities. Psychoses may also develop in the form of delusions or hallucinations.

Nursing interventions include providing for safety from self-harm and balanced psychologic and physiologic functioning. The first-line treatment for mania is the use of **psychotropic medication**, including mood stabilizers or anticonvulsants and lithium.

Providing a safe environment with minimal stimulation is also critical. Persons with major manic behavior often need to be hospitalized because of exhaustion and the need to reinstate a treatment plan including medication compliance. Clients in the community who become manic can become extremely resistant to help because of their grandiose and expansive thinking. In addition, clients may be sexually inappropriate; they may speak so loudly and rapidly that it is impossible to get a word in, or they may be bordering on the brink of exhaustion. At any of these times, it will take a team approach that involves mental health professionals as well as other community persons who can collaborate to prevent both self-harm and harm to others. If the person is thought to be a danger to self or others, you may need to call in the police to assist with transport when hospitalization is needed.

Developing and maintaining a working relationship with professionals in the community becomes essential for a good and positive outcome. Recovery for persons with bipolar disorder requires acceptance of the illness and understanding that medication must not be stopped when a manic cycle begins and the client feels "on top of the world." This can be a lifelong learning process for individuals. Prevention of relapse is a primary goal as symptoms become worse and recovery more difficult with each successive relapse.

## Anxiety Disorders

Anxiety is a normal, healthy aspect of living, alerting a person to take action in the face of danger. Someone who is experiencing mild to moderate levels of anxiety may use voluntary coping skills (getting information, avoiding situations, or seeking resources) that will decrease the anxiety (see Table 15–1). If, however, anxiety levels become unmanageable or the person lacks the coping skills to manage the anxiety, he or she may be at risk to develop any of the anxiety disorders.

Some of the more common anxiety disorders are generalized anxiety disorder, panic disorder (with or without agoraphobia), posttraumatic stress disorder (PTSD), and OCD.

### Generalized Anxiety Disorder

Generalized anxiety disorder (GAD) affects about 3% to 4% of the U.S. population, and it primarily affects women. The person experiencing GAD is often on edge and easily fatigued. Chronic worry that causes one to experience irritabil-

**TABLE 15-1. FOUR LEVELS OF ANXIETY**

| Level | Client's Focus |
|---|---|
| **Mild**—Increase in pulse, blood pressure and heart rate | Alert, able to problem solve |
| **Moderate**—Muscle tension, sweating, increased pulse, blood pressure and breathing rate, peripheral vasoconstriction | Attention focused |
| **Severe**—"Fight or flight" responses, dry mouth | Detailed focus very narrow; no learning can occur |
| **Panic**—Continued increase in symptoms | Focus entirely on internal symptoms |

ity, muscle tension, and sleep disturbance is common. Persons with GAD are likely to present with physical symptoms and other disorders, such as major depression, panic disorder, and substance addictions. Clients do not always seek treatment, may not initially admit to feeling anxious, and may suffer for years until their physical symptoms cause them to seek medical attention. Clients with GAD may self-medicate with alcohol, other substances, or prescription medications.

Nursing interventions involve awareness of the behaviors that may indicate an underlying anxiety disorder. This means going beyond the physical symptoms, exploring a client's history, and focusing on the client's anxieties, fears, and concerns. Another aspect of effective nursing intervention in anxiety is awareness of the nurse's own reactions to the anxious client. Anxiety is contagious, and we can easily become excited and anxious, particularly when others are experiencing high levels of anxiety and panic. Awareness involves taking a deep breath and centering awareness on remaining calm. A nurse's ability to be calm and focused can, in itself, be the most effective nursing intervention offered.

### Panic Disorder

The prevalence of panic disorder is about 1% to 2% of the U.S. population, with women being twice as likely to be diagnosed. Diagnosis of panic disorder may be difficult because of symptoms that mimic a variety of medical problems. These clients may present in a hospital emergency room with what they think is a heart attack, when in reality, it is a panic attack.

A panic attack usually lasts for only a short time (minutes) and begins suddenly with intense feelings of fear and impending doom. Symptoms can include shortness of breath, dizziness, palpitations, trembling, light-headedness, abdominal distress, numbness, chest tightness and pain, and a fear of going crazy. The individual can actually be fearful of dying. Panic attacks are time limited, usually reaching a peak within 10 minutes.

After recurrent attacks, there is a pervasive worry of having another and avoidance of the situations in which previous panic attacks occurred. In addition, a person may develop agoraphobia, which is the fear of being in places from which it might be difficult or embarrassing to escape. Common fears involve being in crowd, waiting in a line, or traveling in a car, bus, or plane. If untreated, panic disorder greatly reduces one's quality of life and ability to perform activities of daily living.

Nursing interventions with panic include first determining that it is indeed panic and not a heart attack as the client may believe it is. This will require assessing vital signs and calmly giving guidance and direction. The person in panic has no decision-making skills as all energy is wrapped up in the fear and the symptoms. Calmly talking your client through the panic, knowing that it is time limited, and reassuring and validating what the client is experiencing are all effective interventions.

Those clients who experience panic and agoraphobia may require referral to mental health professionals to manage their symptoms.

### Posttraumatic Stress Disorder

The incidence of PTSD in the general population is about 7%, with 50% of high-risk populations experiencing PTSD. It occurs at all ages and may include symptoms of depression, chemical dependency, and anxiety.

A real and devastating event or events in one's life cause PTSD. Events that are beyond the individual's control, such as natural disasters; sexual abuse; the horrors of war; or being the witness of trauma, mutilation, or death, may cause PTSD. A primary feature of this disorder is that the person continues to reexperience the event by having recurrent, persistent, and frightening thoughts and memories of the experience.

The manner in which people relive their experiences is through nightmares, obsessive thoughts, or flashbacks that occur at random times. Fear and persistent arousal lead to sleep disturbances and hypervigilance with exaggerated startle response that leads to difficulty concentrating and completing tasks. Symptoms of depression, feelings of emotional detachment and emotional numbness, anger, sadness, and rage may also occur.

PTSD is treated with antianxiety and antidepressant medications. Psychotherapy and group therapy are needed for the individual to work through the experience and regain a sense of security. Recovery is variable, with some people recovering within 6 months. For others, PTSD becomes chronic.

Nursing interventions with PTSD require assessment to determine the magnitude of symptoms. Often referral to mental health professionals allows the client options such as medication and individual and/or group therapy.

### Phobias

A phobia is a severe, persistent, and irrational fear of a specific object or situation. The person is generally aware that the fear is unreasonable, but he or she is unable to control it and will do everything he or she can do to avoid the situation or object that triggers the fear. The objects or situations that cause phobias include animals, lightening, public speaking, and crowds. Phobias generally start in childhood and early adulthood and affect approximately 13% of the population, making them the most common type of anxiety disorder.

Treatment includes the use of antianxiety medications and most often behavioral therapy in which the person is exposed to the feared object or experience and is taught to alter his or her responses.

Nursing intervention involves assessment of the disability caused by the phobia and appropriate referral for treatment.

### *Obsessive–Compulsive Disorder*

Persons of all ages and both sexes (approximately 2% of the U.S. population) are affected by OCD. It is most often diagnosed during the teen years or young adulthood, with frequent co-occurrence of depression and panic attacks. In childhood, it may occur with other neurologic disorders.

OCD is characterized by preoccupation with recurrent, ritualistic thoughts or actions that the individual has difficulty controlling. Obsessions are persistent thoughts, impulses, or images that are intrusive and cause anxiety. Compulsions are the uncontrollable repetitive acts used to relieve the anxiety of the obsession. An example is having the obsession that your hands are always contaminated. The high level of anxiety about that contamination causes the compulsive act of hand washing. The person knows that the thoughts of contamination are irrational, and at the same time, he or she is afraid that they are true. Attempts to avoid either the thought or the action as well as interruptions in the ritual lead to great anxiety.

The antidepressant medications clomipramine and fluoxetine have been most effective in the treatment of OCD. Behavioral and family therapy tend to be the most effective modes of nonpharmacologic treatment.

One aspect of nursing care to remember when working with persons with OCD is to never interrupt their compulsions. To tell them to stop or in any way interfere with the compulsive behavior causes greater anxiety and distress. Let them complete what they are doing and then interact. In cases in which daily living is significantly affected, appropriate referral for behavioral or medication treatment is essential.

## Schizophrenia

Schizophrenia is a thought disorder that is characterized by a disturbance in how one thinks, feels, and relates to others and the environment. This disorder affects 2 million people in the United States and remains one of the least understood and least accepted of the mental illnesses. It is now known that schizophrenia is a neurobiological disorder of the brain. This knowledge has led to major advances in the treatment of schizophrenia. Newer antipsychotic medications offer individuals treatment with fewer side effects, which contributes to better compliance and treatment outcomes. The *DSM–IV–TR* diagnostic guidelines for schizophrenia identify nine categories of illness: schizophrenia, schizophreniform disorder, schizoaffective disorder, delusional disorder, brief psychotic disorder, shared psychotic disorder, psychotic disorder due to a general medical condition, substance-induced psychotic disorder, and psychotic disorder not otherwise specified.

The positive symptoms of this illness are any variety of the following: delusions, hallucinations, disorganized speech, and disorganized or catatonic behavior. The negative symptoms of this illness are flat affect, lack of drive to perform, and lack of interest or ability for follow-through. Social and occupational dysfunctions are caused by positive or negative symptoms. Depending on the degree of functioning of the client, community management of the client can involve many facets.

Medication management is a priority, as are housing and economic management. Health issues and safety concerns may need to be addressed in relation to issues of paranoid or delusional thinking, hallucinations, lack of self-care, and vulnerability. Box 15–6 outlines nursing interventions specific to schizophrenia.

## COMMUNITY-BASED NURSING CARE GUIDELINES

### Box 15-6 ▶ Nursing Interventions Specific to Schizophrenia

Clients with schizophrenia may exhibit unusual or bizarre behaviors; they may have very limited communication; and they may demonstrate altered thinking. These behaviors may make developing a therapeutic relationship particularly challenging.

**Interventions for Developing a Relationship**

Approach in a calm, genuine, and accepting manner
- Spend short periods of time with the client, even if they interact very little.
- Demonstrate interest and concern for how the client perceives their illness.
- Speak clearly and distinctly with short sentences and with one thought per sentence.
- Encourage the client to identify and discuss feelings and concerns.

**Ongoing Assessment Factors to Observe**
- Disturbance in the client's thought processes including the presence of hallucinations or delusional thinking
- Response and adherence with medication regimen as well as assessment of side effects from medications
- Behavioral changes in hygiene, isolation or withdrawal, and lack of motivation
- Suicide assessment

## CLIENT SITUATIONS IN PRACTICE

### ▶ Assessing the Mentally Ill Patient

Mary Smith is a 29-year-old woman who has never been married. The history she provides is somewhat vague; however, she says that she comes from the West and that her family is very dysfunctional. She makes several references to rape and her crazy family, but there are no further details offered.

She says that she was diagnosed as bipolar when she was a teenager. Mary was taking lithium for several years, but how long she took it and how much are unclear. She dropped out of school when she was a junior because she says that the voices she was hearing in her head made it too hard to concentrate on her studies. She was diagnosed with schizophrenia and was prescribed Haldol. She took the Haldol for awhile, but because she didn't like the side effects, she was off medications for most of her 20s.

She has seen a doctor in the last month and is currently taking 200 mg of Seroquel. She recently became homeless for a time, but then she was able to find an apartment. I first met Mary in a group for the homeless at our clinic.

### What further information would you pursue?

The issue of being raped would be an important one to consider in terms of when and what degree of assault. The diagnosis of schizophrenia and bipolar disorder would lead to questions about hallucinations or delusions and mood swings, as well as her level of functioning. What symptoms is she having and to what degree are they affecting her?

It would also be important to assess her use of her medication Seroquel. Is she taking it as prescribed? Is she having any side effects? Does she feel it is helping?

On my first community visit to Mary, I found her living in a relatively safe part of the city, in a secure building. Her room was on the top floor, which meant a four-flight walk. Her apartment was a room, about 8 x 10 feet, with a small closet with no door. She had a sink, stove, and refrigerator and two large windows that faced another building about 5 feet away. Mary had many drawings hung on the walls, and she had also painted her windows. She was pleasant and friendly. Mary was dressed in a tee shirt that did not cover her protruding stomach and blue plaid pants. She proceeded to talk about all the things she was planning to tell me and in doing so became disorganized, moving from topic to topic: "I feel great. I'm having a good day. Do you suppose we could get some milk? Could you pray for me? I am joining that rape support group, you know. My refrigerator is working good, and I have bread."

I asked Mary, "Is there any man trying to hurt you now? Are you afraid?" Mary replied, "No, oh, no, I am not dating. There is a nice man down the hall; he helped take out my garbage the other day. How do you like my apartment, isn't it nice? I really want to stay here . . . ."

### What are the major safety issues for Mary?

Mary is proud of having her own apartment, meager as it is. She displays disorganized thinking. The biggest concern is for Mary's vulnerability because she is pleasant and friendly and talks to anyone. Although she appears to have been the victim of sexual assault in the past, her state of mental health does not protect her from sexual assault in the future.

### What behavior would you reinforce?

We decided to take a walk to a nearby grocery store. On our walk back to her apartment, I encouraged Mary to be sure to take her medicine as prescribed and to see me again in 3 days.

### What steps would you take?

Because my visit was on a Friday, I left the crisis line phone number with Mary in case she needed someone over the weekend. On Monday morning, I phoned a service called Early Intervention to get Mary a mental health case manager. I will also make referrals for Mary for day treatment and social programs where she can interact with others safely. After letting her psychiatrist know of my concerns, we arranged for an appointment with Mary and her psychiatrist to reevaluate her medication. My biggest concern for Mary is her vulnerability and her safety.

## Borderline Personality Disorder

Borderline personality disorder is manifested by highly manipulative actions that an individual uses to get his or her needs met. Frequent eruptions of anger are common when expectations are not realized. The client has strong underlying fears of abandonment and exhibits concrete thinking, with all things categorized as being right or wrong, good or bad.

Borderline personality disorder, as with all personality disorders, often becomes evident by the emotions evoked by the client's behaviors. If you are experiencing a strong emotional reaction to a client, feeling angry, frustrated, or agitated, you are possibly dealing with someone with borderline characteristics. Box 15–7 outlines the behaviors.

There is a term called "**staff splitting**" that involves the manipulative behaviors of clients with borderline personality disorder. It occurs when a client with borderline personality disorder pits staff members against each other. An example of this is when a client tells you what a horrible thing another staff member did to him or her, or that you are the only person in the whole world who understands him or her because you are the best nurse to ever live. Secretive feelings about a client, feelings like you are the only one who understands him or her, or staff conflict over how to treat a client are examples of the effects of manipulation by a client with borderline personality disorder. When these issues arise, it is necessary to take a team approach to problem solving. The team's responsibility is that of processing the issues and then planning a cohesive approach to care that involves clear boundaries: which nurse does what, when, and how.

A major safety issue may be the establishment of the behavioral contract. This is a verbal or written agreement between you the caregiver and the individual experiencing self-harming behavior. The contract is most often a written document that can be put in the chart to verify that both you and the client agree on a plan for safety. See Box 15–8 for a summary of nursing interventions and Box 15–9 for guidelines in writing a behavioral contract.

### ASSESSMENT TOOLS

#### Box 15–7   Assessment Criteria for Borderline Personality Disorder

- Highly manipulative actions used to get needs met, with frequent eruptions of anger when expectations are not realized
- Repeated feelings of boredom and emptiness that lead to the seeking out of repeated intense and chaotic interpersonal relationships
- Extremes in emotional reactivity; major mood swings that change from minute to minute, hour to hour, or day to day
- Impulsive behavior that is often self-damaging including cutting, burning, excessive sexual encounters, or binge drinking
- Chronic suicidal behavior such as threats with our without actions and self-mutilating behaviors such as cutting and burning areas of the body

## COMMUNITY-BASED NURSING CARE GUIDELINES

**Box 15–8** ▶ Common Nursing Interventions in Borderline Personality

- Involve all members of the team working with the client to address the manipulative behaviors.
- Approach the client in a therapeutic manner, being non-judgmental in your manner.
- Become aware of your reactions, such as when you are feeling very positive or negative about the client. Observe what client behavior patterns cause your feelings.
- Seek clinical supervision to deal with your feelings.
- Present a direct matter-of-fact approach when setting limits.
- Model appropriate problem-solving behaviors.
- Reinforce appropriate behaviors.
- Be patient, persistent, flexible, and trusting.
- Assist client to delay gratification.
- Contract for behavioral change.

---

▶ **Box 15–9.**  The Client Contract ◀

The client contract is usually a written contract. It is a way of helping the client be accountable for his or her behaviors, particularly in the area of safety.

**Contract for Safety**
1. When I (the client) feel disturbed, I will go to a friend or family's house where I can air my (intense) feelings.
2. I will call the Crisis Center if I can't stop thinking about harming myself.
3. While I'm receiving care, I will refrain from using verbal or physical threats.
4. When I feel like lashing out, I will try to identify other ways to cope, such as
   a. Removing myself from a conflicting situation by going to another room or taking a walk away from the area.
   b. Stepping back and counting to 5 very slowly.

Signed _____
        Client

Signed _____
        Nurse

## Eating Disorders

Anorexia nervosa and bulimia nervosa primarily affect White women in the middle to upper socioeconomic groups in industrialized countries, with typical onset between the ages of 12 and 22. Young women in Western society are vulnerable to these disorders because of the societal emphasis on youth, dieting, weight, and body shape.

The development of eating disorders is believed to have its psychologic base in issues of coping, self-esteem, and perfectionism. The major problem is not with food but rather with issues of self-esteem, control, management of intimate relationships, and developmental expectations. The degree of regulation and use of food are expressions of the individual's difficulty in managing these issues. By focusing on food, the person's time is consumed, so that making decisions and facing the challenges and issues of life can be avoided.

### Anorexia Nervosa

The anorexic client presents with poor self-image, eagerness to please, concrete all-or-none thinking, and extreme perfectionism. As the anorexic loses weight, her fear of fatness increases and she loses her ability to read her body's signals.

The primary goal of treatment for anorexia nervosa is to restore the anorexic to her normal weight. Nutritional rehabilitation, psychosocial intervention, and medication management with use of the selective serotonin reuptake inhibitors (SSRIs), a class of antidepressants, are most often employed with eating disorders in both inpatient and outpatient settings. The family dynamic is an important consideration due to the fact that alcohol or substance abuse, rape, incest, verbal abuse, and neglect are common issues of people with eating disorders.

Nursing interventions revolve around developing a therapeutic relationship that allows for disclosure of the eating disorder and support for ongoing treatment. There are both inpatient and outpatient eating disorder programs. Another intervention strategy is that of obtaining information and referral resources for the client and family and supporting their efforts toward recovery.

### Bulimia Nervosa

People with bulimia tend to be of normal weight and engage in the binge–purge cycle. Bulimic clients are often tense and anxious before bingeing. During bingeing, bulimics feel a temporary sense of relief. Shortly after bingeing, the anxiety begins to mount, and the urge to purge occurs. Purging behavior most often involves vomiting, with a release of tension and a pervasive sense of relief.

The primary goal of treatment for bulimia is to reduce or eliminate binge eating and purging behaviors. As with anorexia nervosa, nutritional rehabilitation and psychosocial interventions are effective.

## Substance Abuse

The economic costs to society of substance abuse exceed $300 billion per year. This number includes alcohol and drug-related loss of productivity as well as drug-related crime. The cost to the individual who is addicted and family members, friends, and society as a whole is immeasurable. When a person becomes addicted, emotional and maturational growth ceases. All actions of the addicted individual are focused on the drug of choice: how to get it, when to use it, how to get more of it. Substance abusers may lose all moral and legal judgment, engaging in behaviors such as prostitution and selling of drugs.

Three major unconscious psychologic defenses are used by persons who are addicted: denial, rationalization, and projection. Denial is the addicted person's insistence that he or she does not have a problem despite concrete evidence to the contrary. Contrary evidence such as driving under the influence (DUI) arrests, missed days of work, and obvious concerns of others are ignored and denied. Rationalization is a means of justifying one's addictive behavior. An example is the statement that "I am not an alcoholic or cocaine addict because I only use on weekends." Projection is the blaming of external forces, such as a nagging wife, stressful job, or impossible boss, as a reason to use and abuse substances. These defenses affect the addicted individual, those who are part of the individual's family and social system, as well as society as a whole. As health care professionals, we must not be afraid to recognize and confront the use of these defenses and educate the individual struggling with substance abuse, as well as the family members about their importance in the dynamics of substance abuse.

Nurses need to be aware of the signs and symptoms of drug and alcohol use and abuse. Addicted persons present in every setting in health care and may present with intoxication or withdrawal at any time. Drug and alcohol withdrawal may lead to a medical emergency in some cases. See Box 15–10 for signs and symptoms of drug and alcohol intoxication and withdrawal.

The symptoms of substance disorders include the consistent use of alcohol or other mood-altering drugs until the client is high or intoxicated, or he or she has passed out. There is the inability to stop or cut down use, despite wishes to do so or negative consequences from use. There is denial that substance use is a problem despite feedback from significant others stating that the abuse is negatively affecting them. The abuse continues despite recurrent and persistent issues with physical, legal, vocational, social, or relationship problems directly related to the chemical use. Addicted individuals also consume a substance in greater amounts and for longer periods than intended.

## Treatment

Recovery and abstinence from drug or alcohol addiction is a lifelong process that requires a complete change in one's life. Old routines that activate drug use and alcoholic behaviors have to be replaced with new and productive patterns of coping. Without the use of the substance, individuals must confront long-standing anger, resentments, and unresolved grief. Changing friends, where one lives, and with whom one socializes are all aspects of the challenges of recovery. Resources for recovery tend to be highly structured with an emphasis on self-awareness, limit setting, group therapy, skill development, and family treatment. They may include behavioral and family therapy and various group therapy options, such as involvement in a social skills group; loss and grief group; developing-structured-support group; mental illness/chemical dependency (MI/CD) group, for those with a dual diagnosis; and self-help groups. Self-help groups such as Alcoholics Anonymous (AA), Cocaine Anonymous, and Narcotics Anonymous use a 12-step program to help the addict develop a different lifestyle and lend support to those in recovery. Box 15–11 lists the 12 steps of AA, providing a road map for recovery and a life of abstinence.

> ▶ **Box 15–10.** Symptoms of Drug and Alcohol ◄
> Intoxication and Withdrawal

All conditions of drug and alcohol intoxication and withdrawal present a medical emergency and may require hospitalization.

- Alcohol Intoxication: impaired judgment, slurred speech, double vision, dizziness, volatile emotional changes, stupor, and unconsciousness

   Alcohol Withdrawal: anxiety, insomnia, tremors, and delirium tremors (DTs), which include confusion and convulsions (a hospital emergency)

- Sedative-Hypnotic and Anxiolytic Intoxication: slurred speech; slow, shallow respirations; cold, clammy skin; weak, rapid pulse; drowsiness and disorientation

   Sedative-Hypnotic and Anxiolytic Withdrawal: anxiety, insomnia, tremors and convulsions that may occur up to 2 weeks after stopping use

- Opioid Intoxication: sedation, hypertension, respiratory depression, impaired function, constipation, and constricted pupils with watery eyes and hypertension

   Opioid Withdrawal: restlessness, irritability, panic, chills, sweating, cramps, watery eyes with dilated pupils, nausea, and vomiting

- Cocaine Intoxication: irritability, anxiety, hyperactivity, hypervigilance, slow and weak pulse, shallow breathing, sweating, and dilated pupils

   Cocaine Withdrawal: agitation, depression, and suicidal ideation; usually requires hospitalization.

- Amphetamine Intoxication: agitation, hyperactivity, and paranoia, dilated pupils, headache, and chills

   Amphetamine Withdrawal: prolonged periods of sleep, disorientation, and major depression

- Hallucinogen Intoxication: bizarre behavior with mood swings and paranoia, nausea and vomiting, tremors, and panic with aggression; and possibly flushing, fever, and sweating

   Hallucinogenic Withdrawal: depression, irritability, and restlessness

 **Mental Health Assessment**

Establishing a framework for mental health assessment is a vital component of working with clients who are at risk. It can be particularly challenging to gather information from a client whose thought processes and communication skills are impaired. You will be called on to be creative and sensitive in your approach. Utilizing a framework such as the one outlined in Box 15–12 can help you stay focused and aware of the basic information that is important to assess.

### Establishing the Therapeutic Relationship

As a community health nurse, the major goal is the establishment and maintenance of the therapeutic relationship. In hospital and clinic nursing, we may see

> ▶ **Box 15–11.** The Twelve Steps of Alcoholics Anonymous ◀

1. Admitted we were powerless over alcohol—that our lives had become unmanageable
2. Came to believe that a Power greater than ourselves could restore us to sanity
3. Made a decision to turn our will and our lives over to the care of God *as we understood Him*
4. Made a searching and fearless moral inventory of ourselves
5. Admitted to God, to ourselves, and to another human being the exact nature of our wrongs
6. Were entirely ready to remove our shortcomings
7. Humbly asked Him to remove our shortcomings
8. Made a list of all persons we had harmed and became willing to make amends to them all
9. Made direct amends to such people wherever possible, except when to do so would injure them or others
10. Continued to take personal inventory and, when we were wrong, promptly admitted it
11. Sought through prayer and meditation to improve our conscious contact with God as we understood Him, praying only for knowledge of His will for us and the power to carry that out
12. Having had a spiritual awakening as the result of these steps, we tried to carry this message to alcoholics, and to practice these principles in all our affairs.

———
Source: Alcoholics Anonymous World Services, Inc.

clients for one or more 8-hour shifts over a week's time, or for a 15-minute clinic visit. As a community health nurse, you may see the client for 1-hour visits, but you may see this client over time for 6 months, a year, or even longer. By being in the community, we have the unique pleasure of meeting the client on his or her turf, which can offer us a much more holistic view of our clients. Two concepts that are vital to this process are partnership and connection.

Partnership means collaborating, mutual relating, and relationship building with the client to effect the best outcome for him or her. To do so, the nurse needs to connect with his or her clients in a trusting, nonjudgmental, and nonconfrontational manner. **Professional relatedness** involves understanding, mutual relating, self-awareness, reliability, and respect for privacy.

The process of understanding involves avoiding imposing one's own will on a client and being open to the client's experience, such as what makes him or her happy, sad, scared, or anxious. Nurses should consider how life is for their clients, what impact their environments have on them, and what relationships they have. What do they care about, and what is their source of joy, fun, and peace? This process of understanding involves the professional responsibility of educating oneself to the culture of those with whom you relate. Culture as we first consider

## ASSESSMENT TOOLS

### Box 15–12 Framework for Mental Health Assessment

**Client Description and Current Life Situation**

Name, age, sex, race, marital status, current employment/means of financial support, current living situation

**Sources of Information**

Client, family, friends, health care worker, other associates

**Presenting Problem**

The major issue/s affecting the client at this time

**Current Functioning**

Mental status including appearance and self-care, attention, concentration, orientation, relating through eye contact and facial expression, thought content, delusions, hallucinations, preoccupations
   Ability to have insight and judgment
   Stressors, coping ability, and supports

**History Including Mental Health History**

Developmental, familial, and social history
Issues of trauma, losses, and abuse

**Physical Health**

Current health and significant health history

**Current Medications**

Psychotropic and other medications; known drug allergies; use of alternative substances

**Chemical Health**

Current use, history of use, history of chemical dependency treatment, family history

---

it may involve one's ethnic origin. Chapter 3 provides information on the topic of culture. It also may be important to learn about the culture of poverty as many of our clients may be in poverty. See Box 15–13 for additional information on the culture of poverty.

Self-awareness involves being aware of what one does not know as well as being aware of oneself. Part of making assumptions is the process of not knowing or being aware. By making assumptions, we block reality and awareness, thinking that we know what our clients need and want without asking them. In terms of oneself, we need to be aware of our personal language and expression. Professional self-awareness is the act of self-reflection, as well as the humble act of being open to learning, to the environment, and to the impact that we as professionals have on our clients.

Mutual relating means being flexible and open in our approach, being honest, relating on the client's level, having a sense of humor, and using self-disclosure appropriately. This does not mean disclosing private and personal information, but rather, it involves sharing common ground such as hobbies or interests.

---

## ▶ Box 15–13.  Culture of Poverty ◀

It is essential to understand ethnic origins as well as class origins. Because so many of our mentally ill clients live in poverty, it becomes essential to understand the culture of poverty. Many nurses who serve mentally ill clients come from middle-class backgrounds and may have difficulty understanding why their clients act the way they do. There are norms within the three economic classes: wealthy, middle class, and poor. We need to understand our origins and expectations as a basis for understanding the different classes.

**Social Values of the Wealthy**

Political connections
Investment of money
Prestige

**Social Values of the Middle Class**

Work/getting ahead
Order/cleanliness
Responsibility

**Social Values of the Poor**

Survival/making it day to day
Relationships

**Characteristics of Poverty**

Jobs are about getting enough money to survive, not about climbing a career ladder
Academic achievement is not prized
Belief that fate and destiny exist over the consideration of choice
Polarized, concrete thinking where options are not considered and everything is right or wrong, black or white
Time orientation is on the present, with the focus on now
Little or no consideration of future consequences

*(continued)*

▶ **Box 15–13.** Culture of Poverty *(Continued)* ◀

**Implications for Nurses**

It becomes our ethical responsibility to not judge others based on our social values. We must educate ourselves and learn the values of the people with whom we serve. The following example illustrates this point:

When your client spends all her money the day she receives it with no consideration for the month's rent due in 2 weeks (present time orientation), has a messy disorganized home that is noisy (part of the chaos of crisis living), continually makes excuses for her children's misbehavior (because maintaining a relationship with her son is most important, and who knows better than she about her son's behavior), you will understand that she is operating out of the values of her class. And you will become aware of your middle class values that are in direct conflict because it is out of the question to not save your money to pay rent (responsibility with future orientation), your apartment is most often clean, organized, and quiet (order and cleanliness values), and you always hold your children accountable for their misbehavior (Who's responsible? Holding son accountable).

---

Adapted from Bridges Out of Poverty.

---

## CLIENT SITUATIONS IN PRACTICE

### ▶ Developing a Trusting Nurse–Client Relationship

I was working with Dottie, who was very quiet and was considered "treatment resistant" by our team. Dottie had been a resident of the local homeless shelter for more than a year, but until recently, no one really knew anything about her. Dottie would come and go and did not engage in any outreach efforts. Being the new kid on the block, I was appointed to try to see what I could do to connect with her. After a couple of meetings with Dottie, I learned that she liked to knit, but she had always wanted to crochet and had never learned. I asked her if she would mind if I brought a crochet hook and some yarn to our next meeting, and she said that would be fine. I taught her how to crochet, and in the period of several weeks, we talked and she opened up to tell me about the tragic loss of three of her family members to a man who robbed their home when she was 15, the physical and sexual abuse that she endured in her first marriage, and the loss of her grandmother, who was her main support and friend.

---

 ## Community Mental Health Agencies and Related Services

Community support services are public and privately funded resources to assist persons who are **seriously and persistently mentally ill (SPMI)** and SMI. The resources promote mental health, prevent mental illness, and serve the needs of the mentally ill. Some of the services provided include crisis intervention, mental health treatment, case management, advocacy, and supportive services for living and working. Three areas of support, including community mental health agencies, housing, and human needs support, are discussed here.

Community mental health agencies are funded primarily through public dollars and offer a variety of services. As a community mental health nurse, you may be employed by one of these agencies and refer any variety of services to your clients. If you are not connected to an agency through employment, it is important that you learn what community mental health agencies exist, what services they offer, and how they can best serve your clients. Some of the following services are offered through community mental health agencies:

Individual psychotherapy

Group therapy

Mental health assessment, diagnosis, and treatment

Chemical health assessment, diagnosis, and treatment

Medication management

Vulnerable adult protection

## Housing

Housing options can be battered women's shelters, homeless shelters, halfway houses, transitional housing, and supportive housing. Shelters for battered women offer safety to women and their children who are in abusive living situations. These shelters offer services to both mothers and their children, including school transportation and case management for women seeking safe housing. Homeless shelters are of two kinds: overnight shelters with check-in from 5:00 to 8:00 pm and checkout by 7:00 am to 24-hour shelters where people can stay in during the day. Halfway houses and transitional housing are both temporary housing but are generally longer-term living situations than shelters for persons who are not ready to live independently. Supportive housing is long-term housing that offers intensive case management to clients who are unable to live independently. This type of housing is ideal for persons with chronic mental illness who are unable to live independently or with family support. The greatest difficulty with housing services is the acute shortage of supportive housing options available for people with mental illness.

## Human Needs Support

Human support services for the mentally ill include self-help groups, clothes closets, food shelves, services to immigrants and victims of abuse and crime, legal assistance, job training and placement, education programs, advocacy programs, and programs for ex-offenders. It is your responsibility when working with mentally ill clients in the community to become knowledgeable of the resources offered in your community. Once you know the resources, you are able to refer clients when appropriate as well as knowing when you need to go outside of your community to get what is needed. More than likely, you will experience frustration with lack of services; this can be your opportunity to work to effect political awareness and change.

## Challenges to Successful Implementation

The decade of the 1990s brought with it both federal and state resources that focused on the study of the brain in terms of the development and implementation of magnetic resonance imaging (MRI), positron-emission tomography (PET), and computed tomography (CT). These technologies have contributed to the understanding and validation of mental illness, but there is more to be done.

As is outlined in the *Healthy People 2010,* which lists objectives for mental health, the overriding goal is to improve mental health and ensure access to appropriate, quality mental health services (DHHS, 2000). The 14 objectives developed to accomplish this goal by 2010 are found in Box 15–14.

The *Healthy People 2010* objectives for mental health clearly speak to the major mental health issues facing life in the United States at this time. We as professional nurses need to advocate for mental health legislation that promotes the well-being of our clients. Affordable housing as well as structured housing options for our clients is a must. Insurance coverage for mental health services and manageable copays for medications are all-important issues.

Another challenge to successful implementation of community mental health is the current nursing shortage, as well as the challenge posed by working in the community. The independent nature of community mental health nursing is not for every nurse. The fears of being out in the community, outside the constraints of a hospital or clinic, can be frightening. The individuals with whom we work can live in areas of poverty where it is not always safe. Those with mental illness may be violent.

Another major challenge to community mental health nursing can be the lack of facilities for referrals, decreases in funding with cuts in services, and heavy caseloads. There is a need for teamwork and trust among team members that, if missing, makes this work very, very difficult.

Despite the multitude of obstacles facing community mental health nursing today, there is no more exciting area in which to work. The federal government is setting mental health as one of its priorities, and the 21st century has once again brought deinstitutionalization to the forefront, moving the mentally ill back into the community. This is both an exciting and challenging time for community mental health nursing as more people are served in the community. We as nurses are better able to know these clients holistically and within the context of their lives and their stories.

## Conclusions

The evolution of mental health care has exploded in the last 2 decades. Understanding the origins of mental illness has contributed to major breakthroughs in medication management and treatment. These advances have also helped to eliminate some of the myths about mental illness. Essential to good care are strong communication skills that allow for flexibility and acceptance of a variety of behaviors. The magnitude of mental illness lends itself to assessment in every setting where a nurse is employed. As nurses, we must be able to look beyond the physical issues and consider our clients' stories and how they are coping. The gift of relationship is what community mental health nursing is all about. Being in a relationship with our clients, their families, and other mental health professionals, we are able to collaborate and achieve the best possible outcome for our client's mental health.

# HEALTHY PEOPLE 2010

Box 15–14   **Objectives for Mental Health**

MENTAL HEALTH STATUS IMPROVEMENT
1. Reduce the suicide rate.
2. Reduce the rate of suicide attempts by adolescents.
3. Reduce the proportion of homeless adults who have serious mental illness.
4. Increase the proportion of persons with serious mental illnesses who are employed.
5. Reduce the relapse rates for persons with eating disorders, including anorexia nervosa and bulimia nervosa.
6. Increase the number of persons seen in primary health care who receive mental health screening and assessment.
7. Increase the proportion of children with mental health problems who receive treatment.
8. Increase the proportion of juvenile justice facilities that screen new admissions for mental health problems.
9. Increase the proportion of adults with mental disorder who receive treatment.
10. Increase the proportion of persons with co-occurring substance abuse and mental disorders who receive treatment for both disorders.
11. Increase the proportion of local governments with community-based jail diversion programs for adults with serious mental illnesses.

STATE ACTIVITIES
12. Increase the number of states and the District of Columbia that track consumer satisfaction with the mental health services they receive.
13. Increase the number of states, territories, and the District of Columbia with an operational mental health plan that addresses cultural competence.
14. Increase the number of states, territories, and the District of Columbia with an operational mental health plan that addresses mental health crisis interventions, ongoing screening, and treatment services for elderly persons.

Source: U.S. Department of Health and Human Services (2000). *Healthy people 2010: Understanding and improving health* (Chapter 18). Washington, DC: U.S. Department of Health and Human Services, Government Printing Office.

(www.who.int/whr/1999/en/report.htm)

# What's on the Web

The American Psychological Association (APA)
**Internet address:** _http://apa.org_
This professional and scientific organization for the practice of psychology has several brochures and fact sheets for consumers and health professionals. Write or call APA Public Affairs, 750 First Street, NE, Washington, DC 20002–4242; (899) 374-3120.

The National Alliance for the Mentally Ill (NAMI)
**Internet address:** _http://www.nami.org_
This site has a medical information series that provides clients and families with information on several mental illnesses and their treatments. NAMI state affiliates provide emotional support and can help find local services. Find your local NAMI on the Web site under State and local NAMIs.

The National Institute of Mental Health (NIMH)
**Internet address**: _http://www.nimh.nih.gov_
This site offers information and publications on all the mental health disorders. Contact the Information and Resources and Inquiries Branch, NIMH, Room 7C–02, MSC 8030, Bethesda, MD 20892-8030; (800) 421-4211.

The National Mental Health Association (NMHA)
**Internet address:** _http://www.nmha.org_
The NMHA publishes information on a variety of mental health issues. NMHA also provides referrals and support. Write or call the NMHA Information Center, 1021 Prince Street, Alexandria, VA 22314-2971; (800) 969-6642.

## References and Bibliography

American Psychiatric Association. (2000). _Diagnostic and statistical manual of mental disorders_ (4th ed., text rev.). Washington, DC: Author.

Armstrong, E. (1999). Role of the community nurse in caring for people with depression. _Nursing Standard. 13_(35), 40–44.

Beebe, L. H. (2002). Problems in community living identified by people with schizophrenia. _Journal of Psychosocial Nursing and Mental Health Services, 40_(2), 38–45,52–53.

Chan, S., Mackenzie, A. Tin-Fu, D., & Leung, J. K. (2000). An evaluation of the implementation of case management in the community psychiatric nursing service. _Journal of Advanced Nursing, 31_(1), 144–156.

Coombs, R. (2000). Home front. . . community psychiatric nursing. _Nursing Times, 96_(23), 5406.

Edwards, D., Burnard, P., Coyle, D. Fothergill, A., & Hannigan, B. (2001). A stepwise multivariate analysis of factors that contribute to stress for mental health nursing working in the community. _Journal of Advanced Nursing, 36_(6), 805–813.

Friend, B. (1999). Community spirit . . . community psychiatric nurse. _Nursing Times, 95_(47), 69–72.

Godin, P. (2000). A dirty business: Caring for people who are a nuisance or a danger. _Journal of Advanced Nursing, 32_(6), 1396–1402.

Herz, M. I., & Marder, S. R. (2002). _Schizophrenia, comprehensive treatment and management._ Philadelphia: Lippincott Williams & Wilkins.

Hughes, H. (1999). Follow-up after an attempted suicide. _Nursing Times, 95_(46), 50–51.

Jordon, S., Hardy B, & Coleman, M. (1999). Medication management: An exploratory study into the role of community mental health nurses. _Journal of Advanced Nursing, 29_(5), 1068–1081.

Jordon, S., & Hughes, D. (2000). Learning curve. Community teamwork is key to monitoring the side-effects of medication. _Nursing Times, 96_(15), 39–40.

Kaminski, P., & Harty, C. (2000). Ignorance is not bliss . . . tackling the problems of stigma associated with mental illness. *Nursing Times, 96*(2), 28–29.

Long, A., Baxter, R. (2001). Functionalism and holism: Community nurses' perceptions of health. *Journal of Clinical Nursing, 10*(3), 320–329.

Marland, G. R., & Sharkey V. (1999). Depot neuroleptics, schizophrenia and the role of the nurse: Is practice evidence based? A review of the literature. *Journal of Advance Nursing, 30*(6), 155–162.

McCann, T. V., & Baker, H. (2001). Mutual relating: Developing interpersonal relationships in the community. *Journal of Advanced Nursing, 34*(4), 530–537.

Nehls, N. (2000). Being a case manager for persons with borderline personality disorder: Perspectives of community mental health center clinicians. *Archives of Psychiatric Nursing, 14*(1), 12–18.

Payne, R. K., DeVol, P., & Smith, T. D. (2001). *Bridges out of poverty, strategies for professionals and communities.* Highland, TX: Aha! Process, Inc.

Ross, T., Pollock, L., & Tilly, S. (1998). Community psychiatric nurse: What does it mean? *Mental Health Nursing, 18*(1), 10–14.

Struthers, J. (1999). An investigation into community psychiatric nurses' use of humor during client interactions. *Journal of Advanced Nursing, 29*(5), 1197–1204.

U.S. Department of Health and Human Services and National Institutes of Health. (1999). *Mental health: A report of the surgeon general.* Rockville, MD: Author. Retrieved from www.surgeongeneral.gov/substanceabuse

U.S. Department of Health and Human Services. (2000). *Healthy people 2010: Understanding and improving health* (Chapter 18). Washington, DC: U.S. Government Printing Office. Retrieved from www.health.gov/healthypeople/Document/

U.S. Department of Health and Human Services. (2001). *Mental health: Culture, race and ethnicity—A supplement to mental health: A report of the surgeon general.* Rockville, MD: U.S. Department of Health and Human Services, Substance Abuse and Mental Health Services Administration, Center for Mental Health Services. Retrieved from www.surgeongeneral.gov/substanceabuse

# LEARNING ACTIVITIES

## JOURNALING: ACTIVITY 15–1

In your clinical journal, discuss a situation you have encountered in one of your clinical experiences with a client who is having difficulties with a mental illness.
- Describe your feelings and reactions to what you see and hear.
- Reflect on your preconceptions and compare them to what you see when working with individuals with mental illness.
- What was the most important thing you learned about mental illness?

## JOURNALING: ACTIVITY 15–2

Contact a community mental health center in your community and find out about the volunteer opportunities available for a nursing student. When you have found something that appeals to you, volunteer for a month, several months, or longer. Keep a journal about your experiences as a volunteer.

### PRACTICAL APPLICATION: ACTIVITY 15-3

Visit a homeless shelter and meet the staff to discuss the issues and services available for the homeless.

### PRACTICAL APPLICATION: ACTIVITY 15–4

With a group of students, assist with the serving of a meal in a homeless shelter. Before you go, identify an article in a nursing journal about homelessness, poverty, or mental illness and homelessness. While at the shelter, have at least one interaction with one of the people you are serving (eg, ask someone if you can sit down and have a cup of coffee and visit with him or her.) After the interaction, discuss the following:

- What are your feelings and reactions to what you said and heard?
- What did you expect that this experience would be like, and what did you actually experience?
- What did you learn from speaking to the person with whom you interacted?
- What evidence of mental illness, if any, did you see in any of the residents at the shelter?
- Discuss the article you read and how it relates to what you saw.
- Identify the most important thing you learned during this experience.

### PRACTICAL APPLICATION: ACTIVITY 15–5

Contact a mental health nurse working in a community setting. Interview him or her and ask the following questions:

- What are your primary responsibilities as a nurse in this setting?
- What are the challenges and benefits of this type of work?
- What are the goals and missions of your agency?
- Would you recommend this type of work to a new graduate?
- What kind of additional education would be beneficial in preparation for doing this type of work?

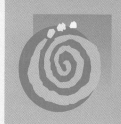

# IMPLICATIONS FOR FUTURE PRACTICE

**A**ny nurse, whether he or she has practiced for years or is just entering the profession, needs to think ahead. What are the implications for the future in community-based nursing care? How can you best prepare yourself to give quality care in your future practice?

Chapter 16 reviews current health care practice and anticipated future trends. The role of the nurse in the future, including educational preparation and advanced practice nursing, is discussed at length. Cost containment will remain a prominent deciding factor in health care delivery, but it must also be weighed in relation to the client's receiving quality care. The implications of technologic development and the information age, and their profound impact on everyday nursing care, are discussed. All of these trends are considered in light of the shift in demographics in the United States.

With a knowledge base of basic concepts, development of skills, and an understanding of how to apply this knowledge and skill to community-based nursing care, you will be ready to practice as a nurse of the present and future.

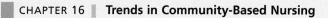

CHAPTER 16 | **Trends in Community-Based Nursing**

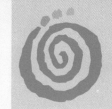

# CHAPTER **16**

# Trends in Community-Based Nursing

Roberta Hunt

## Trends in Health Care

Forces affecting health care in the future will also affect the role of the nurse. One can only speculate about what that future will be. According to Lindeman (2000), some broad changes can almost certainly be predicted in the future of health care, including the following:

▶ Emphasis on cost containment resulting from market-driven economic policy
▶ Advancements in technology
▶ Knowledge explosion
▶ Demographic shifts

Schools of nursing will have to revamp their curricula to meet these changing requirements. Content related to cost containment will be essential. It will be a given that nurses are technologically competent. This means not only computer competent, but also able to keep up with new ways of accessing and using information. The knowledge explosion requires that nurses develop skills in evaluating the legitimacy, efficacy, and importance of information and new treatments. All of these changes will occur within the context of changing demographics as nurses care for a population that is older, more diverse, and living with more chronic conditions.

This chapter discusses trends and concerns about current and future health care that concern nursing care, cost containment, technologic development, the knowledge explosion, alternative therapies, and shifting demographics. These components are addressed within the context of community-based care.

**The Future of Nursing Care**

Several broad competencies will be demanded of nurses in practice in the 21st century. These include critical thinking and clinical judgment skills, effective organizational and teamwork skills, service orientation and cost awareness, accountability for clinical outcomes and quality of care, continuous improvement of health care, population-based approaches to care, an ethic of social responsibility, and commitment to continual learning and development (Bellack & O'Neil, 2000).

Nurses must be prepared to use critical thinking skills to solve problems and make decisions regarding care. They must also be able to make independent clinical judgments. They must be knowledgeable about making age-appropriate referrals to other disciplines and community agencies. Role responsibilities in community-based settings require a mutual decision-making model as nurses work with clients and families.

Because clients will be more ill when they are discharged home, nurses must be more technically advanced in their skills and adept at detailed documentation to ensure payment for services. The need to care for the acutely ill client in an isolated home environment creates an autonomous practice mode for home care nurses. The future will bring a need for competent, skilled nursing practitioners who are comfortable with practicing independently.

Flexibility will be important because cost-containment measures require decreased specialization. Some predict that current demands for care will lead to a decrease in specialization. Administrators are introducing multiskilled health care providers who are cross-trained to practice in a "seamless care" environment, in which practitioners provide care in different facilities or settings. With the trend away from specialization of health care personnel, nurses will be called on to perform more tasks and to cross discipline lines. In home care nursing, this is evidenced by nurses doing venipunctures (a laboratory technician's role) and teaching and monitoring administration of oxygen (a respiratory therapist's role). To prepare for the home care role, nurses must be competent as managers of care and teachers of self-care.

Nurses must become involved in the political, legislative, and regulatory processes of government. Nurses should not only know who their elected congresspeople and senators are, but also educate these officials about research findings so the officials can positively affect future legislation on health care reform (Fig. 16–1). Our profession has made major progress in two of these areas. The issue of delegating duties to nonlicensed personnel has been addressed and continues to need clarification. Today, advanced practice nurses (APNs) can bill directly through Medicare and in most states can prescribe medication.

## Unlicensed Assistive Personnel Performing Nursing Functions

Decreased specialization has resulted in the increased use of **unlicensed assistive personnel** (UAP) for some duties formerly assigned only to RNs. As a cost-containment strategy, many acute care settings are reducing the number of RNs and increasing the number of UAP (Spencer, 2001; Kido, 2001). This change in the composition of the work force, with employees crossing disciplines to deliver care, is a clearly emerging trend. However, the cost savings produced by using more nonprofessional employees and fewer professional staff is not well documented.

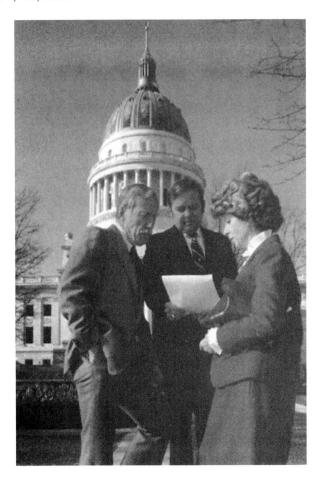

***Figure 16–1.*** ▶ Nurses are invaluable sources of health care information for legislators.

There is, and will be in the future, a danger of liability for the nurse supervising UAP. Chapter 7 covered the importance of the nurse following proper standards for delegation. Increasing use of UAP for nursing functions has caused a great deal of controversy. Nursing professionals may benefit from embracing a flexible position in regard to this issue.

In some communities, lay workers functioning as UAP form the critical link between the underserved or high-risk populations and the formal health care system. Nurses have partnered with community members to identify, support, and provide training and consultation to lay health workers who are members of the community and committed to assisting themselves and their neighbors through outreach networks. In this way, nurses can significantly impact barriers to health care, increase accessibility of needed services, and thus improve the health status of the community (Craven & Hirnle, 2000, p. 28).

## Educational Preparation and Advanced Practice Nursing

If current trends continue, future nurses will perform a wider range of responsibilities. This will require both increased knowledge and skill. For example, community-based care demands a more proficient and autonomous practitioner. The current number of nurses educated at each level of preparation does not support this growing demand. Fifty-two percent of all new nurses graduate from an associate degree program; 44% receive baccalaureate degrees and 4% from hospital-based programs (U.S. Department of Health and Human Services [DHHS], 2000b). The need for nurses with a baccalaureate degree will exceed the supply in the first 2 decades of the 21st century.

Nurse practitioners began to appear in the United States and Canada in the late 1960s in response to a limited supply of physicians. Nurse practitioners most often provide primary care and diagnoses and treat common diseases and injuries. They prescribe medications in all states and Canada.

Currently, there is a great deal of support for APNs or RNs with specialty training at the master's degree level to provide primary care. During the early 1990s, state laws broadened the authority of nurse practitioners by allowing prescriptive authority and third-party billing. As a result, nurse practitioners can establish independent practices paralleling those of primary care physicians.

As early as the 1980s, studies have shown that when comparing the same type of clients, nurse practitioners have as good or better outcomes as physicians. These studies are discussed in Chapter 12.

Specialty areas of nurse practitioners include adult, gerontologic, neonatal, occupational, pediatric, psychiatric, school or college student, and women's health. Nurse practitioners work in both rural and urban areas, from rural North Dakota to New York City. They practice in diverse settings such as community health centers, hospitals, college student health clinics, physician offices, nurse practitioner offices, nursing homes and hospices, home health care agencies, and nursing schools.

There is an established need for practitioners with an interest in research and advanced practice at the master's and doctoral levels. Nursing administrators must be educated and trained in management, finance, and the economic and social implications of our changing population as it affects the health care system.

Trends call for all nurses to be well prepared for the practice roles of today and tomorrow. Nurses must view education as an ongoing process, not limited to a job entry degree. Continuing education is essential as the care delivery system demands more education, including baccalaureate, graduate, and postgraduate degrees. In most areas of the country, the curriculum at each level lays the groundwork for the next level of education, facilitating ongoing nursing education.

##  Cost Containment

The U.S. health care system is the most expensive in the world, using 14% of the gross national product (GNP), yet the country ranks 24th in terms of healthy life expectancy (World Health Organization, 2000). Every industrialized nation except the United States has a national health plan in place that covers all citizens. However, in the United States, health care is not a right but a commodity available to those who can purchase it, sold as a part of a **market-driven economy.** In a market-driven economy, consumer demand drives production regarding what services will be created and consumed and in what quantity. Keeping costs down and profits up is always a key aspect of a market-driven economy. Managed care has increasingly become an important provider of care because its central element is cost containment. Thus, cost containment as an important element of health care is here to stay. Consequently, nurses must continue to be aware of the financial aspects of the work they do, whatever the setting or position, now and in the future.

Cost-containment concerns have resulted in several specific trends in nursing:

- A shift in the provision of nursing care from the acute care setting to the home and community
- Increased need for nurses to be technologically and transculturally competent
- Increased use of nonprofessional caregivers for roles and responsibilities formerly restricted to the practice of RNs
- Increased use of APNs as primary care providers

 ## Technology and Information

### Technologic Development

The health care system of the future will be driven by technology and information. Technology is the tool to extend human abilities. Technology will be used to manage information and make decisions about care. Such technology may include medications, procedures, devices, and electronically based systems that support care delivery. Already clients are wearing programmable medication administration pumps. Nurses will need to program and troubleshoot such machines. These models will evolve constantly. The most promising advances are those related to high-speed telecommunications and portable computers. At present, it is possible to link a desktop computer to a modem and standard telephone line to transmit radiographs, computed tomography images, electrocardiograms, electroencephalograms, and health histories instantly. The potential for improving continuity is obvious. Table 16–1 describes some of the new technologies relevant to nursing care.

Several trends are shaping technology in health care. One trend is that of globalization. This started at the beginning of the 20th century with the invention of the telephone and was expanded at the end of the 20th century with the creation of the Internet. Gradually, the world's borders have dissolved as the world has become one. Thanks to telephones, telecommunications, and telemedicine, nurses are now able to practice across geographic and national borders. Physicians and health care organizations are using globalization to export expertise, a practice that has accelerated because of concerns for cost and profit. Through the construction of systems, health care providers, intermediaries, and consumers are able to collaborate and share information. Further, through technology, we now have the capability to maintain comprehensive health care databases for creating disease management programs and clinical protocols. In addition, through telemedicine and remote-monitoring technologies, health care providers are able to access health information 24 hours a day, 7 days a week (Elfrink, 2001).

For the last 4 decades, clients have been aggressively treated for acute episodes of illness. We have enhanced this capacity through technology. Although "recovery" from an acute situation may result in a long-term chronic condition, technologic assistance is continuing to be developed to enhance care for the rest of a client's life. What occurred in the intensive care unit yesterday may occur at home tomorrow. With the increase in available technology, care can be provided at an ever-higher level of sophistication in the home. If respirators, intravenous therapy, and home dialysis are now common, what will technology allow in the future? It is

---

**TABLE 16–1** • Emerging Technologies for Nursing

| Technology Description | Implications |
|---|---|
| Computer-Based Patient Records—a multimedia archive includes free text, high-resolution images, sound, video and elaborate coding. | This type of system could alert clinicians to patient specific problems and medication, eliminate the problem of illegible notes and prescriptions, streamline the reimbursement and billing process, suggest supplementary patient education materials and reduce staffing needs. It can ensure that clinicians have the quality information needed to make the right decision at the right time |
| Internet and Intranets can be used for client health education, access to patient self-testing, appointments and medication renewal. For health care providers its uses include job posting, and insurance functions. | Internet prescription renewal and appointment making capacity have a long way to go before they can be widely implemented. First issues of privacy, security, confidentiality and validity have to be addressed. |
| Clinical decision making systems are defined in several ways, but all of them empower clinicians through access to expert knowledge, supporting research, and managing administrative complexity. These systems have been documented as the single most important tool for improving the quality of health care. | Organizations must decide which type of clinical decision making system is best for them. The technical and organizational infrastructures must be in place for this type of technology to be effective. |

Adapted from Ball, M. & Lillis, J. (2000). Health information systems: challenges for the 21t century. *AACN Clinical Issues, 11*(3), 386-395.

---

anticipated that advancements in technology will improve the quality and efficiency of client care, raise the general health care status of the nation's population, and reduce the overall cost of health care.

## Knowledge Explosion

The **knowledge explosion** has produced what is often referred to as the information age. Major scientific developments have been occurring so quickly that knowledge overload is common. In the past, clients and families have consulted their nurses, nurse practitioners, or physicians for information regarding health and illness. The health care provider has carried that information in his or her head or has known where to go to explore the question. Now, an almost infinite amount of information is available to anyone who is computer literate. This causes difficulty for the consumer as well as the health care provider. Not only is the amount of information overwhelming, but also it is difficult to discern what is outdated, incorrect, or unproven information and what is not. Therefore, it is important for the health care provider and the consumer to realize that being information literate is an ongoing process (Candy, 2000).

Genetics is one area in which the information explosion is particularly evident. Because of the completion in 2000 of part of the Human Genome Project, which has mapped the human genetic code, treatments will be possible that were not even considered within the realm of possibility 10 years ago. For example, **pharmacogenomics** is the technology of developing and producing medications tailored to specific genetic profiles. The physician or nurse practitioner would give a genetic blood test that would indicate which medication was right for each person. Biotech companies are developing blood tests that reveal disease–gene mutations that forecast an individual's chances of developing a certain condition or disease (Brown, 2000; Henry, 2001).

## Nursing Implications

Computer technology has freed the nurse from some paperwork, allowing more time for client care and teaching about self-care. The expanding implementation of computer-based client records allows the preservation of a client's history from birth to death.

Automation in home care is viewed as a way to improve efficiency. Recent developments in information technology offer a variety of alternatives for documentation. For instance, the use of handheld computers for field staff is a growing trend. Here, the practitioner inputs clinical, financial, and administrative data, and the system produces appropriate reports and forms. These systems are capable of redefining the data content, structure, and preconceptions about clinical information, client assessment, care planning, and care delivery. Nurses chart information directly on a terminal or laptop computer with no need for writing copious notes, charting from memory, or carrying around stacks of papers. Data entry is done through the keyboard, mouse, touch screen, voice activation, bar code, or pen touch. The system can alert nurses about inconsistencies in the data or the need to collect more information, generate a time-based report, or create a task list for each client. A growing number of manufacturers produce this developing technology that integrates data with a central system, facilitates the tracking of specific costs, and allows the client to interact with the system and retrieve information regarding care.

Imagine working as a home health care nurse, transmitting pertinent diagnostic data directly to the attending physician and having a three-way interaction with the client, physician, and nurse instantly. It has become common for nurses to electronically connect with client databases to obtain information from the client's complete nursing, medical, diagnostic, medication, and treatment history. Nurses are also able to order on-line prescriptions or home care equipment.

As a result of the explosion in information, people have access to near-infinite amounts of information. Many diagnostic kits will become available in the consumer market. The nurse may be called on to interpret or explain the results. Misinformation and misunderstanding by the consumer may be possible, which will require another service of the nurse (Hupfeld, 2000).

Are educational programs for nurses preparing students for this future? Are nurses comfortable moving into a present and future dominated by information systems? Educational institutions must have exit criteria that ensure basic computer knowledge. Faculty members benefit from continually updating their skills in computers and other technology. The profession of nursing has to have an impact on the future of home care.

 ## Alternative Therapies

Twenty years ago, **alternative therapies** were considered fringe treatments by most Western health care practitioners. However, consumers wanted more choices for treatment and more control over their care. As a result of possible unpleasant side effects of conventional therapies and a growing skepticism about Western medicine, consumers have turned in larger numbers to alternative therapies. There is a basic distinction between alternative therapies and Western medicine. Western medicine bases care on the disease model and the nature of pathology, whereas alternative therapies address holistic functioning within the social and environmental context, not focusing only on the function of the organs (Reed, Pettigrew, & King, 2000).

Today, alternative therapies are gaining respect and recognition from the general public and medical professionals as more people report positive results. Large numbers of individuals use alternative therapies, as seen in the classic studies done in 1993 and 1998 by Eisenberg and colleagues. These studies reported that one third of persons contacted in a national survey had used unconventional therapy in the past year. Total out-of-pocket expenditure for alternative therapies was estimated at $10.3 billion in 1990, compared with $12.8 billion for all hospital care in the United States that year. In 1998, Eisenberg found that the out-of-pocket expenditure for alternative therapies was $21.2 billion. Alternative therapies are increasingly being valued and used by nurses and other health care providers. In the future, nurses will increasingly be called on to provide knowledge about and use of alternative therapies. Therefore, it is imperative that nurses build their knowledge and skill base about alternative therapies (Box 16–1).

For the person who feels intimidated and dehumanized by the sterility and businesslike environment of most Western medical facilities, the warm, personal caring and concern of alternative practitioners may be therapeutic (Fig. 16–2). Because stress and anxiety are major factors in many illnesses, the soothing environment and supportive attitude of alternative practice and practitioners have contributed to their appeal.

Research provides evidence that alternative therapies do enhance health and promote recovery from illness for both the client and family caregivers (Box 16–2). Those who support only Western methods of health care have ignored or repudiated the value of more traditional or alternative methods. These alternative therapies have persisted and grown because people find them useful. Acknowledging the full breadth of services that individuals use, and working with them, is more productive than ignoring what the client chooses to do in the quest for wholeness and health.

---

## ▶ Box 16–1.  Why Nurses Should Learn About ◀ Alternative Therapies

- Large numbers of individuals are now using alternative therapies.
- As the population becomes more diverse ethnically, more methods of promoting health and treating illness are necessary.
- Alternative therapies have gained legitimacy with governmental agencies such as the National Institutes of Health, which has established an Office of Alternative Medicine.
- Medical educators and physicians are integrating alternative therapies into their practice.

Adapted from Reed, F. C., Pettigrew, A., & King, M. O. (2000). Alternative and complementary therapies in nursing curricula. *Journal of Nursing Education, 39*(3), 133–139.

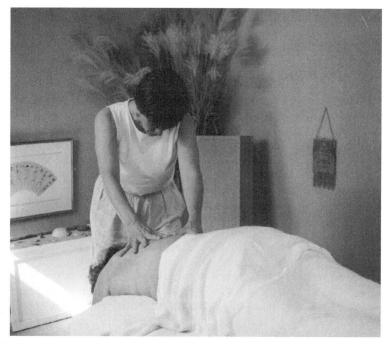

***Figure 16–2.*** ▶ One complementary therapy is neuromuscular and therapeutic massage.

## Nursing Implications

To follow the holistic perspective, nurses must be knowledgeable about alternative therapies. With such knowledge, they can monitor care and treatment and provide information about benefits for clients. The National Institutes of Health has categorized alternative modalities and therapies into major types of modalities seen in Box 16–3. Nurses should attend training in multiple alternative therapies to provide expanded care to their clients.

Nurses can begin to broaden their perspectives about different health care therapies by addressing their own bodies, minds, and spirit issues. It is possible to work successfully with clients who use alternative approaches.

## CLIENT SITUATIONS IN PRACTICE

### When the Nurse Has Not Been Exposed to Alternative Therapies

Lisa is a 29-year-old woman who delivered a healthy, 9-lb, 10-oz baby boy 2 weeks ago. The home health care nurse makes a home visit. Lisa complains about continued perineal discomfort with no unusual discharge or odor. The nurse suggests hydrocortisone cream and suppositories. Lisa says that she wants to avoid steroid creams and asks if there is an alternative. The nurse is concerned but states that she cannot provide her with any other suggestions. The only things that work, she says, are hydrocortisone and time, and Lisa should adhere to the medications that are known to be effective. Lisa is left feeling insecure and unsatisfied, without a remedy for her discomfort.

Aromatherapy, the use of essential oils with diverse medicinal qualities, was shown over a decade ago to help in the treatment of a range of conditions, including perineal discomfort (Dale & Cornwell, 1994). If the home health care nurse had interest and training in alternative therapies, she may have been better equipped to care for her client. When the nurse is willing to acknowledge the client's philosophy and values, the client may be willing to consider what the nurse has to offer for the client's care.

---

## RESEARCH IN COMMUNITY-BASED NURSING CARE

**Box 16–2** ▸ Therapeutic Effects of Massage Therapy and Healing Touch on Caregivers of Patients Undergoing Autologous Hematopoietic Stem Cell Transplant

---

Caregivers play an integral role in providing care to clients with cancer. Stress results from the demands of the caregiver role. Massage therapy is believed to be useful in alleviating caregiver stress. This research examined the effect of massage therapy and healing touch on anxiety, depression subjective caregiver burden, and fatigue experienced by caregivers of clients undergoing autogous hematopoietic stem cell transplant. The sample consisted of 36 caregivers, 13 in the control group and 13 in the massage therapy group, and 10 in the healing touch group. All caregivers completed the Beck Anxiety Inventory, the Center for Epidemiologic Studies Depression Scale, the Subjective Burden Scale, and the Multidimensional Fatigue Inventory before and after treatment. The intervention group received treatment consisting of two 30 minutes massages or healing touch treatments per week for three weeks. Those in the control group received usual nursing care as well as a supportive visit from one of the researchers. The results of the research showed significant declines in anxiety scores, depression, general fatigue, reduced motivation fatigue and emotional fatigue for those who were in the massage therapy group. Anxiety and depression scores were decreased in the healing touch group and fatigue and subjective burden increased but none were significant differences. The researcher concluded that massage may be one intervention that can be used by nurses to decrease feelings of stress in caregivers.

---

Rexillius, S., Mundt, C., Megel, M., & Agrawai, S. (2002). Therapeutic effects of massage therapy and healing touch on caregivers of patients undergoing autologous hematopoietic stem cell transplant. *Oncology Nursing Forum Online, 29(3)*. Retrieved on June 9, 2003 from http://www.ons.org

▶ **Box 16–3.** Major Types of Complementary and ◀ Alternative Therapies

**Alternative Systems** are systems built on theory and practice that have evolved apart from and earlier than the conventional medical approach used in the United States. Examples include homeopathic and naturopathic medicine, and traditional Chinese medicine.

**Mind-Body Therapies** are techniques designed to enhance the mind's capacity to affect bodily function and symptoms. These include the commonly used patient support group and cognitive-behavioral therapy as well as meditation, prayer, mental healing and creative arts such as art, music, or dance.

**Biologically Based Therapies** are those substances found in nature, such as herbs, foods and vitamins. Examples include dietary supplements and herbal products.

**Manipulative and Body-Based Methods** are therapies that are based on manipulation and/or movement of one or more parts of the body. Examples include chiropractic or osteopathic manipulation and massage.

**Energy Therapies** consist of two types. One is biofield therapies that are intended to affect energy fields that purportedly surround and penetrate the human body. Examples are qi gong, Reiki, and Therapeutic Touch. Bioelectromagnetic based therapies involved the unconventional use of electromagnetic fields, alternative current or direct current fields.

Source: National Center for Complementary and Alternative Medicine. National Institute of Health. What is complementary and alternative medicine? Retrieved on June 9, 2003 from http://www.nccam.nih.gov/health/whatiscam/

 ## Shifting Demographics

The number and proportion of older people continues to increase. Since 1900, the percentage of the population older than 65 years has tripled, and growth is expected to continue. By 2030, more than 20% of the U.S. population will be age 65 or older (DHHS, 2001). During the second decade of the 21st century, the postwar baby boom generation will move into the 65-and-older age group. Figure 16–3 shows the change in the percentage of the population in three age groups from 1950 to 2050.

People living longer with more chronic conditions require an increased use of health care resources. It is estimated that nearly 20% of the population lives with disabilities, and this proportion is on the rise. The number of people younger than 18 years with activity limitations increased by 33% for girls and 40% for boys between 1990 and 1994. Among adults ages 18 to 44, there was an increase of 16% in the number with activity limitations (DHHS, 2000a). Without intervention, it is likely that as this group ages, the percentage of the elderly population with chronic conditions will increase exponentially.

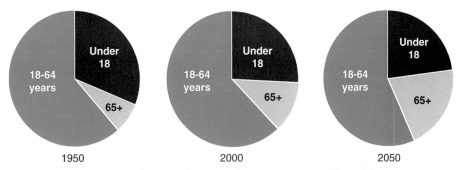

**Figure 16–3.** ▶ Percent of the population in three age groups: United States, 1950, 2000, and 2050. National Center for Health Statistics. (2002). *Health, United States, 2002: Chartbook on trends in the health of Americans.* Hyattsville, MD: Author (p. 19).

Because community-based nursing practice will be central to the care of this large population of aging and chronically ill people, nurses will have to do the following:

- ▶ Develop nurse-centered service models
- ▶ Consider going into independent practice
- ▶ Have competence in home care practices
- ▶ Be knowledgeable about client education techniques for every educational and socioeconomic level
- ▶ Have good organizational skills
- ▶ Be well versed in the aging process and have the skills necessary to care for the aged population

In North America, cultural diversity continues to increase. In 1900, about one out of eight Americans was of a race other than White. By 2000, about one out of four Americans was of a race other than White (Hobbs, & Stoops, 2002).

## Nursing Implications

Providing nursing care to diverse populations has been discussed throughout this text and will increasingly be an issue for nurses. In the future, regardless of the nurse's own ethnic background, the nurse must be proficient at transcultural nursing to be effective in promoting self-care. Nurses will play a major role in addressing health promotion and disease prevention issues for elderly clients. A larger proportion of the nurse's caseload will include individuals with chronic, disabling conditions. Promoting self-care and health promotion and disease prevention with this population entails skills and knowledge that are different from those needed for clients in an acute episode of a resolvable condition.

Continuity is more difficult in cross-cultural nursing. Every decision hinges on the cultural context of the issue. Also, it is often more difficult to enhance continuity with an older client who has a weak support system or multiple chronic conditions that impair mobility or sensory perception than it is for a middle-aged client with a spouse.

Collaboration is even more important when working with diverse populations. Collaboration across disciplines is always challenging, but it is particularly so if the interdisciplinary team members are from several cultural backgrounds.

## Civic Responsibility

The Pew Health Professions Commission's 21 competencies for the 21st century are shown in Box 1–2 in Chapter 1. It is easy to see how these competencies follow the trends discussed in this chapter. The first competency is "embrace a personal ethic of social responsibility and service." Cost containment has changed the delivery of nursing care and forced lay caregivers and clients themselves to be more responsible for self-care. Because health care is a commodity, many individuals (and often entire families) do not have access to care. Thus, a growing number of underserved individuals and families do not have access to health care but could benefit from nursing care. The competency of **civic responsibility** is intended to serve this growing **underserved population.**

One way to develop this competency is through volunteerism. Nurses, students, and nursing faculty must make a sustained commitment to community well-being through direct service. By carefully exploring options, students may find that by volunteering in a community-based setting, they learn more than they would in a traditional clinical setting.

A second way to develop the competency of social responsibility is through experiences that are structured to combine learning and volunteering. **Service learning** experiences can be valuable for the nurse or student to develop empathy, social awareness, and social and cultural competence. Students and nurses can take the initiative to learn while volunteering by taking an internship or independent study in an area of community health that interests them.

## The Future of Community-Based Nursing Care

Cost containment will continue to be a driving force for health care services, challenging nurses to be flexible, autonomous, and creative in their thinking. The current decrease in specialization calls for flexibility in the performance of roles across disciplines and the articulation of nursing as a profession. This requires the nurse to encourage clients and families to maximize their independence and follow through with self-care in all aspects of their lives. The educational preparation of the nurse will determine tasks; however, this may involve a broad range of activities from the simple to the complex. More education will be necessary for some who are required to perform, teach, and oversee complicated care. Further, as in most professions, nurses benefit from continually updating their skills and knowledge related to emerging technology in health care.

### Self-Care

In the future, the number of clients requiring assistance with self-care will grow as the percentage of the population with chronic disease increases. Self-care requires the nurse to recognize that assessment, planning, intervention, and evaluation revolve around the question, "How much care can the client and caregivers safely provide on their own?"

Self-care is especially challenging when the client is older or is from a different culture. The nurse of the future must be equipped to enhance the self-care skills of the client who is likely to be aging, from a different culture, and coping with several chronic conditions.

Self-care in the future will require mastery of an increasingly complex technology. To manage at home with a chronic health problem, the client and family caregiver will have to use complicated monitors and life-sustaining medical equipment, while the nurse uses sophisticated telecommunications devices to access information and transmit client data to the agency, attending physician, or nurse practitioner.

## Preventive Care

The future focus of health care will be on treatment efficacy rather than technologic imperative. This promotes preventive nursing care, as discussed in Chapter 2. Community-based nursing considers all three levels of prevention. Focusing on prevention will be particularly challenging as the percentage of the aging and chronically ill increases. Growing trends in alternative health therapies allow more culturally sensitive options in preventive care.

Health care's focus on cost containment challenges the nurse to use prevention strategies to reduce costs. This is as true in the hospital as in other community-based settings. Rather than being seen as expensive baggage that can be eliminated, nurses need to be seen as the key holding down health care costs by using their expertise in prevention. This concept has been discussed throughout this book. A summary of some different ways that nurses can operationalize the concepts of community-based nursing follows:

▶ Nurses can position themselves as the first link between clients and the hospital, thus developing long-term relationships. This involves periodically contacting clients with chronic problems.
▶ Nurses can develop telephone triage services for the hospital by fielding calls, referring clients to more cost-effective services, and reducing the number of unnecessary visits to emergency departments.
▶ Nurses can be proactive by contacting clients about immunizations and screening programs or fielding calls about medication administration, dressing changes, or proper diet. They can help correct problems before they become serious or identify already serious problems that need immediate care rather than postponed service.
▶ Nurses can develop and implement educational programs on drug counseling, substance abuse, birth control, diet, and prenatal and well-baby care.
▶ Nurses can contact aging clients routinely to identify health problems at early stages and to eliminate some physician visits that are motivated by loneliness and boredom. Nurses can lead self-help groups for this population.

## Care Within the Context of Community

Earlier chapters explained the value of the community in providing health care, and Chapter 3 discussed the cultural aspects of community-based nursing. Nursing care must be provided within this cultural context, taking into consideration the strengths and resources of the client, family, and community. Considering affordable health care, the nurse will provide care in the home within the parameters of the family, community, and client. As the population ages, this challenge will be further complicated by the demands of technology. Acceptance of alternative methods of care will allow care within the context of the client's family and community, including, in many cases, popular and folk healers. Because the racial and ethnic face of the nation is changing, nurses will be required to speak languages other than English or to be knowledgeable about using interpreters. The nurse may need to carry a card explaining to non-English-speaking clients that it is their right to have interpretation services provided at no charge. Nurses should also encourage representatives of minority groups to enter the nursing profession.

## Continuity of Care and Collaborative Care

The hospital of the future may be known as a **health care organization** or an **integrated health care system.** These systems already exist in many parts of the country. More community-based care programs will come from these integrated systems. Another term used is **seamless care**, in which all levels of care are available in an integrated form. Continuity allows quality care to be preserved in a changing health care delivery system. It is an essential component of cost containment and prevents duplication of services, rehospitalization, and inappropriate use of services. An older, more diverse population will provide challenges to the nurse as continuous care becomes the expected norm.

As a result of increased use of alternative therapies, the importance of continuity is evident. It will be essential for traditional and nontraditional providers to respect one another's contributions to the client's care and to communicate and coordinate care effectively.

## Conclusions

Cost-effective and quality health care accessible to everyone remains at the forefront of health care goals for the 21st century. In addition, flexibility will be an important aspect of community-based care. Trends demand nurses to be flexible when performing roles across disciplines while simultaneously articulating nursing as a profession. Ongoing professional development will be imperative to keep pace with the professional demands of community-based nursing.

The nurse of the future must be equipped to care for the client who is likely to be aging, from a different culture, and coping with several chronic conditions. It will be essential for traditional and nontraditional providers to respect one another's contributions to the client's care and to communicate effectively. Trends in alternative methods of healing allow more culturally sensitive options.

The nature and scope of nursing are broader than any one setting in which care is offered. Nursing care has remained constant in its philosophy over the decades. However, nurses must now adapt their care delivery models to include clients in acute care settings, long-term care, ambulatory settings, and the home. Nurses follow the standards of nursing care in all settings. In the future, this will require a more educated and proficient nurse.

# What's on the Web

Alternative Medicine Homepage
**Internet address:**
*http://www.pitt.edu/~cbw/altm.html*
This site, maintained by the Falk Library of the Health Sciences at the University of Pittsburgh, is a starting point for sources of information on alternative therapies.

American Botanical Council
**Internet address:**
*http://www.herbalgram.org*
This site is dedicated to providing current and accurate information on herbal medicine. There is an educational link that consumers may find helpful. On this site are a variety of accredited continuing education modules for professionals interested in learning more about the safety and efficacy of herbal products.

American Medical Informatics Association Nursing Informatics Work Group
**Internet address:**
*http://www.amia-niwg.org*
This organization's goal is to promote the advancement of nursing informatics within an interdisciplinary context. This goal is pursued in professional practice, education, research, and governmental and other service.

Ask Dr. Weil
**Internet address:**
http://www.amia.org/working/ni/main.html
A popular question and answer section is one of the highlights of this site. Dr. Weil is the founder of the Program for Integrative Medicine at the University of Arizona.

Healthworld Online
**Internet address:**
*http://www.healthyupdate.com*
This site provides basic information related to overall health, self-care management, and healthy lifestyles, with a section on alternative and complementary therapies.

Online Journal of Issues in Nursing
**Internet address:**
*http://www.nursingworld.org/ojin*
This on-line publication provides a forum for discussion of current issues in nursing.

National Center for Complementary and Alternative Medicine (NCCAM)
NCCAM Clearinghouse
P.O. Box 7923
Gaithersburg, MD 20898
Telephone: (888) 644-6226
TTY/TDT: (888) 644-6226
Fax: (301) 495-4957
**Internet address:** *http://www.nccam.nih.gov*
The NCCAM at the National Institutes of Health (NIH) conducts and supports basic and applied research on complementary and alternative therapies. This site disseminates information on complementary and alternative interventions to practitioners and the public. This is an excellent site for current, reliable information based on research.

## GENERAL WEB RESOURCES

adam.com
**Internet address:** *http://www.adam.com*
This is a commercial site that provides health and wellness information.

Aetna InteliHealth
**Internet address:**
*http://www.intelihealth.com*
This site provides physician-reviewed, consumer-friendly articles; on-line communities; and a medical dictionary. The "Ask the Doc" feature is popular.

American Heart Association
**Internet address:**
*http://www.americanheart.org*
This Web page contains information related to heart health, support group links, licensed products and services, and science and research. There is an excellent client and caregiver education area, "Congestive Heart Failure," at *http://www. americanheart.org/chf*

American Lung Association
**Internet address:** *http://www.lungusa.org*
This site contains information on lung disease in all forms, with special emphasis on asthma, tobacco control, and environmental health.

The Body: An AIDS and HIV Information Resource
**Internet address:** *http://www.thebody.com*
This site is a comprehensive resource with information on the disease processes of acquired immunodeficiency syndrome (AIDS) and human immunodeficiency virus (HIV). It discusses safe sex, support group treatment, mental health, and legal and financial issues from a variety of sites and links.

cancer.gov
**Internet address:**
*http://www.cancernet.nci.nih.gov*
Maintained by the National Cancer Institute, this site has extensive credible information on cancer, reviewed by oncology experts and based on research.

Health on the Net Foundation
**Internet address:** *http://www.hon.ch*
This international initiative has a multilingual search engine for information on health and health care.

Health Promotion Online
**Internet address:** *http://www. hc-sc.gc.ca/hppb/hpo/index.html*
This Canadian site addresses a wide range of health promotion and disease prevention programs. It also offers content in French.

Health Resources on IHP Net
**Internet address:** *http://www.ihpnet.org4/ listserv.htm*
Designed to save time, this site provides direct routes to health information.

Healthfinder
**Internet address:** *http://www.healthfinder.gov*
This site from the DHHS leads to publications, clearinghouses, databases, Web sites, and support and self-help groups, as well as providing reliable information.

*Healthy People 2010*
**Internet address:** *http://web.health.gov/ healthypeople*
This site provides access to all of the *Healthy People 2010* (DHHS, 2000a) documents and initiatives.

Lippincott Williams & Wilkins
**Internet address:** *http://www.lww.com*
Lippincott leads in the world of information resources for nursing, medical, and allied health professionals and students.

March of Dimes
**Internet address:** *http://www.modimes.org*
This organization focuses on issues related to prenatal care and prevention of birth defects, infant mortality, and low-birth-weight infants. The Web site includes information on research, programs, and public affairs.

MayoClinic.com
**Internet address:** *http://www.mayohealth.org*
Sponsored by the Mayo Clinic, this site features reliable information on a variety of health issues with resources for each.

McGill Medical Informatics
**Internet address:** *http://www.mmi.mcgill.ca*
This Canada-wide database for medical teaching and learning has a wide variety of medical information.

Medscape
**Internet address:** *http://www.medscape.com*
This commercial site is a professional site built around practice-oriented information.

National Institutes of Health
**Internet address:** *http://www.nih.gov*
The NIH Web site is an excellent all-around resource for nurses from all specialties. It contains news and events, health information, grants, scientific resources, and links to other sites, including the National Institute of Nursing Research and the W.G. Magnuson Clinical Center Nursing Department.

National Institutes of Health
Warren Grant Magnuson Clinical Center Nursing Department
**Internet address:** *http://www.cc.nih.gov/nursing*
This site provides links to federal resources, Internet search engines, and other useful resources.

This nursing-specific site provides information from universities, the Centers for Disease Control and Prevention, and the National Institute of Nursing Research.

National League for Nursing
**Internet address:** *http://www.nln.org*
A resource for nursing education, practice, and research, this site has the latest information about the organization and nursing in general.

National Women's Health Information Center (NWHIC)
**Internet address:** *http://www.4woman.gov*
The NWHIC is a free information and resource service on women's health issues for consumers, health care professionals, researchers, educators, and students. This bilingual site (English and Spanish) contains a wealth of information on health issues that is free of copyright restrictions and may be copied.

OncoLink
**Internet address:** *http://www.oncolink.upenn.edu*
This site is maintained by the University of Pennsylvania Cancer Center. It contains news, education on treatment options, reporting on clinical trials, psychosocial support through an active on-line community, and resources such as associations, support groups, on-line journals, and book reviews.

Planned Parenthood
**Internet address:** *http://www.plannedparenthood.org*
In both Spanish and English, this Web site includes legislative updates, statistics, newsletters, and a library with information on family planning.

PubMed
**Internet address:**
*http://www.ncbi.nlm.nih.gov/entrez/query.fcgi*
This search service of the National Library of Medicine provides access to more than 10 million citations.

RealAge
**Internet address:** *http://www.realage.com*
This commercial site provides news, an on-line support community, and interactive health assessment tools.

Resources for Nurses and Families
**Internet address:**
*http://pegasus.cc.ucf.edu/~wink/home.html*
This site contains resources for families, nurses, and nurse educators.

Sudden Infant Death Syndrome and Other Infant Death (SIDS/OID) Information Web Site
**Internet address:** *http://sids-network.org*
At this site, you will find up-to-date information about SIDS.

Transcultural Nursing
**Internet address:** *http://www.culturediversity.org*
This site's goal is to provide information about transcultural nursing to help other nurses understand behavior and its cultural basis.

U.S. Department of Health and Human Services
**Internet address:** *http://www.dhhs.gov*
This site provides links to numerous health resources from the federal government.

U.S. National Library of Medicine
**Internet address:** *http://www.nlm.nih.gov*
The U.S. National Library of Medicine is the world's largest medical library.

World Health Organization
**Internet address:** *http://www.who.int*
This is the Web site of the international World Health Organization, which is committed to the attainment of the highest possible level of health for everyone worldwide.

## References and Bibliography

Ball, M., & Lillis, J. (2000). Health information systems: Challenges for the 21st century. *AACN Clinical Issues, 11*(3), 386–395.

Bellack, J., & O'Neil, E. (2000). Recreating nursing practice for a new century: Recommendations and implications of the Pew Health Professions Commission final report. *Nursing and Health Care Perspectives, 21*(1), 15–19.

Brown, K. (2000). The human genome business today. *Scientific America, 283*(1), 50–55.

Candy, P. (2000). Preventing "information overdose": Developing information-literate practitioners. *The Journal of Continuing Education in the Health* Professions, *20*(4), 228–237.

Clark, D. (2000). Old wine in new bottles: Delivering nursing in the 21st century. *Journal of Nursing Scholarship, 32*(1), 11–15.

Craven, R. F., & Hirnle, C. J. (2000). *Fundamentals of nursing: Human health and function* (3rd ed.). Philadelphia: Lippincott Williams & Wilkins.

Dale, A., & Cornwell, S. (1994). The role of lavender oil in relieving perineal discomfort following childbirth: A blind randomized clinical trial. *Journal of Advanced Nursing, 19*(1), 89–96.

Eisenberg, D., Davis, R., Ettner, S. L., Appel, S., Wikey, S., Van Rompay, M., & Kessler, R. C. (1998). Trends in alternative medicine use in the United States, 1990–1997: Results of a follow-up national survey. *Journal of the American Medical Association, 280*(18), 1569–1575.

Eisenberg, D., Kessler, R., Foster, D., Norlock, F., Calhins, D., & Delbanco, J. (1993). Unconventional medicine in the United States. *New England Journal of Medicine, 328,* 246–252.

Elfrink, V., (2001). A look to the future: How emerging information technology will impact operations and practice. *Home Healthcare Nurse, 19(*12),751–757.

Heller, B., Oros, M. T., & Durney-Crowley, J. (2000). The future of nursing education: 10 trends to watch. *Nursing and Health Care Perspectives, 21*(1), 9–13.

Henry, C. (2001). Pharmacogenomics. *Chemical and Engineering News, 79*(33),37-42.

Retrieved June 10, 2003, from http://pubs.asc.org/cen

Hobbs, F., & Stoops, N., (2003). U.S. Census Bureau, Census 2000 Special Reports, Services CENSR_4. *Demographic trends in the 20th century.* Washington, DC: U.S. Government Printing Office.

Hupfeld, S. (2000). Through the looking glass: Tomorrow's hospital. *RN, 63*(6).

Kido, V. (2001, November). UAP dilemma. *Nursing Management.* Retrieved on June 9, 2003, from www.nursingmanagement.com

Larsen, P. D. (2000). Community-based curricula: New issues to address. *Journal of Nursing Education, 39*(3), 140–141.

Lindeman, C. A. (2000). The future of nursing education. *Journal of Nursing Education, 39*(1), 5–12.

Lo-Mon, B. (2000). The role of the nurse practitioner. *Nursing Standard, 14*(21), 49–51.

Mawn, B., & Reece, S. (2000). Reconfiguring a curriculum for the new millennium: The process of change. *Journal of Nursing Education, 39*(3), 101–107.

National Center for Health Statistics. (2002). *Health, United States, 2002: Chartbook on trends in the health of Americans* (p. 19). Hyattsville, MD: Author.

National Institutes of Health, National Center for Complementary and Alternative Medicine. (2002). *What is complementary and alternative medicine?* Retrieved June 9, 2003, from http://www.nccam.nih.gov/health/whatiscam/

Reed, F. C., Pettigrew, A., & King, M. O. (2000). Alternative and complementary therapies in nursing curricula. *Journal of Nursing Education, 39*(3), 133–139.

Rexillius, S., Mundt, C., Megel, M., & Agrawai, S. (2002). Therapeutic effects of massage therapy and healing touch on caregivers of patients undergoing autologous hematopoietic stem cell transplant. *Oncology Nursing Forum Online, 29(*3). Retrieved June 9, 2003, from http://www.ons.org/

Spencer, S. (2001). Education, training, and use of unlicensed assistive personnel in critical care. *Critical Care Nursing Clinics of North America, 13*(10), 105–115.

U.S. Department of Health and Human Services. (2000a). *Healthy people 2010* (Conference edition I & II). Washington, DC: U.S. Government Printing Office.

U.S. Department of Health and Human Services. (2000b). *The registered nurse population: Findings from the National Sample Survey of Registered Nurses.* Retrieved November 11, 2002, from http://bhpr.hrsa.gov/

U.S. Department of Health and Human Services. (2001). *A profile of older Americans: 2001.* Washington, DC: U.S. Government Printing Office.

World Health Organization. (2000). *WHO issues new health life expectancy rankings* [Press release]. Retrieved from http://www.who.int/inf-pr-2000/en/pr2000-life.html

# LEARNING ACTIVITIES

## JOURNALING: ACTIVITY 16–1

1. In your clinical journal, identify a future trend in health care. Find at least two articles about this trend and summarize each.
2. Follow the summary with two paragraphs in which you discuss how this trend could change or affect nursing. What are the implications for health care, the nursing profession, and nurses' daily practice? What further education needs come from these implications?

## CLIENT CARE: ACTIVITY 16–2

The year is 2025—the future is here. You are a case manager in a busy, urban nursing clinic. You have a caseload of clients who live in the community where your center is located. You either see your clients in the ambulatory clinic or you communicate with them by computer. Today, one of your clients, Alfred Martinez, who is 64 years old, is having a sigmoid bowel resection with a temporary colostomy by laparoscopic laser surgery at the day surgery center. Home care will be provided by his wife, who will be assisted by their three adult sons on a rotating basis. It is your responsibility to coordinate the disciplines involved in his health care and manage his nursing care.

1. Identify risk factors that must be addressed when you plan for Mr. Martinez's postoperative recovery at home.
2. List five questions you will ask Mr. Martinez when you assess his care needs. Review the questions.
   Do these questions view the client holistically?
   Are they indicative of a contextual approach to identifying the client's needs?
3. Organize topics you will include when you teach Mrs. Martinez and her sons about Mr. Martinez's postoperative care. Compare and contrast current care from the care provided in 1987.
4. State alternative treatments or nursing interventions you included in the plan of care. Determine if they are paid for by a third-party payer.
5. Analyze how technology will assist you in Mr. Martinez's care (eg, in making the assessment, communicating, and implementing the plan of care).

## PRACTICAL APPLICATION: ACTIVITY 16–3

Interview a nurse who has been employed for at least 10 years. Use the following questions as a basis for the interview:

- When did you first start working as a registered nurse?
- What was nursing like when you first started working?
- How has nursing changed in the last 10 years?
- How is nursing different now?
- How many clients did you care for when you first started working as a nurse?
- How are the clients different now than when you first started working as an RN?
- What were your responsibilities for client care when you first started working and how have those responsibilities changed?
- What concerns do you have about how nursing has changed over the last 10 years?
- What is better about how nursing care is provided now?
- Summarize the interview. What did you learn?

## PRACTICAL APPLICATION: ACTIVITY 16–4

Interview an elderly client or family member who has had a chronic condition over a long period of time (at least 10 years). Ask that person the following questions:

- How have health care services changed over the last 10 years (or however long you have had your health condition)?
- What differences are of particular concern to you and why?
- Has your family taken over more of your care?
- What has that been like for you?
- What has that been like for your family members?

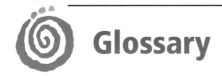

# Glossary

**acculturation:** individuals or groups from one culture learning the ways to exist in a new culture

**activities of daily living (ADL):** normal tasks of daily life

**acute care:** short-term medical or nursing care

**adult foster care homes:** small residential sites that provide housing and protective oversight; also known as board and care homes or family care homes

**advance directive:** written guide that allows people to state in advance what their choices for health care would be if certain circumstances should develop

**advanced practice nurse:** registered nurse who has completed graduate study in a specialty area according to specific academic requirements

**advocacy:** protection and support of another's rights

**affective interventions:** those teaching and nursing interventions that facilitate changes in attitudes, values, and feelings

**affective learning:** changes in attitudes, values, and feelings

**agoraphobia:** fear of being in places from which it might be difficult or embarrassing to escape

**alternative therapies:** interventions that focus on body, mind, and spirit integration; may be used in addition to conventional treatments. Examples include relaxation, imagery, prayer.

**ambulatory care center:** any health care setting that provides a wide variety of services, including those related to medical, surgical, mental health, or substance abuse

**assessment:** a dynamic, ongoing process that uses observations and interactions to collect information, recognize changes, analyze needs, and plan care

**assimilation:** individuals or groups from one culture identifying more strongly with the dominant culture in values, activities, and daily living

**assisted-living facilities:** multiple dwellings that provide help with activities of daily living, such as being reminded to take medication, assistance with dressing and bathing, and meal preparation

**barriers:** factors that may adversely affect a process, (eg, referral process)

**behavioral interventions:** teaching or nursing interventions that assist clients to change their own behavior

**boarding care homes:** homes for the disabled or older person who needs meal service and housekeeping only and can manage most personal care

**brokerage model:** a model of case management that defines the role of the case manager as a coordinator of care mediating between all parties

**care manager:** individual who manages the care of the client

**care of the caregiver:** nursing interventions intended to assist the individual providing care for the client

**case finding:** a set of activities used by the nurse working in community settings that identifies clients who are not currently receiving health care, but who could benefit from such care

**case management:** a systematic process used by nurses to ensure that clients' multiple health and service needs are met. These include assessing client needs, planning and coordinating services, referring to other appropriate providers, and monitoring and evaluating progress.

**civic responsibility:** a personal ethic of social responsibility and service

**client advocacy:** intervening or acting on behalf of the client to provide the highest quality health care obtainable.

**clinical nurse specialist:** a registered nurse with a graduate degree in a specialty or subspecialty area of nursing who usually practices in acute care settings, providing direct or indirect client care

**cognitive interventions:** teaching or nursing actions that enhance the client's ability to intellectually process information

**cognitive learning:** the ability to intellectually process information, including remembering, perceiving, abstracting, and generalizing

**collaboration:** purposeful interaction between nurse, clients, and other professional and community members based on mutual participation and joint effort

**community:** people, location, and social systems

**community assessment:** the process of determining the real or perceived needs of a defined community of people

**community-based nursing:** nursing care within the context of the client's family and community with a prevention focus that enhances the client's ability for self-care; a collaborative effort to maintain continuity of care

**community health problem:** the health need identified in community assessment

**community resources:** a collection of health care providers or supportive care providers who share common interests or a sense of unity

**complementary therapies:** interventions that focus on body, mind, and spirit integration; may be used in addition to conventional therapies. (Examples: relaxation, imagery, prayer.)

**constructed survey:** a time-consuming and expensive method of collecting information about a community with a valid and reliable survey, using a random sample of a targeted population where the data collected are analyzed for patterns and trends

**consultation:** an interactive problem-solving process between the nurse and the client

**continuity of care:** coordination of services provided to clients before they enter a health care setting, during the time they are in the setting, and after they leave the setting

**coordinated care:** the coordination of interdisciplinary sources of care and support to provide successful continuity of care

**coordination:** harmonious adjustment or working together

**cultural assessment:** considers the cultural beliefs, values, and practices of an individual, group, or community to determine needs and interventions within a specific cultural context

**cultural awareness:** self-awareness of one's own cultural background, influences, and biases

**cultural blindness:** lack of recognition of one's own beliefs and practices or of the beliefs and practices of others

**cultural care:** health care in a cultural context, acknowledging the client's cultural beliefs about disease and treatment

**cultural encounter:** direct contact with members of cultural communities

**cultural knowledge:** familiarity with a culturally or ethnically diverse group's world view, beliefs, values, practices, lifestyles, and problem-solving strategies

**cultural sensitivity:** the considerate, respectful, compassionate, empathic, and sensible response to a person or situation

**cultural skill:** the ability to collect relevant cultural data regarding the client's health history

**culture:** a set of values, beliefs, and attitudes that characterizes a group and provides guidance in determining one's behavior

**day surgery centers:** ambulatory services that provide preoperative, operative, and postoperative care on an outpatient basis

**deinstitutionalization:** discharge from an inpatient mental health facility into the community where ongoing treatment can be provided by community-based mental health services.

**delegation:** a management principle used to obtain desired results through the work of others, and a legal concept used to empower one person to act for another

**demographics:** statistics related to age-specific categories, birth and death rates, marital status, ethnicity

**detoxification center:** facility that provides individuals safe detoxification of chemicals. The focus is on immediate health care needs and discharge planning

**developmental family assessment:** determination of family developmental stage and ability to meet the developmental tasks of that stage

**developmental task:** the usual and expected psychosocial, cognitive, or psychomotor skills at certain periods in life; failure to master the developmental task can lead to unhappiness and difficulty with later tasks

**diagnosis-related groups (DRGs):** classification of clients by major medical diagnosis for the purpose of standardizing health care costs

**discharge planning:** coordinating, planning, and arranging for the transition from one health care setting to another

**diversity:** the condition of being different

**documentation:** the process of obtaining and recording information used for communication, reference, and legal issues

**dual diagnosis:** coexistent mental health and other disorder (often an addictive disorder)

**emic care:** care determined by the local or insider's views and values

**employee assistance programs:** provision of assistance to an employee when emotional or physical illness threatens to interfere with the employee's health

**employee wellness programs:** plans that focus on keeping employees healthy and preventing illness and accidents

**environmental assessment:** evaluation of the client's home and neighborhood environment

**epidemic:** disease occurrence that exceeds normal or expected frequency in a community or region

**ethnicity:** cultural differences based on heritage

**ethnocentrism:** belief that one's own cultural beliefs and values are best for all

**etic care:** care determined by the professional's or outsider's views and values

**extended care facilities:** synonymous with nursing homes; provide care for individuals who need daily care generally for the rest of their lives

**extended family:** nuclear family and other related people

**family developmental tasks:** the usual and expected family psychosocial, cognitive, or psychomotor skills at certain periods in life; failure to master a developmental task can lead to unhappiness and difficulty with later tasks

**family functions:** activities or behaviors of family members that maintain the unity of the family and meet the family's needs

**family health:** how well the family functions together as a unit; the family's ability to carry out usual and desired daily activities

**family roles:** expected set of behaviors associated with a particular family position

**family structure:** the characteristics of individuals (age, gender, number) who make up the family unit

**family systems theory:** a theory that says the family is a collection of people who are integrated, interacting, and independent, and that the actions of one member impact the actions of other members

**fee-for-service:** retrospective method of reimbursing medical care where each service requires payment

**financial assessment:** evaluation of a client's ability to pay for service

**function:** subjective and objective evidence of ability to perform activities of daily living

**functional assessment:** determination of level of health defined by one's ability to carry out usual and desired daily activities

**genogram:** an assessment to show family structure

**gerontology nursing:** the nursing care of older adults, particularly those older than 65 years

**health:** state of physical, mental, and social well-being and not merely the absence of disease or infirmity

**health disparity:** differences in health and access to health care by gender, race, or ethnicity, education or income, disability, living in rural localities, or sexual orientation

**health indicator:** reflects the major public health concerns and illuminates factors that affect the health of individuals and communities

**health maintenance organizations (HMOs):** health care systems that provide comprehensive health service delivered by a defined network of providers to their members, who pay a fixed premium

**health promotion:** activities that enhance the well-being of an already healthy individual

**health protection:** environmental or regulatory measures that confer protection on large population groups

**health-illness continuum:** health described in a range of degrees from optimal health at one end to total disability or death at the other

**healthy family functioning:** optimal level of family health as defined by the family's ability to carry out usual and desired daily activities

**holism:** a way of viewing the person as an integrated whole of mind, body, and spirit; reflects the interactive process that occurs in all of us

**holistic assessment:** considers not only physical and psychosocial factors, but also cultural, functional, nutritional, environmental, and spiritual aspects of the client

**home care agencies:** official, hospital-based, or proprietary organizations that provide health care in the client's residence

**home health care:** component of comprehensive health care whereby health services are provided to individuals and families in their places of residence for the purpose of promoting, maintaining, or restoring health

**home infusion therapy:** a broad area of chemotherapy that incorporates intravascular chemotherapy performed by home infusion nurses or self-adminstered by patients or their caregivers.

**home visit:** assessment, diagnosis, planning, and evaluation of nursing care in the client's home

**homeless shelter:** facility that provides food and shelter for individuals without homes

**hospice care:** holistic services provided to dying persons and their loved ones to provide a more dignified and comfortable death

**hospital-based home care agency:** an operating department of a hospital that has no mandates and no tax support to determine which services to provide

**hyperemesis:** protracted vomiting with weight loss and fluid and electrolyte imbalance

**infant mortality rate:** rate of death per 1,000 infants defined as 1 month to 1 year of age

**informant interviews:** asking community residents who are either key informants or members of the general public about their observations and concerns regarding their community

**instrumental activities of daily living (IADL):** ability to plan and prepare meals, travel, do laundry, do housekeeping, shop, and use the telephone

**integrated health care system** (also called seamless care): a health care system in which all levels of care are available in an integrated form.

**interdisciplinary team model:** a model of case management built on the concept of collaboration that allows each professional on the team to offer his or her particular specialty

**lay caregiving:** care provided by families, friends, or other nonprofessionals in the home

**learning domains:** three areas (cognitive, affective, and psychomotor) in which teaching and learning occur

**learning need:** a deficit in knowledge, skills, or attitude that interrupts functioning

**learning objectives:** expected outcome for the client, including a subject, action verb, performance criteria, target time, and special conditions

**lifeways:** beliefs about dress, diet, and other activities of daily living

**living will:** written advance directive specifying the medical care a person desires to refuse should he or she lack the capacity to consent or refuse treatment at some point

**managed care:** health care systems that coordinate medical care for specific groups to promote provider efficiency and control costs

**market-driven economy:** a system in which consumer demand drives production regarding what services will be created and consumed and in what quantity

**medication safety:** concern with taking medication the correct way and avoiding taking medication with other drugs and substances that cause harmful interactions

**minority:** race, ethnic, or cultural group that does not belong to the dominant group

**morbidity rates:** rates of illness or injury

**mortality rates:** rates of causes of death

**need to learn:** perception that information or skill is relevant or necessary for immediate or delayed application

**nuclear family:** mother, father, and children living together

**nurse midwife:** a nurse who provides independent care for women during normal pregnancy, labor, and delivery

**nurse practitioner:** see advanced practice nursing

**nursing centers:** clinics that deliver primary health care, managed and served by nurses, practitioners, and other advanced practice nurses

**nursing functions:** those activities that enable the nurse to fulfill the roles of caregiver, manager, educator, planner, and advocate

**occupational health nurse:** registered nurse employed in a work setting who focuses on the health and well-being of people in the workplace

**official home care agency:** mandated to offer a particular group of services and supported by tax dollars

**outpatient services:** also called ambulatory care centers or clinics; provide a broad range of health care services for the client who does not require inpatient care

**parish nurse:** registered nurse employed by a religious organization to provide nursing care to members of the congregation

**participant observations:** examination of formal and informal social systems at work for the purpose of community assessment

**pharmacogenomics:** the technology of developing and producing medications tailored to specific genetic profiles

**polypharmacy:** the prescription of more than one medication

**power system:** a group of people who determine how control is distributed throughout a community or social system

**preferred provider organizations (PPOs):** a network of physicians, hospitals, and other health-related services that contract with a third-party payer organization to provide comprehensive health services to subscribers on a fee-for-service basis

**pregnancy-induced hypertension (PIH):** hypertensive disorder of pregnancy that includes preeclampsia, eclampsia, and transient hypertension; the second leading cause of maternal mortality in the United States.

**preventive services:** services attempting to avoid disease or injury or minimize the consequences

**primary prevention:** actions that avoid the initial occurrence of disease or injury

**professional relatedness:** professional phenomenon that involves understanding, mutual relating, self-awareness, reliability, and respect for privacy.

**proprietary home care agency:** a freestanding for-profit home care agency; services are provided based on third-party reimbursement schedules or by self-pay

**prospective payment:** payment for health care services in advance based on rate derived from predictions of annual service costs

**psychomotor learning:** physical skills that can be demonstrated

**race:** to characterize a distinct human type by traits that are transmitted by descent

**readiness to learn:** emotional state, abilities, and potential that allow learning to occur

**referral process:** a dynamic process between community resources that ensures continuity of care for the well-being of a client

**rehabilitation centers:** either residential or outpatient facilities providing services to those requiring either physical or emotional rehabilitation. Residence is generally limited to the achievement of goals

**reimbursement requirements:** governmental or proprietary requirements that must be met before a service is paid for

**residential centers:** supervised group facilities with various levels of independence, including, among other levels, retirement communities, assisted living facilities, board and care, skilled nursing facilities, and subacute rehabilitation centers

**respite care:** services to a family or caregivers to temporarily relieve caregiving demands

**retirement communities:** homes or apartments with supportive services provided by the retirement community, providing a community living style for individuals who choose to live with other seniors

**school nurse:** a registered nurse charged with the health care of school-age children and school personnel in an educational setting

**secondary data:** records, documents, or any previously collected information

**secondary prevention:** actions providing early identification and treatment of disease or injury with the purpose of limiting disability

**self-care:** the actions of individuals, families, and communities to preserve and promote their own health, life, and sense of well-being

**service learning:** experiences that are structured to combine learning and volunteering.

**skilled nursing facilities:** provision of nursing, medical, and therapy services for the individual who does not require acute care, but requires ongoing care. Generally transferred to extended care or to home

**sliding fee scale:** payment schedule based on the client's ability to pay for service

**social system:** the various components of a community, including economic, educational, religious, political, legal, and methods of communication

**specialized care centers:** facilities that provide health care for a specific population group

**spiritual assessment:** allows the nurse to determine the presence of spiritual distress or identify other spiritual needs and incorporate them into the plan of care

**spirituality:** a flowing, healing, dynamic balance that allows and creates health and well-being; sometimes involves organized religion

**staff splitting:** manipulative behaviors by which a client pits health care staff members against each other.

**stereotyping:** a mental picture or an assumption about a person based on a characteristic that comes from myths, or generalizations based on the perceived membership in a group

**structural family assessment:** family assessment that maps out the composition of the family, such as a genogram

**subacute rehabilitation centers:** limited time residence; discharge usually occurs when the client has met certain goals

**support services:** services that help people avoid problems or solve problems that interfere with their well-being

**technology:** a tool to extend human abilities

**tertiary prevention:** actions to maximize recovery and potential after an injury or illness

**transcultural nursing:** a body of knowledge and practice for caring for people from other cultures

**transferring:** moving from one tertiary care setting to another

**transitional housing:** temporary service often used between acute illness episodes or a personal housing crisis and permanent housing

**underserved populations:** individuals and families who do not have access to health care

**unlicensed assistive personnel (UAP):** persons without a professional license

**vital statistics:** information related to ongoing registration of births, deaths, adoptions, divorces, marriages, causes of death, and other statistics that reflect the vital signs of a community

**wellness promotion:** to encourage or promote a healthy state

**windshield survey:** motorized equivalent of a simple observation where the observer drives through a chosen neighborhood and uses the power of observation to conduct a general assessment of that neighborhood

**work site health promotion:** programs that focus on the health of employees within business and industry

# Index

Page numbers followed by "f" denote figures, "t" denote tables, and "b" denote boxes

APPENDIX **6-1**

# Implications for Teaching at Various Developmental Stages

| Age | Physical Development | Language (Cognitive) Development (based on Piaget) | Psychosocial Development (based on Erikson) | Nurse's Approach to Teaching |
|---|---|---|---|---|
| Overview of birth to 1 y | | Sensorimotor stage of development | Development task: trust vs. mistrust. Learns to trust and to anticipate satisfaction. Sends cues to mother/ caretaker. Begins understanding self as separate from others (body image). | Involve caretaker in all aspects of care |
| 1–3 y | Begins to walk and run well. Drinks from cup, feeds self. Develops fine motor control. Climbs. Begin self-toileting. Kneels without support. Steady growth in height/weight. Adult height will be approximately double the height at age 2. Dresses self by age 3. | *Preoperational stage* of development. Has poor time sense. Increasing verbal ability. Formulates sentences of 4 to 5 words by age 3. Talks to self and others. Has misconceptions about cause and effect. Interested in pictures. *Fears:* • Loss/separation from parents—peak • Dark • Machines/equipment • Intrusive procedures • Bedtime Speaks to dolls and animals. Increasing attention span. Knows own sex by age 3. | *Developmental task: autonomy vs. shame and doubt.* Establishes self-control, decision making, indepen- dence (autonomy). Extremely curious and prefers to do things himself. Demon- strates indepen- dence through negativism. Very egocentric; believes he or she controls the world. Attempts to please parents. Participates in parallel play; able to share some toys by age 3. | Be flexible. Begin any inter- vention with play period to establish rap- port. Be honest Praise for cooperation. Begin slowly; speak to child. Involve care- taker/parent Let child hold security object. Allow child to play with stethoscope, tongue blade, flashlight before using on child if possible. |

(continued)

| Age | Physical Development | Language (Cognitive) Development (based on Piaget) | Psychosocial Development (based on Erikson) | Nurse's Approach to Teaching |
|---|---|---|---|---|
| 4–6 y | Growth slows. Loco-motion skills in-crease and co-ordination im-proves. Tricycle/bicycle riding. Throws ball but difficulty catching. Con-stantly active, increasing dexterity. Eruption of permanent teeth. Skips, hops, jumps rope. | *Preoperational/thought stage of development continues.* Language skills flourish. Generates many questions, eg, How, Why, What? Simple problem solving. Uses fantasy to understand and problem solve. *Fears* • Mutilation • Castration • Dark • Unknown • Inanimate • Unfamiliar objects Causality related to proximity of events. Enjoys mimicking and imitating adults. - | *Developmental tasks: initiative vs. guilt.* Attempts to establish self like his or her parents, but independent. Explores environ-ment on own initiative. Boasts, brags, has feelings of indestructibility. Family is primary social group. Peers increasingly important. Assumes sex roles. Aggressive, very curious. Enjoys activities such as sports, cook-ing, shopping. Cooperative play. Likes rules. May stretch the truth and tell large stories. | Establish rap-port through talking and play Introduce self to child. Have parent present but direct conversation to child. Games such as "follow the leader" and "Simon says" can be used to elicit elicit necessary behaviors. Explain each intervention in simple language. Ask for child's help help and use flattery. Use pictures, models, or items he or she can see or touch. Reserve genital examination for last; drape accordingly. |
| 6–11 y | Moves constantly. Physical play prevalent; sports, swimming, skat-ing, etc. Increased smoothness of movement. Grows at rate of 2 inches/7 lb a year. Eyes/hands well coordinated. | *Concrete operations stage of develop-ment.* Organized thought; memory concepts more complicated. Reads, reasons better. Focuses on concrete understanding. *Fears:* • Mutilation • Death • Immobility • Rejection • Failure | *Developmental task: industry vs. inferiority.* Learns to include values and skills of school, neighbor-hood, peers. Peer relationships important. Focuses more on reality, less on fantasy. Family is main base of security and identity. Sensi-tive to reactions of others. Seeks approval and recognition. Enthusiastic, noisy, imaginative, desires to explore. Likes to complete a task. Enjoys help-ing others. | Explain all procedures and impact on body. Encourage questioning and active participation in care. Be direct about explanation of procedures, based on what child will hear, see, smell, and feel. (In addition, explain body part involved, and use anatomical names and pictures to explain step by step.) Be honest. |

*(continued)*

| Age | Physical Development | Language (Cognitive) Development (based on Piaget) | Psychosocial Development (based on Erikson) | Nurse's Approach to Teaching |
|---|---|---|---|---|
| | | | | Reassure child that he or she is liked. Provide privacy. Involve parents, but give child choice as to whether parent will stay during exam. Reason and explain. Allow child some choice as to direction of assessment. May be able to proceed as if assessing adult. Praise cooperation. |
| 12–18 y | Well developed. Rapid physical growth (early adolescence: maximum growth). Secondary sex characteristics. | *Formal operations stage of development* Abstract reasoning, problem solving. Understanding of of multiple cause-and-effect relationships. May plan for future career. *Fears:* • Mutilation • Disruption of body image • Rejection by peers | *Development task: identity vs. role confusion.* Predominant values are those of peer group. Early adolescence: outgoing and enthusiastic. Emotions are extreme, with mood swings. Seeking self-identity; sexual identity. Wants privacy and independence. Develops interests not shared with family. Concern with physical self. Explores adult roles. | Respect privacy. Accept expression of feelings. Direct discussions of care of care and condition to child child. Ask for child's opinions and encourage questions. Allow input into decisions. Be flexible with routines. Explain all procedures/ treatments. Encourage continuance of of peer relationships. Listen actively. Identify impact of illness on body image, future, and level of function ing. Correct misconceptions. Involve parent in assessment only if child requests presence. |

*(continued)*

| Age | Physical Development | Language (Cognitive) Development (based on Piaget) | Psychosocial Development (based on Erikson) | Nurse's Approach to Teaching |
|-----|----------------------|---------------------------------------------------|---------------------------------------------|------------------------------|
| 19–30 y | | *Formal operations* | *Developmental task: intimacy vs. isolation.* Intimate relationships are ultimate. | Involve significant other in care and consider how the client's condition affects the relationship. |
| 30–60 y | | *Formal operations* | *Developmental task: generativity vs. stagnation.* Concerned with parenthood, mentoring and guiding the next generation. | Work, family, and children are priorities. Teach with this concern in mind. |
| 60 y to death | | *Formal operations* | *Developmental task: integrity vs. despair.* Reviews life to bring life events into an integrated life theme. | Use life review to help client reduce anxiety and blocks to learning. |

Adapted from Weber, J. (1997). *Nurses' handbook of health assessment* (3rd ed.). Philadelphia: Lippincott-Raven.